ENDORSED BY

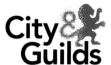

Level 2 Health and Social Care: Core

FOR WALES

■ Anne-Marie Furse,
Maria Ferreiro Peteiro,
Victoria Tibbott

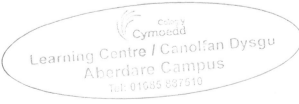

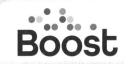

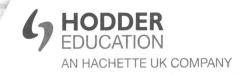

HODDER
EDUCATION
AN HACHETTE UK COMPANY

Every effort has been made to trace all copyright holders, but if any have been inadvertently overlooked, the Publishers will be pleased to make the necessary arrangements at the first opportunity.

Although every effort has been made to ensure that website addresses are correct at time of going to press, Hodder Education cannot be held responsible for the content of any website mentioned in this book. It is sometimes possible to find a relocated web page by typing in the address of the home page for a website in the URL window of your browser.

Hachette UK's policy is to use papers that are natural, renewable and recyclable products and made from wood grown in well-managed forests and other controlled sources. The logging and manufacturing processes are expected to conform to the environmental regulations of the country of origin.

Orders: please contact Hachette UK Distribution, Hely Hutchinson Centre, Milton Road, Didcot, Oxfordshire, OX11 7HH. Telephone: +44 (0)1235 827827. Email education@hachette.co.uk Lines are open from 9 a.m. to 5 p.m., Monday to Friday. You can also order through our website: www.hoddereducation.co.uk

ISBN: 978 1 3983 3440 3

© Anne-Marie Furse, Maria Ferreiro Peteiro, Victoria Tibbott 2021

First published in 2021 by
Hodder Education,
An Hachette UK Company
Carmelite House
50 Victoria Embankment
London EC4Y 0DZ

www.hoddereducation.co.uk

Impression number   10 9 8 7 6 5 4 3 2 1

Year   2025 2024 2023 2022 2021

Cover photo © Gstudio – stock.adobe.com

City & Guilds and the City & Guilds logo are trade marks of The City and Guilds of London Institute. City & Guilds Logo © City & Guilds 2021

Illustrations by Integra Software Services Ltd

Typeset in India by Integra Software Services Ltd

Printed in Slovenia

A catalogue record for this title is available from the British Library.

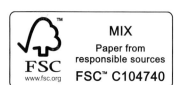

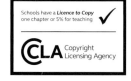

Contents

Introduction

This textbook supports learners studying the City and Guilds Level 2 Health and Social Care Core Qualification approved by Qualification Wales.

People who undertake this qualification may be in school or college thinking about starting a career in health and social care, or they may be already in a job, starting a new career or having worked for some time in the Social Care sector. Whatever your situation, this book is for you.

Working in health and social care, whether supporting children and young people or adults, requires a vast amount of skills and knowledge which you will continue to develop throughout your career. This core qualification will ensure you have the essential skills and knowledge required to deliver quality services to people you support in a way which meets their individual needs. It will give you a great foundation to support your work so that you can move on to further learning and development in the future.

The aims of the qualification are to enable learners to develop knowledge and understanding:

- of the core principles and values which underpin Health and Social Care practice;
- of ways of working in the Health and Social Care sector;
- which informs effective practice within Health and Social Care;
- to support progression onto further study within Health and Social Care.

This book gives you the knowledge you need to complete the units in the Core qualification, whether your focus is on working with children and young people or adults. The subjects covered are:

- principles and values of health and social care
- health and well-being
- professional practice as a health and social care worker
- safeguarding individuals
- health and safety in health and social care.

How your knowledge will be assessed

In order to achieve this qualification you will need to undertake a period of teaching and learning. The book will help you throughout this period. You will then go on to the assessment which consists of:

- three externally set case studies which will be marked by your tutor or assessor
- one externally set and externally marked multiple-choice test

You should have plenty of time and support to help you prepare for your assessments. This book will help you revise your knowledge for both the case studies and the test. You can read more about the different learning features that will help you with assessment in the following How to Use This Book section.

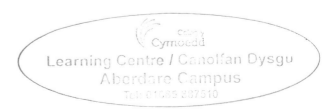

Continuing your learning journey

If you are studying this qualification at school or college and thinking of a future career in care, you may also be undertaking the Principles and Contexts qualification at either Level 2 or Level 3. This book will also help you to achieve this qualification as many of the topics covered overlap. If you then go on to work in social care you will already have completed the qualification required to support your registration as a Social Care Worker.

If you are already working in a health or social care setting, you will also be required to undertake a Level 2 or 3 practice qualification. This book will give you the knowledge you need to underpin your practice and help you achieve your practice qualification. This Level 2 Core qualification is a prerequisite to both the Level 2 and Level 3 practice qualifications.

Whatever route you decide to take in your career in health and social care, this book will give you a comprehensive understanding of the social care sector. It will help you learn how to work in a person-centred way, ensuring the well-being and safety of people you support. It will also help you make informed decisions about your own career ambitions and development.

The authors of the book have many years' experience of working in the health and social care sector and are thrilled that they can pass on their knowledge to support your learning. We hope you enjoy the book and wish you every success in your core qualification and future career.

Picture credits

The author and publishers would like to thank the following for permission to reproduce copyright material.

p.9 © michael spring/stock.adobe.com; p.12 © LIGHTFIELD STUDIOS/stock.adobe.com; p.35 © auremar/stock.adobe.com; p.41 © jovannig/stock.adobe.com; p.47 © Mark Davidson/Alamy Stock Photo; p.56 © Jacob Lund/stock.adobe.com; p.71 © pressmaster/stock.adobe.com; p.80 © Graphicroyalty/stock.adobe.com; p.89 © pololia/stock.adobe.com; p.90 l © Welsh Government – Crown Copyright, r © LIGHTFIELD STUDIOS/stock.adobe.com; p.99 © lovelyday12/stock.adobe.com; p.119 © Public Health England in association with the Welsh Government, Food Standards Scotland and the Food Standards Agency in Northern Ireland – Crown Copyright; p.126 © rocketclips/stock.adobe.com; p.141 © dimasobko/stock.adobe.com; p.145 © Monkey Business/stock.adobe.com; p.156 © rawpixel.com/stock.adobe.com; p.157 l © stanislav_uvarov/stock.adobe.com, r © Evgeniy Kalinovskiy/stock.adobe.com; p.163 l © yAOinLoVE/stock.adobe.com, r © Africa Studio/stock.adobe.com; p.168 © DragonImages/stock.adobe.com; p.170 © natalialeb/stock.adobe.com; p.171 © Alena Ozerova/stock.adobe.com; p.175 © DenisProduction.com/stock.adobe.com; p.180 © mjowra/stock.adobe.com; p.185 © Odua Images/stock.adobe.com; p.189 © DC Studio/stock.adobe.com; p.190 © Social Care Wales; p.199 © Comeback Images/stock.adobe.com; p.204 © Prostock-studio/stock.adobe.com; p.209 © JackF/stock.adobe.com; p.213 © Valerii Honcharuk/stock.adobe.com; p.219 © Jacob Lund/stock.adobe.com; p.221 © mnirat/stock.adobe.com; p.232 © .shock/stock.adobe.com; p.240 © Justinboat29/stock.adobe.com; p.249 © Robert Kneschke/stock.adobe.com; p.251 © Monkey Business/stock.adobe.com; p.257 © fizkes/stock.adobe.com; p.264 © olly/stock.adobe.com; p.273 © Mangostar/stock.adobe.com; p.278 © DragonImages/stock.adobe.com; p.280 © Monkey Business/stock.adobe.com; p.298 © Stephen Barnes/Medical/Alamy Stock Photo; p.300 © mjowra/stock.adobe.com; p.314 © Monkey Business/stock.adobe.com; p.318 © Barselona Dreams/stock.adobe.com; p.321 © DavidBautista/stock.adobe.com; p.323 © Elnur/stock.adobe.com; p.324 © fizkes/stock.adobe.com

About the authors

Anne-Marie has worked in the Health and Social Care field for 37 years. She started out as a registered nurse in learning disability working with adults and children. She then went on to manage community-based residential and day services across North Wales. She set up Progression Training, a work-based training provider, in 2003. More recently, Anne-Marie has also been working with Social Care Wales and City and Guilds to develop the Health and Social Care suite of qualifications. She is a principal moderator and external quality assurer for City and Guilds. Anne-Marie's passion is developing others in order to improve services to vulnerable people.

Vicky has over 15 years' experience working with children and young people in a variety of residential and early years settings before moving into Training and Development. She currently oversees the training and education of staff in an array of Health and Social Care settings, and her centre delivers qualifications in Health and Social Care and Children's Care, Play, Learning and Development across Wales. Vicky worked as a consultant on assessment material which was produced for the new suite of Health and Social Care qualifications in Wales.

Maria commenced her career in Health and Social Care 31 years ago living and working in a lay community in France alongside individuals with a range of disabilities and health conditions. Her journey continued through a variety of services and settings in the UK that included working within and leading provision for young and older adults who have learning disabilities, physical disabilities, dementia, mental health needs, challenging needs and sensory impairments. Maria then embarked on delivering a range of Health and Social Care programmes and qualifications in both college and work-based settings. The experience she gained in work and academic settings led Maria to become a qualified assessor, internal and external quality assurer and the chief verifier for vocational-based qualifications in Health and Social Care and Children and Young People's Services. Maria has combined her experience in the social care sector with teaching adults with mental health needs, learning disabilities and additional needs to drive, which is proving to be both enjoyable and rewarding.

How to use this book

Throughout the book you will see the following features.

Key terms, marked in bold purple in the text, are explained to aid your understanding. (They are also explained in the Glossary at the back of the book.)

> ### KEY TERM
>
> **Safeguarding:** protecting an individual's health, well-being and human rights; enabling them to live free from harm and abuse.

Case studies provide examples of situations, with questions or discussion points which will help you think about the topics covered and how you might apply them in practice. These will prepare you for the case studies in your final assessment.

> ### CASE STUDY
>
> Ianto has limited verbal communication following a stroke and mainly communicates through body language and facial expression. Over the last year or so Ianto has started becoming increasingly withdrawn.
>
> **Discussion points:**
> - What might be the cause of this?
> - What should social care workers do in this situation?

Reflect on it activities will help you to reflect on your own experiences, skills and practice, and develop the skills necessary to become a reflective practitioner.

> ### REFLECT ON IT
>
> Imagine a teenager needs to change his living situation when he turns 18. Explain the approaches that can be used to make this transition a positive one.

Research it activities encourage you to explore an area in more detail.

> ### RESEARCH IT
>
> Think about the media and news stories over the last year, and find examples of stories which reflect a rights-based approach.

Further reading and research boxes offer useful resources and links at the end of every unit.

Short questions to **check your understanding** and multiple-choice questions for **exam practice** appear throughout the book, generally at the end of each LO. These are designed to identify any areas where you might need further training or revision.

> ### FURTHER READING AND RESEARCH
>
> **Weblinks**
> Information about the Social Services and Well-Being (Wales) Act 2014:
> **https://socialcare.wales/hub/resources**

About Units 001/002

The first chapter (Units 001/002) covers knowledge outcomes from Unit 001 Principles and values in health and social care (adults) and Unit 002 Principles and values in health and social care (children and young people).

Text relating to adults only is highlighted in blue.

Text relating to children and young people only is highlighted in orange.

PRINCIPLES AND VALUES IN HEALTH AND SOCIAL CARE (ADULTS, CHILDREN AND YOUNG PEOPLE)

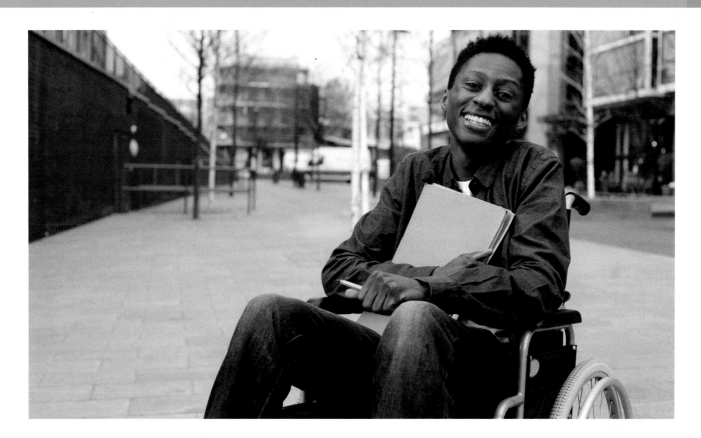

ABOUT THIS UNIT

Guided learning hours: 100

In this unit you will gain knowledge of how legislation, national policies, guidelines and frameworks support health and social care provision. You will gain an understanding of:

- the need to promote equality and diversity
- how person/child-centred and rights-based approaches relate to health and social care
- how appropriate risk taking supports well-being, voice, choice and control.

You will also learn about:

- the importance of effective communication, including the role of Welsh language and **culture**, in supporting health and social care provision
- how periods of change and transition can impact on individuals/children and young people
- how to develop positive relationships within professional boundaries and approaches that support positive behaviour
- how your own beliefs, values and life experiences can affect your attitude and behaviour towards others.

The terms 'individual' or 'people' refers to adults, or children and young people. The term 'person-centred' relates to adults, children and young people.

Learning outcomes – Adults	Learning outcomes – Children and young people
LO1: Understand how legislation, national policies and code of conduct and practice underpin health and social care and support for individuals	**LO1:** Understand how legislation, national policies and codes of conduct and practice underpin health and social care and support for children and young people
LO2: Understand how rights-based approaches relate to health and social care	**LO2:** Understand how rights-based approaches relate to health and social care
LO3: Understand how to use person-centred approaches	**LO3:** Understand how to use person-centred approaches
LO4: Understand how to promote equality, diversity and inclusion	**LO4:** Understand how to promote equality, diversity and inclusion
LO5: Understand how positive risk taking supports well-being, voice, choice and control	**LO5:** Understand how positive risk taking supports well-being, voice, choice and control
LO6: Understand how to develop positive relationships with individuals, their families and carers in the context of professional boundaries	**LO6:** Understand how to develop positive relationships with children and young people and their families and carers in the context of professional boundaries
LO7: Understand the importance of effective communication in health and social care	**LO7:** Understand the importance of effective communication in health and social care
LO8: Understand the importance of Welsh language and culture for individuals and carers	**LO8:** Understand the importance of Welsh language and culture for children and young people
LO9: Know how positive approaches can be used to reduce restrictive practices in social care	**LO9:** Know how positive approaches can be used to reduce restrictive practices in social care
LO10: Understand how change and transitions impact upon individuals	**LO10:** Understand how change and transitions impact upon children and young people
LO11: Understand how own beliefs, values and life experiences can affect attitude and behaviour towards individuals and carers	**LO11:** Understand how own beliefs, values and life experiences can affect attitude and behaviour towards children and young people

LO1 UNDERSTAND HOW LEGISLATION, NATIONAL POLICIES AND CODE OF CONDUCT AND PRACTICE UNDERPIN HEALTH AND SOCIAL CARE AND SUPPORT FOR INDIVIDUALS/ CHILDREN AND YOUNG PEOPLE

GETTING STARTED

There are numerous pieces of legislation that affect people working in health and social care services in Wales. In order to be committed to following legislation, it will help you to know the aim of legislation.

Think about why there is legislation in Wales.

- Who is the legislation there to help?
- How might people benefit from the legislation?

Think about what might happen if there was no legislation.

UK and international legislation or laws are established by governments and are in place to support our rights and protect us from being discriminated against. They also guide workers as to how they should work, and what they should and shouldn't do. They are there to protect workers and the people they support.

AC1.1 Principles and values of the Social Services and Well-Being (Wales) Act 2014

The Social Services and Well-Being (Wales) Act outlines the way in which care services are provided in Wales.

Aims of the Social Services and Well-Being (Wales) Act

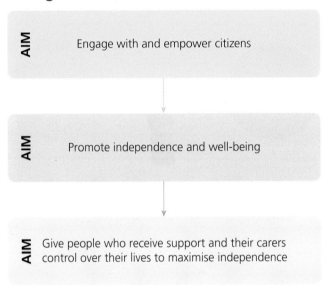

▲ Figure 1.1 Aims of the Social Services and Well-Being (Wales) Act

The Act puts the individual and their **carers** right at the centre of any health and social care services.

REFLECT ON IT

Well-being

What does well-being mean?

- List all the things that you think constitute well-being.
- What impact will this definition of well-being have upon practice?

Well-being can be in relation to any of the following:

- physical, mental and emotional health
- education, training and recreation
- domestic, family and personal relationships
- social and economic circumstances
- protection from abuse and neglect
- being part of communities and society
- securing rights and entitlements
- a suitable home.

In relation to adults, well-being also includes:

- control over day-to-day life
- participation in work.

In relation to children and young people, well-being also means:

- physical, intellectual, emotional, social and behavioural development.

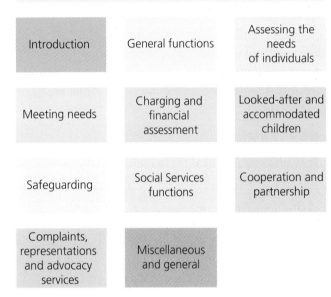

▲ Figure 1.2 Parts of the Social Services and Well-Being (Wales) Act

In order to ensure well-being, an **assessment** of need should take place when someone is in need of care and support. Where appropriate, an assessment for a carer can be combined with this. The individual or carer can then be signposted to other services that can help and prevent them from needing further support, such as drug rehabilitation or bereavement counselling.

KEY TERMS

Carers: a person who provides or intends to provide care for an adult or child. For the purposes of the Act, the person is not a carer if they provide care under a contract or as voluntary work.

Well-being: a person's health, happiness and ability to achieve goals and develop.

Assessment: a way of finding out what help and support a person needs. This will be different for each person.

If the individual's needs cannot be met by **preventative services**, a **care and support plan** should be developed with them in order to meet their needs. Every care and support plan will be different as no two people are the same.

A care and support plan must identify personal outcomes and set out the best way to achieve them. See AC3.11/3.12 for more information about this type of plan.

The Act gives people more control over their lives and gives them a voice when deciding what support they need and what is right for them in order to ensure well-being. It states that everyone should work together to support the individual in the best possible way.

KEY TERMS

Preventative services: these include services which will help people to be as independent as possible, or to prevent a situation from getting worse, for example, dietician involvement for somebody with an eating disorder. Preventative services aim to reduce the amount of help and support people might need in the future.

Care and support plan: this is developed by a social worker, the individual who needs support and their family/carer. It identifies what matters to the individual, and what help the individual needs in order for them to be as independent as possible, to ensure their well-being, achieve personal outcomes and support their development.

CASE STUDY

David's son is coming out of hospital after a serious road traffic accident. He has been left with long-term injuries. David is unsure of what support he will have but thinks it will include help with shopping and travelling to appointments. David is not sure how long his son will need this extra support.

Discussion points:

- Under the Act, would you consider David to be a carer?
- At what point would David be considered a carer and needing support?

Key principles of the Act

There are five key principles of the Act. These should guide you in everything you do at work. They should help in the planning of services as well as helping workers to support people in their daily lives.

The key principles are shown in Figure 1.3.

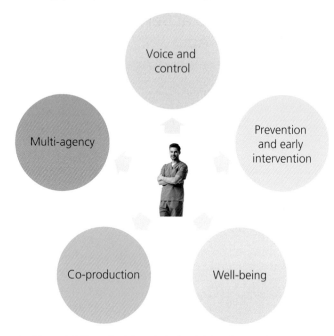

▲ Figure 1.3 Key principles of the Social Services and Well-Being (Wales) Act

Voice and control

Everybody needs to be able to have control over what happens in their life and what care and support they receive. Their voice needs to be heard and listened to. By giving people a voice and control over their lives, you can ensure that any care and support that is planned puts the individual at the centre of any decision making as equal partners.

Services should be aiming to support individuals to become as independent as possible and achieve the things that matter to them. They should be a valued part of their community, supported by family and friends.

Sometimes people need help to exercise their rights and to speak up about what they want. This could be because of their age, communication difficulties, learning disabilities, dementia, confidence levels, autism or because they are vulnerable. An advocate is somebody who can help individuals in situations like this. Under the Act, everybody has a right to an advocate if they need help exercising voice and control.

Children and young people in particular may need support to be heard and have control over their lives. Whilst adults have parental responsibility, professionals need to listen to children and young people and ensure their views and wishes are taken into account in any decisions made.

We will look at advocacy in more detail Learning Outcome 2.

REFLECT ON IT

Think about a time in your life when you felt you didn't have control or people weren't listening to you. How did this make you feel? What did you do in this situation?

Imagine if you have had no control over most of your life and other people have made decisions for you. This could be about things such as:

- where you live
- who you live with
- what you wear
- what and when you eat
- what activities you do.

Many services have been planned like this for a number of years. The Social Services and Well-Being (Wales) Act is designed to change this so that people are in control of their own lives.

Prevention and early intervention

The Act ensures that people can ask for help when they need it. Putting help in place early enough ensures people get the support they need to lead fulfilled lives without the situation getting worse and further help being required.

This can also be important for carers: sometimes they can feel isolated and not able to cope, so prevention and early intervention will help the carer get the support they need to ensure their own well-being.

Childhood and adolescence is a crucial time for physical, emotional, social and intellectual development. Giving children and young people the support they need will contribute to their development and help to prevent difficulties in the future.

CASE STUDY

Nia was very withdrawn and depressed following the death of her father. Bereavement counselling was provided, which helped Nia come to terms with the death.

Discussion point: What are the benefits of this early intervention?

Well-being

Well-being is about supporting people to achieve health and happiness in every part of their life. This makes people feel good about themselves, relaxed and safe. Everyone has a responsibility to ensure their own well-being but sometimes people need help with this. Well-being can influence our mental health as well as the development of children and young people.

Think about well-being in your own life.

- What does this mean to you?
- What makes you happy and fulfilled?
- What is important to you, and how does this improve your own well-being?

CASE STUDY

Alys had been feeling unhappy since finishing her art course in college. She was bored with staying at home all the time, and was becoming fed up as she thought her disability was preventing her from getting a job.

Discussion point: How could Alys be supported to improve her well-being?

The arts can help people improve their well-being. They can help people feel more relaxed and therefore improve emotional health. Creativity helps people's **self-esteem** and helps self-expression. It can:

- reduce social isolation by helping people to make friends
- help people to become more involved in their communities.

KEY TERM

Self-esteem: the value a person places on themselves – what they think and feel about themselves. Low self-esteem refers to a person not feeling very positive about themselves or their abilities.

Different things are important to different people, so supporting well-being isn't the same for everyone. That is why voice, control and well-being go together. It is important to listen to people and give them a chance to say what is important to them, in order to ensure their well-being.

Co-production

Co-production is where individuals and carers who need support and professionals work together as equals in order to plan and design services. Co-production:

- focuses on what people can do and builds on their strengths
- helps to build support networks within communities and develops relationships of trust
- is about shared power and shared responsibility
- ensures everyone feels valued and has a sense of identity as everyone is equal.

Think about people you support. Is there anything you can do to improve co-production?

If you don't support people at the moment, think about how you see co-production working in practice.

Multi-agency

The Act strengthens joint working between professionals such as social services, health services, housing and the voluntary sector. This improves the quality of services to ensure individuals' well-being. It makes sure the right services are available in local communities to meet individuals' needs.

RESEARCH IT

Research your local area to find out what services are available to help individuals.

CASE STUDY

The five principles of the Act

John has had a stroke which has resulted in him not being able to walk or speak. A team of carers are supporting John when he comes out of hospital.

Discussion point: How can each of the five principles be put into action to help improve John's life?

REFLECT ON IT

Think about somebody you support.

- Write down some examples of how you implement the five principles, giving examples of each.
- Can you make any improvements which would help the person lead a better quality of life?

RESEARCH IT

Look at examples of putting the principles into practice on the Social Care Wales website at:

https://socialcare.wales/hub/hub-resource-sub-categories/principles-of-the-act

---

AC1.1 Principles and values of the Social Services and Well-Being (Wales) Act 2014 and the Children Act (1989 and 2004)

The Social Services and Well-Being (Wales) Act is relevant to adults and children. In addition to the principles explained above, the Act also talks about looked after and accommodated children.

The Act supports children and young people in the following ways:

- Ensuring children and young people live with their families in a safe, nurturing environment.
- Supporting cooperation between schools and other agencies.
- Supporting assessment of children's and young people's needs including development needs.
- Ensuring appropriate additional care and support for disabled children.
- Enabling preventative services such as parenting programmes to support families.
- Care and support plans must ensure stability and permanence for children and young people.
- Supporting educational attainment for all children and young people.
- Helping young people prepare for adulthood by ensuring successful transitions to post-18 living arrangements.

- Enabling young people to remain in care until they are 21 or 25 if they are still in education.
- Improving governance of adoption services.

In addition to the Social Services and Well-Being Act, the Children Act is designed to safeguard children and young people from harm and abuse and promote well-being. It ensures children and young people who the court decides are in need of additional services are supported in the following ways:

- The child's welfare is the paramount consideration.
- The wishes and feelings of the child must be considered in line with their age.
- Physical, emotional and educational needs must be considered when deciding what support a child needs.
- Consideration must be given to any harm or abuse they have suffered or are at risk of suffering.
- Capability of parents in meeting the child's needs.

CASE STUDY
CHILDREN AND YOUNG PEOPLE

Osian has been in care since he was 12. He is now 16 and is looking forward to his future. His aims are to get an apprenticeship as a joiner and eventually have a flat of his own.

He has lots of friends in the town he lives in as he is in the local football team. Osian visits his family regularly, who live about 30 miles away.

Discussion point: How can Osian be helped to achieve his goals?

KEY TERM

Pathway plan: this is drawn up between a social worker and a young person leaving care or transitioning to adult services. It defines what help the person needs and how they will be prepared for this transition.

AC1.2 How the principles underpin health and social care and support practice

It is important to understand legislation including the Social Services and Well-Being (Wales) Act, as this will guide you to put the individual you support at the centre of everything you do.

When thinking about the Act, you need to remember the following:

- Individuals have as much control as possible in the services they receive. Some people may have full control, others may need help with this, for example, people with dementia or children and young people.
- **Safeguarding** is a theme that runs throughout the Act.
- You must always ask individuals what they want and listen to their views.
- You must support people to be able to express their views, for example, provide alternative methods of communication if they have difficulties with speaking.
- You must also listen to other people who are important to the individual, for example, parents, carers, advocates.
- If people need support you can't provide, they will need support to access this.
- You will need to work as part of a team to support the individual or young person.

KEY TERM

Safeguarding: protecting an individual's health, well-being and human rights; enabling them to live free from harm and abuse.

REFLECT ON IT

Think about someone you support: list three improvements you could make in order to implement the principles of the Act.

CASE STUDY
ADULTS

Olwen and Dai both have dementia.

Olwen is 83. Her first language is Welsh. She is married to Gwynfor who is a farmer. They still live on the farm and Iwan, their son, also works on the farm. Gwynfor is struggling to cope with Olwen's dementia.

Dai is 62 and has early onset dementia. He lives on his own and his daughter, who lives in London, is worried that Dai isn't safe in his own home.

Discussion point: How might Olwen's and Dai's care and support plans be different?

CASE STUDY
CHILDREN AND YOUNG PEOPLE

Ben is 15 and his mother has just died suddenly. Ben, who is an only child, lived with his mum on the outskirts of Cardiff. Ben's aunt lives in Powys, and she has contacted social services as Ben needs somewhere to live.

Freya is 15 and lives with her mum and John, her mum's partner. Her mum and John both misuse substances. John has recently come out of prison. Social Services were called by a neighbour as they were worried about Freya because they thought she was being neglected. She has become very thin and told the neighbours that John wanted her to get illicit drugs for him from a local dealer.

Discussion point: Give examples of how Ben's and Freya's care and support plans might be different.

AC1.3 Codes of conduct and professional practice, including who these apply to and how they can be used

Apart from legislation, there are also codes of practice that describe the **standards** of professional conduct and practice required of those employed in health and social care in Wales. These standards are useful resources for workers as they outline expectations and good practice. They can be used to support self-reflection and self- or team development. The links to these documents are at the end of this chapter.

The Code of Professional Practice for Social Care

The Code states that workers must:

1 Respect the views and wishes, and promote the rights and interests, of individuals and carers.
2 Strive to establish and maintain the trust and confidence of individuals and carers.
3 Promote the well-being, voice and control of individuals and carers while supporting them to stay safe.

4 Respect the rights of individuals while seeking to ensure that their behaviour does not harm themselves or other people.
5 Act with integrity and uphold public trust and confidence in the social care profession.
6 Be accountable for the quality of your work and take responsibility for maintaining and developing knowledge and skills.

In addition to sections 1–6, if you are responsible for managing or leading staff, you must embed the Code in their work.

The NHS Wales Code of Conduct for Healthcare Support Workers in Wales

This guidance is very similar to the Code of Professional Practice for Social Care but it explains how to implement it in a healthcare setting. It says healthcare workers must do the following:

- Be accountable by making sure you can always answer for your actions or omissions.
- Promote and uphold the privacy, dignity, rights and well-being of service users and their carers at all times.
- Work in collaboration with your colleagues as part of a team to ensure the delivery of high quality safe care to service users and their families.
- Communicate in an open, transparent and effective way to promote the well-being of service users and carers.
- Respect a person's right to confidentiality, protecting and upholding their privacy.
- Improve the quality of care to service users by updating your knowledge, skills and experience through personal and professional development.
- Promote equality: all service users, colleagues and members of the public are entitled to be treated fairly and without bias.

Code of Practice for NHS Wales Employers

This code tells employers how to support workers to implement the Code of Conduct for Healthcare Support Workers. It ensures that:

- people know their roles and responsibilities
- training and education are provided.

The Practice Guidance for Residential Child Care for Workers Registered with Social Care Wales

This practice guidance builds on the Code of Professional Practice for Social Care. It is a guide for residential child care workers about what is expected of them. It:

- describes what is expected of workers
- supports workers to deliver a quality service
- ensures **child-centred care and support**.

The practice guidance tells you how to:

- ensure good communication with children and young people
- ensure confidentiality
- work with family members
- ensure professional boundaries and relationships
- protect children's and young people's rights
- know your own limits
- support children and young people to develop their own personal plans
- promote quality of life
- contribute to meeting the health and education needs of children and young people
- support young people to plan for the future
- keep in contact with young people leaving care
- work as part of a team
- complete records and reports
- support children and young people to comment and complain about a service if they are unhappy with it
- ensure children and young people are safe
- ensure health and safety
- develop your own knowledge and practice
- contribute to improving the service to children and young people
- act in a professional manner at all times.

The Practice Guidance for Domiciliary Care Workers and the Practice Guidance for Adult Care Home Workers

Domiciliary care workers or adult care workers should read this practice guidance in conjunction with the Code of Professional Practice for Social Care. In addition to the guide, a useful app can be found at https://socialcare.wales/resources, which is specifically designed for domiciliary care workers.

Both guides cover the following areas of practice:

Person-centred care and support	- good communication - confidentiality - meeting Welsh language needs - working with families and carers - professional boundaries - rights and protection.
Good domiciliary care practice or good adult care home practice	- expectations of workers - knowing your limits - personal plans - delivering care and support - carrying out tasks delegated by another professional - working in people's homes - working at a distance from your manager - working in teams - maintaining records and reports - comments and complaints.
Safeguarding individuals	- understanding safeguarding - supporting individuals to keep themselves safe - female genital mutilation - preventing people from being drawn into terrorism.
Health and safety	- meeting health and safety and security requirements - medication - safety and well-being - supporting health and safety.
Learning and development	- keeping up to date - supervision and appraisal - supporting the learning of colleagues.
Contributing to service improvement	- use of resources - raising concerns.
Good conduct	- professional registration - gifts and donations - social media - supporting positive behaviour.

KEY TERMS

Standards: these tell you how you should work to ensure quality and implement the legislation. They are the minimum requirements, and may include codes of conduct and practice and regulations.

Child-centred care and support: making sure children and young people receive care and support that meets their individual needs.

Domiciliary care workers: provide care and support to people in their own homes.

AC1.4 How the codes of conduct and professional practice underpin the principles and values of health and social care and support

The codes of conduct and professional practice inform social care workers on how to ensure that person/child-centred care and support is provided to enable the well-being of individuals.

All workers are required to register with Social Care Wales as a social care worker. If you haven't done this yet, your employer will support you with this. In order to register you have to undertake this core qualification – City & Guilds Health and Social Care: Core – and also agree to abide by the standards laid down in the codes of practice.

REFLECT ON IT

Look at the first six standards of the Code of Professional Practice for Social Care above.

- Think about how you implement each of these into your work.
- Can you see the similarities here with the five principles of the Social Services and Well-Being (Wales) Act?

Accountability for your work is required under the standards. This means you must be open and honest. You must tell your employer immediately if something has gone wrong, and they have a responsibility to inform other authorities if required.

You need to give a full account of what has happened so things can be put right and you can learn from your mistakes. This is known as a '**duty of candour**'. It can include things such as:

- medication errors
- giving wrong information to someone
- a breach of confidentiality
- not following organisational policy
- not following up on complaints or concerns raised by an individual or their family
- not reporting safeguarding concerns
- incorrect use of equipment

KEY TERM

Duty of candour: being honest when something goes wrong.

Using social media correctly is another area where you need to think about how you implement the codes of practice. Social media can be very useful to enable you to communicate and keep in touch with people. However if used inappropriately, it can blur the boundaries between professional relationships.

The Code of Practice says you must establish trust and confidence in your professional relationships, and respect privacy and confidentiality. When using social media, this means you:

- must not discuss people you support
- should not accept 'friend' requests from people you support or their families
- must respect the privacy and dignity of the people you support and that of your colleagues.

Check your privacy settings: everything you post has the potential to be spread to a wider audience if you don't have appropriate privacy settings.

LO2 UNDERSTAND HOW RIGHTS-BASED APPROACHES RELATE TO HEALTH AND SOCIAL CARE

GETTING STARTED

We looked at the Social Services and Well-Being (Wales) Act in the last section. A rights-based approach ensures you put the Act in practice in your daily work as you ensure people's rights are upheld by:

- supporting individuals including children and young people to have a voice
- supporting them to have control over their own lives
- treating everyone as equals through co-production.

Think of some ways you can ensure that individuals' rights are met.

AC2.1 Key elements of a rights-based approach

Think about your own life. What rights do you have which are important to you?

We all have many rights in our day-to-day life which have developed over time through changes in legislation in our democratic society. The following rights are considered as important:

- choice
- protection
- confidentiality
- equality
- dignity and respect
- education
- consultation.

A **rights-based approach** ensures that services are provided in a way which puts individuals, children and young people at the centre of planning and delivering services. By working in this way you are ensuring rights are upheld and individuals have support from advocates if they need it.

When you support people in health and social care settings, you will find that individuals are often vulnerable and services in the past haven't always worked in this person-centred way. Over time the culture in our society has recognised the importance of everybody being treated as equals while recognising **diversity**, in a rights-based approach.

RESEARCH IT

Think about the media and news stories over the last year, and find examples of stories which reflect a rights-based approach.

KEY TERMS

Rights-based approach: ensuring that individuals' rights are upheld in their day-to-day lives.

Diversity: individual differences we have from each other, such as religious belief, race, gender.

AC2.2 How legislation and national policies underpin a rights-based approach

REFLECT ON IT

Think about the Social Services and Well-Being (Wales) Act. How does this ensure a rights-based approach?

The Social Services and Well-Being (Wales) Act is the main piece of legislation relating to health and social care provision in Wales. As we have seen, its aim is to ensure vulnerable people are central to everything you do in order to ensure their rights are met. There are other pieces of legislation, shown in Table 1.1, that ensure these principles underpin the way services are delivered.

Legislation	Explanation of this legislation
Equality Act 2010	Protects people from discrimination and unfair treatment on the basis of personal characteristics including: • age • disability • pregnancy and maternity • gender • gender reassignment • sexual orientation • race • religion or belief • marriage or civil partnership.
Human Rights Act 1998	Describes the rights that everybody in the UK is entitled to, such as the right to freedom, right to marry and start a family, right to life and many more. For more information, see Unit 006, AC1.4.
UN Convention on the Rights of Persons with Disabilities	This is an international agreement which protects the rights and dignity of people with a disability. It covers areas such as right to employment, health and accessibility, and states that people with disabilities should be treated equally.
Welsh Language Act 1993 **Welsh Language Measure 2011**	The Welsh Language Act ensures that public bodies should, as far as practicable, treat the English and Welsh language equally in the conduct of public business in Wales. The Welsh Language Measure updates this legislation and introduces standards which public bodies must achieve. For more information, see AC8.2 and AC8.3 in this unit.
Mwy na Geiriau	Translated as 'More than words', this is a framework for Welsh language in health and social care services. It ensures that people who need services in Welsh automatically receive them without having to ask. This is called the '**active offer**'. For more on *Mwy na Geiriau*, see AC8.3 in this unit.

▲ Table 1.1 Legislation affecting adults, children and young people

The legislation in Table 1.2 relates to the care of adults.

Legislation	Explanation of this legislation
UN Principles for Older Persons 1991	This statement of principles ensures that older people in the UK have their basic needs met, as well as other rights such as having a right to work, education and for their dignity to be respected.
Declaration of rights of older people in Wales 2014	Wales has led the way in ensuring that the rights of older people are met. The first Older People's Commissioner was appointed as a result of this declaration to uphold older people's rights in Wales.
Mental Health Act 1989 Code of Practice for Wales 2008	The Mental Health Act is the main piece of legislation that covers the assessment, treatment and rights of people with a mental health disorder. The Code of Practice for Wales gives guidance to professionals about how to implement the Act and also on medical treatment for mental health. For further information, see the links at the end of the chapter.
Mental Health (Wales) Measure 2010	The Measure sets standards for assessment, treatment and advocacy in mental health care.
Mental Capacity Act 2005 The Mental Health Act Code of Practice for Wales	This Act is designed to protect and empower people who may lack **mental capacity**. Where people cannot make a decision or lack capacity, whoever is making a decision on their behalf must do so in the individual's best interests. The Mental Health Act Code of Practice for Wales explains how the Act should be implemented in Wales. It sets standards for hospital admissions, care and treatment, safeguarding and leaving hospital. For further information, see the links at the end of the chapter.

▲ Table 1.2 Legislation affecting adults

Legislation	Explanation of this legislation
Deprivation of Liberty Safeguards/Liberty Protection Safeguards	Deprivation of Liberty Safeguards (DoLS) is an amendment to the Mental Capacity Act. It protects an individual's liberties if there are any restrictions applied under the Mental Capacity Act in order to keep them safe. The Liberty Protection Safeguards (LPS) will replace DoLS in April 2022. They have the same aim as DoLS but the assessment has been strengthened and there is a greater involvement for families. The safeguards have also been extended to cover 16 and 17 year-olds, whereas DoLS required a court order to safeguard young people of this age. LPS will also cover people in domestic settings such as their own home, shared lives or supported living, whereas DoLS is just for people in hospital, nursing or care homes. For more information, see Unit 006.
Welsh Government Strategic Framework for the Welsh Language in Health and Social Care 2013	This framework builds on *Mwy na Geiriau* and looks at how Welsh language will be promoted in health and social care. It looks at topics such as service planning, responsibility, professional education and Welsh in the workplace. For more information, see AC8.2, 8.3 and 8.4 in this unit.

▲ Table 1.2 Legislation affecting adults *(continued)*

Table 1.3 contains legislation which relates to children and young people.

Legislation	Explanation of this legislation
Children Act 1989 and 2004	The Act provides the legal basis for how social services and other agencies deal with issues relating to children. The main principles of the Act are to: • allow children to be healthy • allow children to remain safe • help children to enjoy life • assist children in their quest to succeed • help make a positive contribution to the lives of children • help achieve economic stability for children's future. For more information, see Unit 005, AC1.1.
UN Convention on the Rights of the Child 1990	There are a number of human rights granted to children under this international agreement. They cover areas such as civil, political, economic, social and cultural rights of children of every race, religion and ability.
Welsh Assembly Government's Seven Core Aims for children and young people 2000	The Seven Core Aims was adopted by Welsh Government as a commitment to ensure the rights of children. Figure 1.4 shows the areas covered by these seven aims. For further information, see the links at the end of the chapter.

▲ Table 1.3 Legislation affecting children and young people

KEY TERMS

Active offer: providing a service in Welsh without someone having to ask for it.

Mental capacity: the ability to make an informed decision, and to be able to weigh up the options and consequences.

REFLECT ON IT

Which of the legislation in Tables 1.1, 1.2 and 1.3 is relevant to adults or children and young people you support? Think of examples of how you can put each of the relevant legislation into practice.

1 Early years	2 Education and learning
3 Health, freedom from abuse	4 Play, sport, leisure and culture
5 Participation in decision making	6 A safe home and community
7 Not disadvantaged by poverty	

▲ Figure 1.4 Seven core aims for children and young people

We have seen that there is plenty of legislation in Wales which underpins a rights-based approach. It will guide you in your work to ensure you uphold the rights of the people you support.

AC2.3 How legislation impacts on a rights-based approach in practice

Social care workers have a responsibility to implement the legislation and codes of practice in everything they do. This ensures they adopt a rights-based approach by giving people voice and control, respecting people's choices and ensuring their rights are upheld.

CASE STUDY
ADULTS

Sali has dementia. She is leaving hospital after a stroke and is moving into a care home.
Discussion point: How might legislation impact on Sali?

CASE STUDY
CHILDREN AND YOUNG PEOPLE

Huw is 8 years old and lives with his mum. He has regular visits from social services, who regard him as vulnerable due to his mum's alcohol and drug dependency. He hasn't met all his developmental milestones and has been struggling in school.
Discussion point: How might legislation impact on Huw?

AC2.4 The term 'advocacy' and how it can support a rights-based approach

Advocacy is used in health and social care settings to help stand up for people's rights when they are unable to do so themselves. The advocate works in partnership with the individual, getting to know the person and what is important to them. The advocate would then ensure that the adult's, child's or young person's voice and views are heard and that they are treated with respect. They will also support the individual to understand their rights, to help them make an informed choice.

An advocate can help somebody to:

- access services
- exercise their rights
- express their views
- explore and make informed choices
- make a complaint
- move care settings
- attend meetings and medical appointments
- liaise with other professionals or do this on their behalf.

The Social Services and Well-Being (Wales) Act and the Mental Capacity Act require local authorities to provide an independent advocate if a person in care needs one.

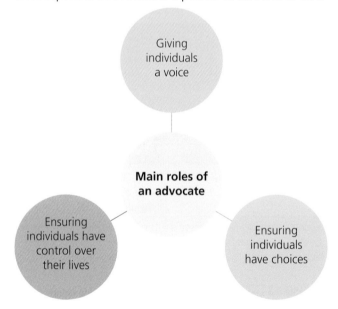

▲ Figure 1.5 Main roles of an advocate

Advocacy promotes social inclusion, equality and social justice. The advocate is independent from other services so is free from conflict of interest.

The advocate should support **self-advocacy** where possible. This means enabling people to stand up for their own rights themselves by giving them the support and information to do this. Where someone doesn't have the capacity to do this, the advocate can act on their behalf.

To ensure accountability, advocates also have a code of practice and charter that they have to work to.

REFLECT ON IT

- Think about how advocacy can support a rights-based approach.
- List key words that demonstrate this, such as **empowerment** and accountability.

KEY TERMS

Advocacy: a service which provides representation to people for purposes relating to their care and support.

Empowerment: supporting people to take control over their own lives and make their own decisions.

CASE STUDY

Discussion point: Thinking about the case studies above, how might an advocate be able to help Sali or Huw?

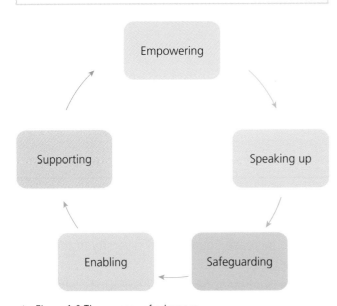

▲ Figure 1.6 The purpose of advocacy

RESEARCH IT

Look at the advocacy charter online to learn more about the role of an advocate:

www.advocacymatterswales.co.uk/about-us/advocacy-charter/

AC2.5 Ways in which individuals, children and young people and their families or carers can be supported to make a complaint or express a concern about their service

Think of an occasion when you were dissatisfied or unhappy about a service you received, such as:

- having to wait too long for an appointment at your General Practitioner (GP) surgery
- the food you were served at a restaurant being too cold or the wrong item
- poor customer service when buying a new mobile phone.

Think about how you felt and what happened.

- Did you take any action?
- If so, what did you do? If not, why not?
- How did it make you feel afterwards?
- Why do you think you felt this way?

Now think about somebody you support.

- Would they need any help to complain if they faced a similar situation?
- How might you be able to help them?
- If they didn't have support to complain, how might they feel?

A rights-based approach recognises when things go wrong and when services are not delivered in a way that they should be. Individuals and their families should have information about how to make a complaint.

Making a complaint can be a scary prospect for many people. Often, we worry that we will offend someone by making a complaint, and this may stop us from making one. Individuals you support may feel the same way when they make complaints. However, you should remember that complaints can lead to improved practice, so it is crucial that you make individuals feel that their concerns and complaints are welcomed and taken seriously.

When supporting someone to make a complaint, you should:

- listen to what they have to say and check your understanding is correct
- ensure the individual has access to the complaints procedure and knows what their rights are
- not disagree with the person but accept their feelings
- thank them for bringing it to your attention and reassure them you will either take action or pass it on to your manager

- pass it on to your manager and agree what action should be taken
- ensure someone feeds back to the individual who has made the complaint
- ensure it is recorded in line with policies and procedures.

If a person needs an advocate in order to make a complaint, ensure they have access to one.

Check your understanding

1 What do the terms 'voice' and 'control' mean?

2 What should be completed when people need care and support?

3 Identify three principles of the Social Services and Well-Being (Wales) Act.

4 Define the term 'well-being'.

5 State two potential impacts of reduced mobility on well-being.

6 List three examples of how you can put the Act into practice when supporting people with dementia.

7 Explain how promoting positive routines, such as set meal and homework times, might support children's and young people's well-being and development.

8 What is meant by the term 'accountability'?

9 Give three examples of breaches of the Code of Professional Practice for Social Care.

10 Outline three reasons why sharing social media contact details with individuals is considered to be poor professional practice.

11 How can an advocate help an individual, child or young person?

12 Why is it important that you support people to make complaints if they are not happy with the service they are receiving?

Question practice

1 How does the Human Rights Act support individuals' rights?

   a It protects individuals from discrimination.

   b It promotes equality.

   c It describes the rights of people with disabilities.

   d It describes the rights everybody's entitled to.

2 What is the most important reason for working in a person/child-centred way in a care setting?

   a to uphold the rights of individuals/children accessing care and support

   b to meet current health and safety requirements

   c to increase equality and diversity in the care setting

   d to promote a feeling of community within the care setting

3 How does the Social Services and Well-Being (Wales) Act aim to support rights-based approaches?

   a It promotes voice and control.

   b It safeguards children.

   c It identifies protected characteristics.

   d It ensures decisions are made in the best interest of the individual.

4 What term is defined by the following description?

'Involving people and communities in the design and delivery of services. Doing things with, rather than doing things to, people.'

a well-being

b co-production

c multi-agency working

d early intervention prevention

5 Why is co-production important when working in partnership with others?

a to make the service cheaper to deliver

b to meet the requirements of current safety legislation

c to improve the reputation of children and young people's settings

d to ensure positive outcomes for the child or young person accessing care

6 What term is defined by the following description?

'Being healthy, feeling good about your life, feeling safe and being able to learn new things as well as being able to grow up happy and being looked after.'

a welfare

b well-being

c looked after children

d rights-based approach

7 Which of the following statements is TRUE?

a You must not ask individuals what they want.

b You must sometimes listen to individuals.

c You will need to work as part of a team to support the individual.

d Individuals have some control in the services they receive.

8 What term is defined by the following description?

'Treating everyone with fairness and respect and recognising the needs of individuals.'

a equality

b inclusion

c judgement

d discrimination

9 Which of the following is covered by the Code of Professional Practice for Social Care?

a Always report disclosed personal information.

b Promote the rights and interests of individuals.

c Protect your own personal well-being in care settings.

d Control the involvement of other care professionals.

10 Which legislation supports rights-based approaches?

a Health and Safety at Work Act

b UN Convention of the Rights of the Child

c Reporting of Injuries, Diseases and Dangerous Occurrences Regulations

d Control of Substances Hazardous to Health Regulations

11 Which two actions would an independent advocate take to support an individual/child or young person?

a Help them express their views.

b Help them make informed choices.

c Give them advice on the best options.

d Tell them what actions they should take.

12 What is the role of an independent advocate where there is a safeguarding concern related to a young person who lives in a residential care setting?

a to decide the best outcome for the young person

b to state their view on the young person's situation

c to prioritise the young person's family or carer's views and needs

d to support the young person's voice and represent their interests

LO3 UNDERSTAND HOW TO USE PERSON-CENTRED APPROACHES

GETTING STARTED

- Think about what makes you an individual and different from your family, friends and others you know. It could be your personality, your beliefs or your interests.
- Now imagine how you would feel if your beliefs were not taken into account by the people who know you. Why would you feel this way?
- Imagine how you would feel if you had the same beliefs as a member of your family and because of this you were both treated in exactly the same way rather than as different individuals. Why is it important to be treated like an individual?

AC3.1 The importance of 'person and child-centred approaches'

Your values are unique to you: they make you who you are and influence what you do and how you do it. Your values represent what you believe to be important to you; they also guide you on how to live your life and the decisions you make.

The care and support that you provide is underpinned by a set of values. These are commonly referred to as 'person-centred' or 'child-centred' values, which means placing the individual or person you support at the centre or heart of everything you do. By making sure

that these values underpin your work, the support you provide will be focused on:

- the individual, and represent their unique needs, wishes and preferences
- enabling the individual to be in control of their life, including how they want to live it
- enabling the individual to plan for the care and support they would like (including changes that may arise in the future).

Person- or child-centred approaches actively involve individuals with care or support needs in the planning and provision of their care. Working in a way that embeds person-centred values is crucial for ensuring individuals are in control of their care or support.

Person-centred/ child-centred values	What they mean in relation to providing care and support
Rights *Helping individuals to understand and access their rights*	This means supporting and encouraging an individual to understand what they are entitled to. For example, ensuring: • individuals' rights are met • there are no barriers to stop them from accessing their rights. Having a disability or using a wheelchair should not be a barrier to joining in activities, and fear of upsetting a worker should not be a barrier to making a complaint. Not being able to read or read English should not be a barrier to signing a form. You should do the following: • Support individuals to access their rights and ensure activities allow everyone to participate. • Make sure that individuals are aware of the process for making complaints. • Support individuals to make a complaint if they need to. • Support anyone who cannot read to understand what they are signing before they do so.
Choice *Enabling individuals to make choices*	This means supporting, encouraging and empowering an individual to make their own choices and decisions. Individuals should choose how they would like to be supported and be given information about what options are available in order to make informed decisions. For example, you should tell individuals about the different care and support services that are available in their local area, so that they can decide which ones are best for them.

▲ Table 1.4 Person-centred values when providing care and support

Person-centred/ child-centred values	What they mean in relation to providing care and support
Privacy *Allowing individuals to have privacy*	This means showing respect for an individual's personal space and personal information. For example, this could include: • knocking on the door of an individual's room before entering • making sure that individuals can spend some time alone if they want to • giving individuals privacy if they request it when family members visit • enabling them to carry out personal care privately if they want to.
Independence *Supporting individuals to be independent*	This means supporting an individual to be in control of their life by doing as much for themselves as they are able to. This could, for example, include: • encouraging an individual to find out about the range of services that are available to them to enable them to remain living in their own home • assessing the risks that individuals face but ensuring that they understand these and are able to live as independently as possible • teaching a young person new skills that would help them prepare for adulthood.
Dignity and respect *Treating individuals with dignity and respect*	This means treating people well and showing respect for their views, opinions and rights. Respect for individuals involves: • taking into account their differences and valuing them as individuals with their own needs and preferences • promoting an individual's sense of self-respect by ensuring they do not feel humiliated or embarrassed in any way. Although you are there to support them, individuals should still feel that they are in control of their lives. Treating them with dignity and respect is a big part of this.
Care *Providing care to individuals*	Providing care is of course the key person-centred value that underpins your role. But, more specifically, it means providing care and support in a way that is consistent, sufficient and meets the needs of the individual. For example: • One of your responsibilities will be to support an individual with their meal times. • However, in order to make sure that you provide good quality care and fulfil this duty adequately, you will need to ensure that the meal is prepared in a way that meets their dietary and nutritional requirements and is enjoyable. You may also need to support them in eating and drinking.
Compassion *Showing compassion and kindness*	This means providing care to an individual in a way that shows kindness, consideration, empathy, dignity and respect. For example, this might mean taking time out from a busy shift to sit with an individual who has received some sad news.
Courage *Speaking up for individuals*	This means providing care and support in a way that is morally acceptable, such as: • doing the right thing for the individuals you support • constantly improving and changing ways of working for better efficiency • speaking up if you have concerns about practice at work or about an individual (including when an individual is being abused but is too scared to report it).
Communication *Communicating effectively with individuals*	Good communication is key to providing high quality care and support and to effective team working. It includes actively listening to what the individuals have to say, and is necessary for building strong relationships with them and colleagues.
Competence *Working effectively and efficiently with individuals*	Being competent in your job role means: • having the knowledge, skills and expertise to provide high quality care and support • understanding the needs of the individuals you support and providing effective care to meet their needs. For example, this could include applying the knowledge and skills you have learnt in relation to moving and handling to assist an individual to move safely from one position to another.
Partnership *Working together with individuals and others*	This means working together, alongside the individuals for whom you provide care and support. This will ensure that they are at the centre of the care you provide and are in control of the care they receive. Partnership also includes working with individuals' families, your colleagues and those outside the organisation. This is essential for the provision of high quality person-centred care.

▲ Table 1.4 Person-centred values when providing care and support *(continued)*

AC3.2 The terms 'co-production' and 'voice, choice and control'

These terms are central to person-centred approaches, and underpin the Social Services and Well-Being (Wales) Act.

Co-production

Co-production means professionals and individuals, children and young people working together as equals in order to plan how the individual is supported. Look back at Learning Outcome 1.1 for further information.

There are many examples in your daily life where you see co-production in action:

- When you go to the hairdressers, you might discuss with the hairdresser the style you would like. The hairdresser may make suggestions but it is your decision, with the hairdresser's guidance if you want it.
- In work you may be in a meeting with an individual you support where you are discussing a new way of doing things, and between everyone, you agree a way forward.

Think about people you support:

- In which areas of their lives can you see co-production in action?
- Are there any areas where you can improve co-production?

Voice

The term 'voice' in the context of person-centred support means enabling the individual to speak up or make their views known. It means respecting their rights and listening to them.

If individuals cannot speak, then you should find alternative ways to enable them to make their views known, such as alternative communication methods or support from an advocate.

People who are vulnerable are sometimes not given a voice due to discrimination. For example, a person with a disability who uses a wheelchair may not be given a choice because people wrongly presume they cannot make a choice.

Choice and control

Choice and control is about enabling people to make choices and have control over their lives.

CASE STUDY

Sian, who has an acquired brain injury following an accident, has just moved from her parents' home into a supported living project. As she now has no speech and significant memory problems, the workers at Sian's new home wanted to give Sian a voice, choice and control as she didn't seem to make many choices.

It was very difficult to know what Sian wanted to do, as she tended to go along with whatever was happening. Every time Sian went out, workers gave her the car keys to hold and said 'Here's the keys'. After a few months Sian went to the key hook and took the keys to the worker. They immediately took Sian out.

Over time they built up the number of objects they used to reference different activities. For example, when they cooked or baked, they gave Sian a wooden spoon and said 'Would you like to cook?' When they did some drawing, they gave Sian some pencils and said 'Would you like to draw?' Sian had a box which contained all these objects of reference. She also had her own house key which she hung on the hook.

Eventually Sian would go to her box and choose what activity she would like to do that day without any prompting.

The staff in this case study gave Sian a voice, and they enabled her to have a choice and control. Sometimes people who have never been given a choice don't know how to make one. They don't realise if they choose something then something else will follow as a result of their choice. This often has to be taught, starting with small steps such as choosing tea or coffee.

It can sometimes take many months for the person to understand they have a choice. Workers should persevere though, as while somebody choosing their own drink may seem like a very small step, it could be the first choice that person has ever made. This could lead them to make more choices and have more control over their own lives.

Discussion point: Discuss ways in which you can support someone to make choices and have greater control over their lives.

AC3.3 The importance of knowing an individual's, child's and young person's preferences and background

We all have our own preferences and background, which are a unique mix of our experience, history, culture, beliefs, preferences, family, relationship, informal networks and community. These are central to the way we manage our lives, the way we think about the future, and our own well-being.

It is important to know the background of children and young people as it has a big influence on the child. This can include:

- their parents' background
- childhood experiences, for example, whether they have been at risk of neglect or abuse
- whether they have lived with their parents or have been in care
- whether they have had consistency in their life or have been in a number of different placements or schools with lots of different carers.

REFLECT ON IT

Make a list of all the people who are important in your life and who know you well. For each person, write down one aspect that they know about you. For example, this could be something about your background, family, likes, interests.

- Why are these aspects of your life important to you?

Now think about an individual you know who has care or support needs. Write down what you know about them.

- How well do you think you know them?
- Why is this?
- Is there anything else you think you need to know about them?
- How could you find out?

As we have discussed, the needs of the individuals that you support should be at the centre of the care and support you provide. In order to make sure this happens, first you will need to find out as much as you can about the individual you will be supporting. You must not only understand what support they think they will need, but also their personal history to enable you to understand them as a person. This in turn will enable you to meet their needs and allow them to live their life as they want to.

There are different ways you can build up a picture of who the individual is and what makes them the person they are. In order to find out more about the individuals you support, you will need to explore different ways to find out this information.

Finding out about an individual's history

By speaking to individuals about their history, you will be able to understand more about the experiences that have informed the person they are.

- You can do this by asking them about their childhood and family background. This is very important, especially when you work with older people. Remember that all individuals have a history, and they may even be eager to share it with you. You could ask if they would like to show you any photographs or tell you any memories. By doing this, you are valuing the person you support as an individual, and showing a genuine interest.
- Where people can't tell you themselves, other people involved in their lives who know the individual well, such as their family, friends, teachers and advocates, may also be a useful source of information.
- You could support children and young people to draw pictures or write a story about their history.
- Watching children playing can give us clues about their history.
- Reading people's care and support plans will help as these should have some background information about an individual.

Think how you feel when someone asks for your opinion, how you are feeling, what your likes and dislikes are, or invites you to talk about your own history. Do you feel that the person asking cares about you and your opinion? Do you feel that they are interested in who you are as an individual? Similarly, asking people about their history will not only allow you to provide better support but will also make the individual feel respected and valued, and not simply feel like another person that requires care.

The individual's preferences

These may be based on the individual's beliefs, values and culture. You can find out about an individual's beliefs by asking them what they view as important, and their culture by asking them (and others who know them well) questions about this and the associated practices they follow. This might affect how they communicate with others, what they eat and what they wear. If somebody is unable to tell you their preferences, you can show them choices so they can pick the one they like. Pictures could be used to support children and young people or people who are unable to communicate verbally to help them express their preferences.

When supporting children and young people, we need to remember that they may have less experience than adults so may need to be shown a number of different options before they can decide what they prefer.

Somebody with dementia may be confused, so you may need to remember what they preferred when they were less confused or they may wish to try out a different option. It is important to remember that people's preferences may change over time and we should account for this.

REFLECT ON IT

Finding out about a person

Reflect on someone you do not know very well. This may be a neighbour or a colleague from work. Imagine you would like to find out more about their beliefs, their values and their culture.

As you do not know them very well, you may find this a little difficult. How could you make this easier? Think about

- how you approach them
- what you are going to say
- the reasons why you are asking them personal information.

The individual's wishes

You can find out about an individual's wishes by asking them about their hopes and dreams for the present and the future. Others who know the individual well may also be helpful when drawing up a picture of the individual's wishes.

The individual's needs

An individual's needs will be assessed and detailed in the care and support plan. You may contribute to this in team meetings. You will also find out on a day-to-day basis through supporting and talking to individuals if their needs have changed.

- **Health** – whilst supporting individuals you may notice they aren't feeling very well or you think their health seems to have deteriorated. By discussing this with them, you can get a better picture so you can pass this information on to your manager.
- **Social interactions** – individuals you support may need help with developing relationships, for example, they may need support to find out what activities are in their community to help them make new friends, or they may need support with communication when interacting with others.
- **Religious and cultural backgrounds** – religious and cultural needs will be detailed in care and support plans. If individuals are from a different culture or religion, finding out about their traditions and beliefs will help you support them better.
- **Educational and employment background** – this information should be detailed in the care and support plan. Finding out about someone's background helps you get to know the person better. People often enjoy talking about their past, for example, someone with dementia may remember a lot about their past so may enjoy discussing their working life with you.
- **A child's development** – knowing what milestones children should reach will help you support children's development according to their age. If a child has any developmental delay, this will be recorded in their care and support plan. For more on child development, see Unit 004.

REFLECT ON IT

Individuals' history

Reflect on why knowing about an individual's history is important when providing care and support.

- What can an individual's history tell you about the person behind the individual?
- How can this help you when supporting them with a task, such as taking part in a cooking activity, or when supporting the individual to socialise with others?
- How would you show the individual that you are taking into account their history?

AC3.4 Ways of working to establish the preferences and backgrounds of individuals, children and young people, what matters to them and the outcomes that they want

Areas of support	What to do
Support an individual with their personal hygiene	Ask the individual or people important to them what support they require with their personal hygiene.
	Provide the individual with the opportunity to choose whether they would like a bath or shower, and whether they would like their hair washed.
	Show respect for an individual's culture and beliefs by asking them if there is a personal hygiene routine they prefer to follow, such as using running water when washing.
	If a person cannot communicate verbally, show them different options or try different things and see what they like and do not like.
	Try to support young children to develop their skills whilst ensuring their hygiene needs are met, for example, teaching them to clean their own teeth whilst ensuring they are cleaned thoroughly.
Support an individual with preparing a meal	Find out the individual's requirements for eating and drinking; whether there are some foods they are unable to eat (due to their beliefs), and their likes and dislikes for food and drink (personal preference). For example, they may prefer to eat only vegetarian, vegan, halal or kosher food.
	Find out whether the individual has any allergies or food intolerances, such as a nut allergy, or being gluten intolerant. This is something you may need to check with medical professionals caring for them and others that know them.
	Promote an individual's independence by enabling them to do as much for themselves as they can when preparing a meal.
	Ask the individual where they would prefer to eat. Do they prefer to eat in the kitchen, lounge or their own room? You should respect their choice.
	Look at an individual's care plan to see if there are any special dietary requirements.
	When supporting children and young people, think about what is age-appropriate for them so you can ensure they can help as much as possible whilst ensuring their safety.
Support an individual with attending a GP appointment	Ask the individual how they would prefer to travel to their GP appointment. For example, by taxi or bus?
	Ask the individual or people important to them what support they require from you. Do they want you to: • travel with them only • attend the appointment with them • speak up for them?
	Promote an individual's right to make their own informed choices by ensuring they understand the information that has been communicated to them by their GP.
	Look at an individual's care and support plan as there may be special considerations when attending a GP. For example, the person may get nervous or upset.
Support an individual with activities	Ask the individual or somebody important to them what activities they would like to do and what support they would like. This could be daily activities, such as cooking and shopping, or recreational activities, such as gardening and going to the gym.
	Find out whether there are any activities the individual would like to do but hasn't tried yet, such as bowling, or learning a new skill such as sewing or painting.
	Promote an individual's independence by encouraging them to lead the activity – give only as much support as required and ensure that you do this by going at their own pace.
	Encourage the individual to reflect on their participation in the activity and discuss what they thought worked well. Ask them what they enjoyed, what they didn't like or what they think could be improved.
	Find out what the individual has enjoyed in the past.
	Look at the individual's care and support plans to see what activities they enjoy.

▲ Table 1.5 Examples of how to establish needs and preferences, and apply person-centred values

RESEARCH IT

Finding out about the individual

Develop a written plan for the different methods you can use to find out about an individual who accesses the care and support provided in the care setting where you work. Once you have agreed these with your manager, put them into practice.

- Did you find out anything you didn't know about the individual?
- How did you find the process?
- If you did this again, would you use the same methods? Why, or why not?

AC3.5 The term 'behaving towards people with dignity and respect' and why this is central to the role of the health and social care worker

As we have seen, person-centred support is all about treating people with **dignity** and **respect.**

Think of a time when somebody showed little or no respect for you.

- How did this make you feel?

Imagine if people you came into contact with on a regular basis showed a lack of respect.

- How would this make you feel over a period of time?
- How do people show you respect?

Treating someone with dignity and respect makes them feel valued and supports their well-being. It helps people's confidence and self-esteem. In your role it is important that you treat people with dignity and respect at all times. This will help build positive relationships and an environment where individuals have voice, choice and control over their lives

There are many ways you can treat individuals with dignity and respect. These include:

- listening to them
- showing you are interested in them, their lives and background

- providing them with the information they need
- respecting personal space and possessions
- removing any barriers to communication
- understanding their point of view even if it differs from your own
- ensuring they know their rights
- supporting them to manage pain
- supporting them to make choices and involve them in decisions about their care and support
- addressing the person in the way they wish to be addressed – they may not like having their name shortened or being called by their first name, but prefer people to use their title and surname
- ensuring food looks and tastes appetising
- handling personal care activities sensitively
- promoting social activities.

KEY TERMS

Dignity: this focuses on the value of everybody as an individual. It involves respecting people's choices and opinions, and not making decisions for people.

Respect: this means taking into account other people's feelings, rights and wishes. It is about being thoughtful, courteous and compassionate to the other person.

AC3.6 AC3.10 Reasons for establishing consent with an individual when providing care or support and why this is important

Establishing **consent** with an individual for an activity or action can only be successful if you:

- work together with the individual – this ensures their rights are respected and their preferences supported
- are flexible in the methods you use – some individuals may be able to consent verbally, others in writing. If they cannot give consent verbally, you will need to watch body language or facial expression to see if they are ok with the situation.

When establishing consent with an individual for an activity or action, it is important to comply with the following best practice guidance:

- Respect the individual's views about the activity or action; for example, discuss when it is to be carried out.
- Listen to the individual and find out about their preferences about the activity or action.
- Discuss or explain what carrying out the activity or action will involve; for example, tell them about the number of staff required to support the activity and the process to be followed. If the individual cannot understand, pictures of the activity might be more appropriate. Demonstrations of what is going to happen might help.
- Provide the individual with relevant and accurate information; this could also be in response to any questions or concerns they may have.
- Support the individual to make their own decisions and respect these; for example, discuss the related benefits, drawbacks and consequences, and respect their decisions even if you disagree with them. If somebody is confused or has communication difficulties, you will need to be more aware of body language and use alternative communication strategies to support choice, for example, giving the individual some objects or pictures that can help them decide which option is best.
- Do not try to persuade the individual into making a decision, even if you think it is in their best interests.
- If the individual lacks capacity, then you should speak to their advocate, guardian or family member if they don't have an advocate, but make sure that in the first instance, you consult the individual. Also make sure that you support those with language and communication difficulties to communicate their consent, and seek the assistance of translators and communication aids.

Remember:

- If you are unsure about anything, refer the individual to someone who does know (such as a medical professional or your manager or senior person). This means the individual has access to the most correct and accurate information available.
- Exercise confidentiality when you are communicating information, especially to those other than the individual. You may be dealing with sensitive and private information, so it is important that you are sure the individual is happy for the information to be communicated to others.

Establishing consent

This is not a process that is completed at the beginning of a shift or once a day: it is an ongoing process that takes place for every activity or action you complete with an individual. This is because an individual's preferences, like yours, may change from one day to another and this must be respected. For example: just because an individual chose to have a shower yesterday morning does not mean they want to have a shower every morning; they may prefer to have a bath instead, or to have a wash at night before going to bed.

You will only know if you have consent by asking. Not asking will prevent you from providing good care and support.

Communicating consent

How is consent communicated? **Informed consent** occurs when individuals are asked for their consent or agreement based on the information they have received about the benefits, risks and consequences. However, how do individuals give or communicate their consent?

You will find that this will vary, depending on the types of things for which you are requesting consent. For example:

- It might be done verbally (verbal consent) when you ask an individual whether they are happy to have lunch, or would like to take part in a group activity, and they tell you that it is okay.
- You may need written consent, such as when individuals are agreeing to serious medical procedures, when they agree for someone to be their advocate or when consent is required around financial matters.

KEY TERMS

Consent: when someone agrees to something. You will need to obtain 'consent' or permission from an individual, or their representative if the individual is unable to.

Informed consent: when an individual decides to consent when they have been fully informed about the benefits, risks and consequences.

However, you will also find that consent is not always communicated. It may often be implied. For example, if you ask an individual who is in bed whether they would like to get up and get dressed, and they sit up in bed and look at their wardrobe, then they are implying that they are ready to do so. Somebody may give you a thumbs up or nod. It is important that you are aware of these different methods and the situations in which it is important to gain more formal written consent.

The above text applies to everybody, regardless of age. However, when supporting children and young people, you must also think about their age and capacity to make or be involved in decisions.

Children and young people have a right to choose to be involved and work on things that are important to them. A parent/guardian/carer/worker has a duty of care to everyone, so must ensure that children and young people are involved in decision making appropriate to their age and/or abilities and what is in their best interest.

Shared decision making might be appropriate for some decisions, if the person needs support and guidance due to their age. In order to support children and young people to make choices, parents or carers will usually help children with this. If parents are deemed as not suitable, for example, if they have serious mental health issues, an advocate can help them to ensure they understand the choices available where possible and to make sure their voices are heard if the child doesn't have the capacity to have the final say on decisions.

RESEARCH IT

For further information on supporting young people to participate in things that are important to them, research the Children and Young People's Participation in Wales Good Practice guide at:

https://gov.wales/sites/default/files/publications/2019-06/good-practice-guide.pdf

Research the Mental Capacity Act and consent. What does it say about how consent must be established when providing care or support to an individual? This is a useful link:

www.nhs.uk/conditions/social-care-and-support-guide/making-decisions-for-someone-else/mental-capacity-act/

Discuss your findings with a colleague and make notes on your discussion.

AC3.7 AC3.6 Ways of working that support person and child-centred approaches

Applying person-centred values in day-to-day work is a key part of being able to provide high quality care and support. Working in this way can also have a significant impact on the quality of individuals' lives and can make a positive difference. By implementing legislation and codes of professional practice, you are ensuring that you will work in a person-centred way.

REFLECT ON IT

Working in ways that embed person and child-centred approaches

Imagine you are an experienced worker and have been asked by your manager to write some guidance for a new member of staff about why it is important to work in a way that embeds person-centred values.

Write down how you would explain what person-centred values are.

- Which ones do you think are the most important?
- Why?

CASE STUDY

Person-centred working in practice

Kian is a **Shared Lives carer** and is married with two children. Stacey has physical disabilities and lives with her parents. She is joining Kian and his family this weekend as they are planning a camping trip to take place the following week and have invited Stacey. As Stacey has never been camping before, she is keen to find out more about what Kian's family are planning, and she agrees to discuss the trip with Kian and his family over afternoon tea.

Kian begins by showing Stacey photographs of previous camping trips they have done together as a family. Kian asks Stacey to take her time to look through these, and as she does so, he asks one of the children to tell Stacey where it was taken and what is happening in the photograph.

Kian has been observing Stacey closely and he can see that she is looking a little upset and so once they have finished looking through the photographs, he asks her if she can help him with the washing up. Stacey agrees, and while the two of them are in the kitchen, Kian asks Stacey what she thinks about camping. Stacey explains that she's feeling very anxious because she has never been camping before.

Kian asks Stacey if she would prefer to camp in their garden first, so that if she doesn't like it she could always go back in the house. Stacey thinks that would be a great idea. They agree that they will do that the next time Stacey comes to stay. If she likes it, they could maybe go for one night somewhere close to home before they try going for a weekend or a little further away. Kian tells her not to worry though, as if she doesn't like it they won't go.

Discussion points:

- The person-centred values applied by Kian.
- Examples of how Kian takes into account Stacey's individual preferences, wishes and needs.
- The impact of Kian's person-centred approach on Stacey.

KEY TERM

Shared Lives carer: someone who opens up their home and family life to include someone with support needs so that they can participate and experience community and family life. The individual may stay with them for the weekend, or they may even go on holiday together.

AC3.8 AC3.7 The term 'active participation'

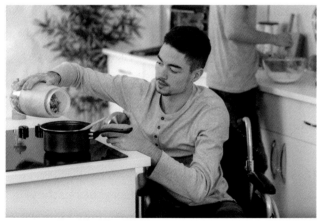

▲ Figure 1.7 Participating in everyday activities independently

Active participation is a way of working that regards individuals, children and young people as active partners in their own care or support rather than passive recipients. Active participation recognises each individual, child or young person's right to participate in the activities and relationship of everyday life as independently as possible, according to their age and stage of development.

Active participation is a person-centred way of working that can lead to improved care and support. This is because it recognises an individual's:

- rights – for example, to participate in activities fully, to maintain relationships in everyday life as independently as possible
- abilities – for example, to be an active partner who is involved in their own care or support rather than a passive recipient who is not involved and on the receiving end of care or support
- potential – for example, to be in control over their care or support and influence how their care or support needs are met.

Active participation means supporting individuals to live their lives as independently as possible. This does not mean doing things for them, but instead helping them to do things for themselves as much as possible. This might mean enabling them to go out shopping on their own or taking part in a social group.

Being able to do things for yourself and being active members of your society and community can impact positively on your life through increased social interactions, the achievement of your own personal goals and living independently. It can also have many positive impacts on your health such as feelings of well-being and increased self-esteem.

Just think about how you feel when you have achieved a goal. Perhaps you ran a 10k race and achieved a finish time that you had aimed for. Or maybe you successfully cooked a dish that you had been trying. Such achievements can give us feelings of well-being and thus impact positively on our health. Likewise, there are many benefits of active participation for individuals who have care or support needs.

KEY TERM

Active participation: the Code of Professional Practice for Social Care defined active participation as a way of working that regards individuals as 'active partners in their own care rather than passive recipients. Active participation recognises each individual's right to participate in the activities and relationships of everyday life as independently as possible'.

REFLECT ON IT

Reflect on the benefits of active participation in Figure 1.8. Now think about the difference each of these benefits would make to your life.

- What impact could it have if you felt good about making your own decisions?
- How can an increase in confidence benefit you?
- Why is being in control of your life important?
- Why is important for your unique needs and preferences to be taken into account and understood?

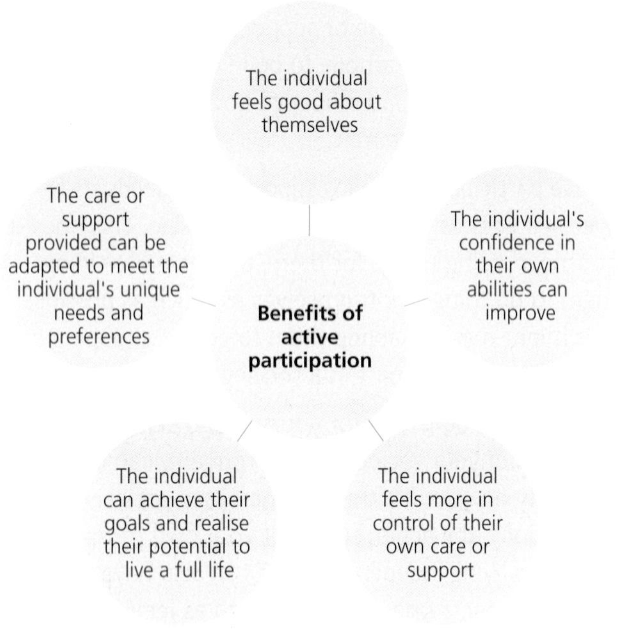

▲ Figure 1.8 The benefits of active participation

AC3.9 AC3.8 The importance of supporting individuals to engage in activities and experiences that are meaningful and enjoyable

The more active and enjoyable a life we lead, the greater our sense of well-being. When supporting individuals to engage in activities, we need to ensure it is meaningful and enjoyable to the person. We can do this by:

- building on their strengths so they are more likely to succeed
- thinking about what the individual enjoys doing – if they carry out an activity they don't enjoy, they are less likely to be motivated to do it again
- ensuring the activity meets their personal goals – if somebody has the aim of living more independently, it would be more meaningful to learn skills that help them achieve this goal, such as cooking
- supporting the person to become more active in their local community – this gives a sense of belonging which helps well-being
- thinking about how activities can meaningfully support relationships and friendships – will particular activities increase an individual's social life?

CASE STUDY
ADULTS

Gwen has moved into a residential care home for people with dementia.

Discussion points:

- How might the team support Gwen to engage in activities which are meaningful and which she enjoys?
- What activities or experiences might they suggest to Gwen?

CASE STUDY
CHILDREN AND YOUNG PEOPLE

Neelam, who is 15 years old and in care, lacks motivation and confidence. She doesn't have any hobbies or interests.

Discussion points:

- How might workers encourage active participation with Neelam?
- What meaningful activities might they suggest?
- How can they ensure she enjoys these activities?

The more you enjoy an activity, the more likely you are to want to do it again. If you feel you are achieving something, you will want to carry on so that you can achieve even more. You often receive some sort of reward for carrying out an activity; for example:

- If you cook a meal, you can enjoy eating it.
- If you do some art, you might produce a nice painting to put on your wall.

If individuals really lack motivation, it is worth thinking about how they will benefit from the activity. What is in it for them? Will something good happen at the end of the activity? This will ensure it is more meaningful for the person and there is a greater chance they will enjoy doing it. For example, think about a hobby you have or an activity you enjoy.

- Why do you enjoy doing the activity?
- How do you benefit from it?
- How would you feel if you had to do an activity you really did not enjoy?

AC3.10 AC3.9 How person/child-centred approaches are used to support active participation and inclusion

When supporting people to become more active participants in their lives, you need to make sure they are an active participant. You need to ask the individual what they would like to do, how they would like to develop their skills, what new experiences they would like to try.

You could try the following:

- Sit down with the individual and plan the day or week with them.
- Do some goal planning with the individual by asking them what they would like to achieve in the future, and how they would like to work towards this.
- Ask the individual if there are any activities they could do in the past but can't now because of an illness or disability. Agree with them what support or aids they might need to help them carry out this activity again.
- Look on the internet with the individual to see if there are things in their local communities they would like to try.
- Look at magazines and books at images of different hobbies, and see if the individual is interested in any of them.
- Plan with the person what support they need to carry out activities of daily living, such as cleaning, cooking or shopping. Activities may need to be changed or broken down into small steps so that they can be involved in parts of the activity.

CASE STUDY

Owain has lived in a community setting with a number of other young men for three months. Owain has learning disabilities and autism, and even though he can speak, he rarely does. He has a number of behaviours which challenge the team who support him. He often hits out at people if they become too close and screams for no apparent reason. He spends a lot of his time sitting on the floor by the radiator, banging his head against it. He usually has his arm over his face so people can't see him.

Jack is Owain's new keyworker, and wants to encourage him to participate more in meaningful activities.

Jack decides he is going to encourage Owain to help cook a meal, as he always seems happy when it is meal times. The first time Owain goes into the kitchen, he swipes at the plates on the drainer and smashes them all on the floor. Jack cooks the dinner while Owain watches.

The next day Jack ensures the crockery is in the cupboard and uses the plastic plates. He cooks a tin of beans and then gives hand-on-hand support to Owain to tip the beans onto his plate. He shows Owain how to put the lever down on the toaster. Owain does this activity with Jack three times a week, and always cooks either beans or spaghetti on toast or soup.

In the beginning, when eating their dinner Owain sits with his arm over his face and hits Jack if he gets too close. Over the next six months, Owain goes from hand-on-hand support to stirring the beans, then to cooking the beans independently and making the toast. He sits at the table and doesn't have his hand by his face. He also chats to Jack without hitting him. Owain even progresses to using ceramic plates without smashing them. He loves doing the washing up afterwards and especially enjoys splashing the water.

Discussion points: This case study shows that everybody can actively participate in their daily lives regardless of their ability.

- Why do you think this activity was a success?
- Think about people you support; are there any activities that they don't currently do in their own home that they might be able to try?
- What support will they need? Can this support be reduced over time?
- Can the task be broken down into small steps and then more steps gradually added, as the person becomes more confident with the task?

AC3.11 The term 'parental responsibility'

Parental responsibility is a term defined in the Children Act 1989 as:

all the rights, duties, powers, responsibilities and authority which by law a parent of a child has in relation to the child and his property.

This means that where someone has parental responsibility for a child or young person, they have to provide a home for the child and protect them from harm. They can make decisions about the care and upbringing involving the child or young person where appropriate, and about consent to medical treatment.

It is usually parents that have parental responsibility. If parents split up, the mother automatically has parental responsibility. The father will still have parental responsibility if he is or has been married to the mother or he is named on the child's birth certificate. If he does not automatically have parental responsibility after splitting up with the mother, he would need to apply to the courts for it.

When a child is receiving care, a local authority can have parental responsibility.

If a child's parents have died, a relative can be appointed as a guardian. They will then take on re-sponsibility for the child. This can be agreed with an individual before they die and written into their will. Alternatively, a relative can apply to be a guardian after a parent's death. This would need to be agreed by the court.

REFLECT ON IT

The Children Act says that those with parental responsibility can make decisions about a child or young person's care. The Social Services and Well-Being (Wales) Act says that children and young people should be given choices and voice and control over their own lives.

- How do you think these two views are balanced?
- Are there times when a parent can make decisions about a child or young person without their agreement?
- Are there times when the child or young person can make decisions without the parent?

When considering what decisions a child or young person can make or contribute to, a number of factors need to be taken into account:

- age
- cognitive ability
- understanding of the decision and its consequences
- whether it is a safeguarding issue
- what the decision is and the impact it can have on the child or young person.

Any decisions made on behalf of the child or young person should always be in their best interests.

AC3.11 **AC3.12** The purpose of personal plans

An individual receiving care will usually have different types of **personal plans**.

A care and support plan is usually written by local authority social workers together with the individual, child or young person and any significant other people, such as family members or spouses. They contain:

- information such as what services will be provided to meet the individual's needs
- the amount of budget available to pay for these services
- a decision on whether the person will have an advocate to support them and ensure their rights are met.

Care and support plans should be person-centred. They ensure that any package of care is designed around the person's individual needs so that they remain as independent as possible and have voice, choice and control over their lives.

If an individual receives services from an organisation, either in their own home, residential accommodation or a day service, they will usually have a personal or care plan. They can be in any format the individual understands. There can be a written part and a visual part if that is easier for the individual to understand, or there could be a voice recording of the plan if they cannot read.

Personal plans will provide:

- information for individuals of the agreed care and support and the manner in which this will be provided
- details of what is important to the individual, their likes and dislikes
- a clear and constructive guide for workers about the individual, child or young person, their care and support needs, and the outcomes they would like to achieve
- goals or outcomes that are important to the person and that they want to achieve – these can be short-term goals which link to long-term goals
- a basis for ongoing review

- a means for individuals and workers to measure progress and whether their personal outcomes are met.

Personal plans are holistic, which means that they should address all the needs of an individual including personal, social, emotional, spiritual, cultural, intellectual and medical needs. They should be updated regularly as an individual's, child's or young person's needs and goals change.

KEY TERM

Personal plan: this looks in detail at what support a person needs in order to achieve their goals.

LO4 UNDERSTAND HOW TO PROMOTE EQUALITY, DIVERSITY AND INCLUSION

GETTING STARTED

Supporting equality, diversity and inclusion in health and social care settings is essential for delivering good, safe, quality care and creating a positive, caring and fair environment. Making sure that people are treated equally and fairly, in a way that takes into account their individual needs, is an essential part of your role.

Think about how you would describe yourself to someone who didn't know you. You might like to do this in terms of your age, background, physical appearance, personality, likes and dislikes.

Now think about three people you know very well, such as your friends or family. For each person, describe what they have in common with you. For example, you might share the same interests or enjoy going to the same places. Why is it important to you that you share similar interests?

For each person you have described, think about how they are different from you. For example, they might be from different backgrounds, live in a different area or speak a different language.

- Why do you think these differences are important?
- Do you value how they are different to you?
- Do you appreciate their differences? In what ways?

AC4.1 The terms 'equality', 'diversity', 'inclusion' and 'discrimination'

Diversity

Diversity means different types and variation. This could refer to different people, or things. In a health and social care setting for example, you will come across people from different or 'diverse' backgrounds and needs. They may be different, for example, because of where they come from, how they dress or their age.

Recognising the importance of diversity allows you to:

- provide high quality care and support that is person-centred
- build trusting working relationships that enable individuals to feel safe
- develop your understanding and respect for the differences that exist in people.

Remember that you are responsible for ensuring that the individuals you support feel that you respect their differences and for treating them as unique people. In this way, they will develop a real sense of belonging.

Living alongside people who are from different backgrounds and contribute different experiences can be a positive experience, because each person brings their own culture, beliefs and experiences. You have the opportunity to learn about new and different aspects of their cultures. This is true whatever your nationality, religion, race, gender or sexuality, and this information can lead to new ideas and beliefs about living together.

We are living through a pivotal time in history, a social revolution, especially with regard to the Black Lives Matter movement and rights of lesbian, gay, bisexual, transgender and queer (LGBTQ) people. Awareness of the importance of diversity and equality led to same-sex marriage being legalised in the UK in 2014, as well as increasingly open discussion of women's rights, issues around historical abuse and the slave trade. These discussions are now occupying an important place on the political stage, and are crucial to social change.

It is important for your role that you try to have a positive and open attitude towards diversity, as you will come across different people from various backgrounds. As you meet people who are different from you, it is important that you respect their rights to have different values, beliefs and cultures.

Equality

Equality means treating people fairly and valuing them for who they are. It means not thinking of anyone as less important than someone else. In a health and social care setting, this also means making sure that everyone has access to the same rights and opportunities.

Person-centred approaches ensure that you:

- recognise that each person is different
- understand how they are different
- treat them in a way which respects their differences.

If you do not recognise the importance of equality, you will not be able to support people's rights, and as a result they will not feel that they are being treated equally. We looked at legislation in LOs 1 and 2 which ensures that people are treated equally.

Treating all individuals fairly and respectfully is one of the essential behaviours expected from all workers. Remember though that treating people equally does not mean treating them all the same. A worker who supports three individuals who live together would need to find out from each one how they want to be cared for. Do not assume that these individuals all have the same preferences in their daily routine: you would need to ask what time they would like to get up in the morning, and whether they prefer to have a shower or bath.

Inclusion

Inclusion means being included or involved, for example, being part of a wider group, or a group of friends. In a health and social care setting, this means ensuring that all individuals are able to be included or to partake in everyday life regardless of any differences. This can create a sense of belonging.

Most people like being around friends and family, and enjoy the feeling of being part of a bigger group of people who may share our interests and hobbies. This may be in real life where we meet with friends and family in person, on the internet through social media.

The term 'inclusion' is linked closely to equality and diversity, because without considering inclusion, you will not be able to treat people fairly and respect their differences. Inclusive care refers to individuals:

- having a purpose or meaning to their lives, for example, a paid job, being part of a group of friends
- being able to play an active part in the community where they live, for example, accessing any local sports facilities that are available, or meeting others who live in their local community

- being valued and respected, such as being asked for their views, or having their preferences taken into account
- having their differences accepted, for example, by not being left out of activities because of their differences (this means making sure that someone with a hearing impairment is not left out of conversations)
- being included and feeling that they belong in any setting
- being empowered, feeling that their contributions are valued and that they have a role in society.

As a care and support worker, you will need to create a sense of inclusion. You should always make sure that you include everyone and find ways to ensure that individuals are involved and feel valued.

Social inclusion

Social inclusion means providing opportunities for individuals to participate and be involved in their wider communities so that they feel included, have a role and are part of society. This might be through:

- accessing public transport
- socialising with friends
- accessing a course at a local college
- participating in a local cultural event.

Discrimination

Discrimination means treating people unfairly or unlawfully, for example, because they have a disability, or are of a different race, gender or age.

Unlike equality, diversity and inclusion, discrimination is a negative behaviour. People may be 'discriminated against' and treated unfairly for many reasons. Discrimination can happen when:

- people are labelled because of the characteristics they have, such as being ridiculed because of facial features or hair colour
- people are viewed as the same because of an assumption or generalisation about the group they belong to which is untrue (this is called **stereotyping**); for example, thinking that all individuals with mental health needs are dangerous

- people are judged because of a preconceived and untrue opinion. 'Prejudice' occurs when you make assumptions about people that are not based on facts or reason, such as thinking that older people cannot learn new skills.

Labelling, stereotyping and prejudice can all lead to discrimination. Discrimination is a negative behaviour because it can:

- disadvantage people – an individual may not be offered a job because of their characteristics
- disempower people – an individual's confidence will be affected if they are not accepted for themselves or their beliefs
- disable people – an individual's physical, mental, emotional and social well-being will be affected if they are prevented from accessing the services, care or support they require.

All those who access, live and work in care settings have a right not to be discriminated against. This type of positive behaviour is known as anti-discrimination.

KEY TERM

Stereotyping: a set idea that may be widely held about what someone or something is like.

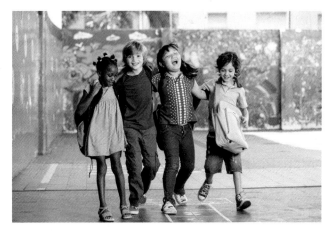

▲ Figure 1.9 Making sure that all individuals are treated equally and fairly

AC4.2 The term 'protected characteristics'

Protected characteristics is a term that appears in the Equality Act 2010. The characteristics it refers to are aspects of a person's identity. There are certain characteristics that are protected under the Act to ensure people are protected from negative treatment. There are nine characteristics which are protected:

1 age
2 disability
3 gender reassignment
4 marriage and civil partnership
5 pregnancy and maternity
6 race
7 religion or belief
8 sex
9 sexual orientation.

The legislation means that people cannot be discriminated against because of one of these characteristics.

REFLECT ON IT

- How might this legislation be relevant to your role?
- How is it relevant to people working in health and social care, such as during recruitment and ongoing employment?
- How is it relevant to people you support?
- Can you imagine times when individuals, children and young people may need support with issues relating to protected characteristics?

AC4.3 AC4.2 Ways in which person/child-centred approaches promote equality, diversity and inclusion

As we have seen already, person-centred approaches involve treating people with dignity and respect, and recognising their uniqueness and individual needs. Giving people a voice, choice and control means ensuring they are involved in all aspects of their lives as much as possible.

People who are significant in our lives might have many differences to us. There is a saying that 'opposites attract'. Often when a partner has a different personality from you, this can be really helpful to provide balance. For example, if one person is an impulsive person and their partner is very considered, this can be helpful in a relationship. By respecting each other's approaches, a happy balance can be found. This example shows how we can respect people's individuality, as we all have something to offer in relationships and to our communities regardless of our background and who we are.

Think about important relationships in your life.

- How do you treat each other with dignity and respect?
- What differences do you have, and how do you support this diversity?

There are many examples of how person-centred approaches are being used to develop services and promote equality and inclusion. Individuals who use services are often involved in recruitment of staff and staff training. Some services have service users on their board of governance or working in the office. Supporting people to make everyday choices about their lives on a day-to-day basis ensures that you are promoting equality, diversity and inclusion.

As we have already seen, diversity means recognising, valuing and respecting the differences that exist so that individuals and workers can continue to be celebrated as unique. Diversity is therefore very important in the work setting. It involves promoting person-centred values, such as:

- showing respect for the individuals that you support and valuing their importance
- showing respect for people's individuality and showing respect towards them; for example, when communicating with them and encouraging them to be their own person
- respecting their rights, such as to choose what they would like to eat and how they would like to dress
- supporting their independence by encouraging them to participate in the activities they enjoy
- respecting individuals' rights to privacy, such as in relation to hygiene
- supporting individuals' rights to make their own choices and making sure they have the information they need to do so

- treating people with dignity, which relates to the first point about treating people with respect, and valuing their beliefs
- working in partnership with others including professionals outside the setting and families and carers.

Each person is different and therefore their 'person-centred values' will be different. For example, some individuals may communicate verbally, others may use signs and pictures to communicate; some individuals may choose not to eat meat; some individuals may enjoy going to worship in a church, others in a mosque.

Developing positive working relationships

You can do this by showing an interest in the differences shown by individuals and your colleagues. For example, you may ask an individual to tell you more about their culture, or find out from your colleague the language they prefer to speak. They will feel comfortable when working with you and start to build their trust in you.

AC4.4 AC4.3 How the cultural, religious and linguistic backgrounds of individuals, children, young people and carers can be valued

Your cultural background influences your personality and your life. This includes your ethnicity, race, socio-economic status, gender, language, religion, sexual orientation and geographical area. People identify with different cultural backgrounds as it gives them a sense of belonging. Cultural identity is an ongoing process as you will be exposed to different sets of beliefs and values throughout your life. Culture is therefore dynamic and complex.

Beliefs

Beliefs can be strong principles that govern the way we live. They can affect how we live, the places we go and the things we eat. For example, the reason that some people do not eat meat might be because they believe that killing animals for food is wrong.

Beliefs may also be religious or political.

Culture

Culture refers to the particular traditions, customs and values that a group of people might share. Often the UK is described as a multicultural society, which means that it is made up of different cultures and groups of people who originate from different places such as Africa, France, India, Italy, Poland, Romania and Russia. Culture can differ between different areas of Wales, for example, people living in Cardiff would probably have a different culture to people living in rural Wales.

Culture can also differ between age groups; the culture in older generations can be very different from younger generations. This can be due to factors such as changes in technology or advances in education. An elderly person may have been brought up with a view that 'children should be seen and not heard'. This may have resulted in them not speaking up or having their own opinions. Young people today are brought up in a way where they formulate opinions early on through influences including social media and being encouraged to debate topics in school.

We can show respect for different cultural, religious and linguistic backgrounds in the following ways:

- Develop cultural awareness – carry out some research on different cultures, their traditions and beliefs.
- Learn to appreciate and value diverse views – listen to other people's opinions and try to see things from their point of view without judging.
- Avoid imposing your own view – discussions on different viewpoints are healthy but we should never force our own opinions on anyone.
- Learn about different cultures – speak to people about their culture and any particular traditions they have. Visit places that are important to different cultures to gain a greater understanding.
- Resist stereotyping – this means giving a label to people because of a characteristic they may have, such as hair or skin colour. Stereotypes imply that all people with that characteristic are the same, which is clearly untrue.

As a worker in health and social care, you must remember the boundaries of your role. Your relationship is a professional one in which your own culture and values have no bearing on people you support.

CASE STUDY

Hiraethog is a residential service for young adults. Every week the workers and Jane, Sam, Lowri, Shivan and Ffion who live in Hiraethog meet up to discuss and share their ideas on activities they would like to do, menus and the general running of the home. They discuss the things that are working well, 'what they like' and what they would like to change or improve.

Today's meeting is focused on how people feel about celebrating Christmas together later on in the year. They have decided to discuss this because people living in the home have different experiences of Christmas. One of the workers begins by supporting everyone to speak up about the different beliefs that are shared among them with respect to celebrating Christmas.

Jane explains how she has always celebrated Christmas since she was a child. Sam, supported by his keyworker, shows the group photographs of him celebrating Christmas with his family, while Lowri and Ffion share the posters they have made to explain the different aspects involved in celebrating Christmas. Shivan says that he doesn't celebrate Christmas because of his religion. He does however begin to show a genuine interest

in the photographs and posters, and asks lots of questions. Ffion then asks whether in the next meeting they can discuss celebrating other festivals such as Chinese New Year and Diwali.

Over the next week Ffion and Shivan begin to put a calendar together of the different celebrations they would like to share as a group. In the next meeting it is agreed that the lounge that everyone shares will not be decorated, to show respect for Shivan who doesn't celebrate Christmas. They agree to have a Christmas tree in the dining room and that they will only decorate the hallway as well as their own individual rooms if they wish to.

Discussion points:

- How are the workers supporting individuals to respect one another's differences?
- How are equality and diversity being promoted?
- How do you think the young people feel by being involved in these discussions?
- How could the support provided by the workers reduce the likelihood of discrimination occurring? Why?

AC4.5 AC4.4 Ways to challenge discrimination or practice that does not support equality, diversity and inclusion

When talking about our work we should be careful of the language we use about people we work with. We should avoid giving people labels, for example, by saying 'I work in learning disabilities'. This label isn't recognising the person as an individual. A better way of saying this would be 'I support people with learning disabilities'. The second example is putting the person first, not the disability.

REFLECT ON IT

Think of other examples of discrimination you may have seen or heard in the workplace or community. As health and social care workers, we should try to model good practice at all times.

People often discriminate because of lack of education or lack of experience. It is your role to challenge this and help educate people to ensure equality and diversity.

It can sometimes be hard to challenge discrimination but we will never make changes in people's attitudes if we don't do so. When responding to discrimination, the following tips may help:

- Don't be angry with the person. It might be they don't realise that their actions are discriminatory. Being angry won't help them see your viewpoint.
- Remain calm, professional and polite.
- Ask them why they think that.
- Explain the alternative non-discriminatory viewpoint.
- If it is a colleague, try to resolve it informally at the time, as that might prevent further occurrences.
- Speak to your manager if you are not sure what to do or the situation doesn't improve.
- Show respect for the other person at all times.

CASE STUDIES

The examples below are all examples of discrimination. Think about each one and how you might have dealt with it. How did each example challenge discrimination and encourage respect, diversity and inclusion? What else could have been done?

1 Emyr has mental health issues and has moved into a small village. While out shopping, he went up to a stranger in the local shop and hugged her. His worker, Theo, suggested they shake hands instead as they didn't know each other. The stranger responded by saying it was OK. Theo discussed this in a non-confrontational way with Emyr and the stranger that some people might not like it and might retaliate. Following that incident, whenever the stranger saw Emyr in the village, she always made a point of offering her hand to shake and to chat to him.

2 Ceri was chatting to Dafydd who is 83. Dafydd said he used to take his car to the rough people at the car wash in the local supermarket. When Ceri asked who he meant, he said the foreigners. Ceri said she didn't think they were rough, and he said they all looked dishevelled. Ceri explained nicely that they had overalls on because they were cleaning cars so possibly wouldn't look too smart.

3 Mari was supporting Ailsa at a summer camp. The other children wouldn't let Ailsa play their game because she uses a wheelchair. Mari suggested to Ailsa that she has a chat with the children, asks them nicely again and tells them that she can join in the game as she can move – her wheels are just like their legs. The children then let her join in and show an interest in how her 'wheels' work.

LO5 UNDERSTAND HOW POSITIVE RISK TAKING SUPPORTS WELL-BEING, VOICE, CHOICE AND CONTROL

GETTING STARTED

Taking risks is part of making choices in everyday life. Not doing so would be a barrier to us achieving what we want to do. Similarly, when workers support individuals' right to make choices about activities, this may involve individuals, children and young people taking risks. This doesn't mean that they will be placed in danger, or be harmed, abused or persuaded not to take risks, but rather that they will be supported to understand what the risks are and how these can be managed. Supporting people to take risks will have a positive effect on their well-being.

List all the risks you have taken over the last few days.

- How would you have felt if you couldn't take those risks?
- Would it have made a difference to your life?
- Can you think of examples of risks that you have taken in your life which had a big impact on your life?

AC5.1 The term 'positive risk taking' and the importance of being able to take positive risks on the well-being of individuals, children and young people

Positive risk taking in relation to person-centred care involves weighing up the benefits and drawbacks to the individual of taking the risk. The greater the potential benefits to the individual, the more important it is to try to find a way of managing the risk safely while supporting the individual to take the risk.

The aim of positive risk taking is to manage risks in a way which improves the quality of life for the person. Not all risks can be managed or reduced, but they can often be predicted.

KEY TERM

Positive risk taking: supporting people to take risks which results in them having a better quality of life.

Supporting positive risk taking has many benefits for individuals.

- It recognises their rights to make their own decisions and to take risks in line with their choices.
- It gives more opportunities for growth and development.
- It enables individuals to become more independent and gives self-confidence. This in turn can improve self-esteem.

By supporting positive risk taking, we build on individuals' strengths, and help them to both learn from their experiences and understand the consequences of their actions. You should work in equal partnership with individuals, being open and honest about the potential risks and benefits so that they can make an informed choice based on the information available.

You should also make sure that everyone's responsibilities are clear and understood. Depending on the risk, it might be good to have plans in place if things begin to go wrong, and to support them to work out why and whether something could be done differently next time. This supports individuals to learn from their mistakes.

When supporting people to take risks, you can follow four steps:

1 **Identify the risks** – this should be realistic, taking into account the individual's strengths and wishes, while identifying what risks may be involved.
2 **Assess the risk** – consider what support may be available to help the individual, what benefits there will be, and whether the person has managed similar activities in the past. The assessment should include the likelihood of harm and the extent of any potential harm. You would need to consider the individual's understanding of the risk; for example, the risk of crossing a road for someone with dementia may be a lot higher. Playing on a climbing wall could be a higher risk for a four-year-old than their ten-year-old brother.
3 **Work out ways to manage the risk – duty of care** needs to be taken into account here, so if the risks of negative consequences are high then you have a duty of care to protect the individual.
    - You need to look at ways of reducing the risk to an acceptable level. Remember, the aim is to improve individuals' quality of life.

- The risk assessment should be recorded so that there is evidence for how you have supported the person to assess the risk. Contingency plans should be developed as part of the risk assessment.
- Individuals should be supported to develop skills of resilience so they can think about problems that may occur and know how to deal with them.
- There should be joint accountability and ownership of decisions. Workers should support individuals to look at alternatives so the activity could take place in the safest way possible. If decisions need to be made for individuals who lack capacity, this should always be in their best interest.

4 **Review** – once the activity has taken place, a review should occur with the individual, child or young person. This should include a reflection on what went well, what could have been done differently, what you have learnt and whether any future action should take place.

KEY TERM

Duty of care: a moral and legal obligation to ensure the safety and well-being of others.

AC5.2 Rights that individuals, children and young people have to make choices and take risks

Assessing the risks and their impact is crucial when supporting individuals' right to make choices, because it involves a careful balance between supporting their right to make their own choices while maintaining their safety. A thorough risk assessment is not only a useful tool, but is also a legal requirement for maintaining individuals' safety while they do the activities that they enjoy.

You are required by law to support individuals to make choices and uphold their rights.

- Health and safety legislation (which we will look at in Unit 007) requires you to ensure people are safe.
- The Social Services and Well-Being (Wales) Act ensures you put safeguards in place to protect people.
- The Human Rights Act also gives individuals rights to make choices and take risks.
- The Mental Capacity Act identifies whether a person is deemed to have capacity. If they have capacity then they have the right to make choices, even if these are viewed as an unwise decision.

By carrying out a risk assessment and supporting people to participate in activities they choose to while ensuring it is as safe as possible, you will meet the requirements of legislation and your own organisation's policies and procedures.

CASE STUDY
ADULTS

Tom, a domiciliary care worker, goes to see Ray, an elderly person with dementia. Ray wants to spend £50 on a bet in the Grand National horse race. Tom knows Ray doesn't have lots of money and cannot really afford £50.

Discussion points:

- What rights does Ray have?
- What responsibilities does Tom have?
- What action should Tom take?

CASE STUDY
CHILDREN AND YOUNG PEOPLE

Anya is 13 years old. She is in residential care because her mum couldn't look after her any longer due to her drug addiction. Anya has always had a support worker with her when going out. She asks staff if she can go to the local shop on her own.

Discussion points:

- What rights does Anya have?
- What responsibilities do the workers have?
- What action should the workers take?

AC5.3 How balancing rights, risks and responsibilities contributes to person/child-centred approaches

We all take risks in our lives. New experiences, relationships and involvement in our communities all involve an element of risk taking. They also offer us opportunities for independence, confidence, well-being and autonomy. Putting the individual's needs first in a person-centred approach means we support the individual to take balanced risks.

People with disabilities or mental ill-health, older people, and children and young people are often not encouraged to take risks. This might be because people don't think they are safe to do so. Children often learn through risk taking in play and seeing what works and what doesn't. You might have heard the phrase, 'wrapping somebody up in cotton wool'. You might do this because you want to keep people safe and you think it is your job to do so.

However, you are putting your own opinions into the situation. You are not recognising that the person has a right to take risks, as long as they are supported to ensure their safety if appropriate. The focus should be more on what people can do, not what they cannot. Otherwise, your own actions are disabling when they should be enabling.

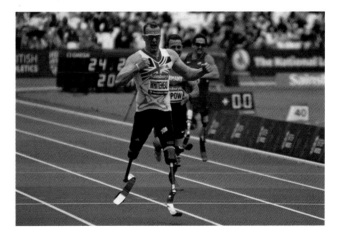

▲ Figure 1.10 Richard Whitehead, MBE

Richard Whitehead, MBE (see Figure 1.10), is a world recordholder for the marathon and half-marathon for athletes with a double amputation. He has competed in athletics at the Paralympic Games and also competes in sledge hockey. He has completed 40 marathons in 40 days. He is also a motivational speaker. He says even though he was born with no legs below his knee, his parents taught him to live a life without limits. They 'enabled' him as opposed to 'disabled him'. No doubt he took many risks along the way. He has however gone beyond many people's expectations and achieved great things.

REFLECT ON IT

Think about your own life.

- Can you think of any significant risks that you have taken?
- Did these actions benefit you?
- Did you learn from them?
- Imagine if you weren't able to take those risks; maybe your parent or partner stopped you from doing so. How would you feel?

We take risks all of the time. These can be small day-to-day risks or bigger risks, such as moving away to start a new job. Some of these have a positive benefit to our lives and some don't. Sometimes we make mistakes, but this is often how we learn. We usually don't make the same mistake again, or we might do it differently next time to get a better result.

By supporting people to take calculated risks you are ensuring their well-being, inclusion and choice, and enabling control over their own lives.

AC5.4 Considerations needed when supporting individuals to take positive risks

AC5.4 Considerations needed when supporting children and young people to take positive risks including their stage of development and life experiences

When supporting people to take risks you should consider all relevant circumstances, including:

- the individual's strengths
- their age
- their abilities
- support networks
- the benefits of the risk
- the hazards
- the nature of the risk
- what understanding the person has of those risks
- safer alternatives
- your duty of care to ensure people's safety
- what experiences children and young people have had in their childhood (are they streetwise or have they had a sheltered childhood?)
- whether the child or young person has been able to do things for themselves in the past (or have their parents done everything for them?)
- what has or hasn't worked in the past with the person.

Children develop an awareness of risk at different stages of their lives.

Age	Awareness of risk
Birth to 3 years old	Children's natural curiosity means they are a high risk as they have no sense of danger.
4–6 years old	Children are less likely to put things in their mouths, but they continue to explore with little thought to danger.
	They start to have some self-control so may begin to identify risks; for example, they should know a fire is hot by the age of 6.
7–9 years old	Children begin to recognise common dangers but often act before they think; for example, road safety.
10–15 years old	Young people in this age group may give the impression that they understand the risks although they often don't.
	Teenagers are often high risk takers. This can be because of peer group pressure; for example, drink and drugs.

▲ Table 1.6 Stages of development and risk taking

When thinking about supporting people to take risks, there are lots of considerations you can make to enable them to do it more safely. This way you are protecting yourself by maintaining your duty of care and working in a person-centred way, but are also supporting individuals, children and young people to take calculated risks.

AC5.5 What is meant by 'best interest decisions'

'Best interest decision' is a term used in the Mental Capacity Act 2005. It refers to decisions made on behalf of a person who lacks capacity to make their own decisions. If somebody or a multi-disciplinary team is making decisions on behalf of a person, they must do this in the best interest of the person.

People making best interest decisions could be:

- the person or team caring for the person
- a social worker
- doctors or other healthcare staff
- a **lasting power of attorney (LPA)** – these are people who have been identified by an individual to act on their behalf should they lose capacity. An LPA could be put in place to make decisions relating to health, finances or both.

In order to check whether an individual has capacity, you must make an assessment, following strict principles and codes of practice to do this as set out in the Mental Capacity Act. An individual may be deemed as having capacity on day-to-day decisions such as what to wear, but not on big decisions such as where they invest their money. In the areas where they do have capacity their wishes should be listened to.

When any decisions have been made, it is still important to involve the individual as much as possible to try to find out their views and wishes. Advocates should be involved for major decisions to ensure the decision is in the individual's best interest.

When making best interest decisions, you need to consider the following:

- Will the individual regain their capacity, and if so, can the decision be put off until then?
- How can the individual participate in the decision making?
- The individual's past and present wishes – they may have made a statement when they had capacity about what medical treatment they do and don't want.
- The individual's beliefs and values.
- Is there anyone else you need to consult, for example, family?
- The advantages and disadvantages including medical, social, emotional and welfare.
- What are the alternatives?
- Is there an alternative way which is less restrictive of the individual's rights and freedom of action?
- Will best interests change over time?
- Does the person have a power of attorney?

KEY TERM

Lasting power of attorney (LPA): covers decisions relating to health and care, finances or both. An individual would set up a lasting power of attorney to ensure they will be supported if they lose capacity in the future. The LPA agreement states the decisions (health- and/or finance-related) that individuals are happy for other people to make on their behalf, and also who they want to make those decisions.

Check your understanding

1 What does courage mean, in relation to providing care and support?

2 What does being competent in your job role mean?

3 What does it mean to support an individual's independence?

4 Why do you think personal plans are important?

5 If you were receiving care services, how would you like your personal plans to be produced? How would you want others to be involved in this?

6 How do person-centred approaches help an individual?

7 What does active participation mean?

8 How do you establish consent with someone who cannot speak?

9 What does diversity mean?

10 How can you ensure that you treat everyone equally?

11 How can you recognise the cultural backgrounds of individuals, children and young people?

12 Define positive risk taking.

13 If individuals, children or young people need support with decision making, what rights do they have when making choices?

14 How do you balance duty of care, rights and positive risk taking?

Question practice

1 What is the most important element of person-centred care planning?

   a to give the individual access to a complaints process

   b to prevent the individual from deciding on the plan by themselves

   c to provide the individual with information on support available

   d to ensure the individual remains central to the plan that affects them

2 Which of the following is a person-centred approach?

   a choosing what an individual you support would like to wear

   b giving two options for the individual to choose from

   c giving the individual their clothes

   d asking the individual what they would like to wear

3 Which of the following **best** describes active participation?

   a involving people in activities they can do

   b supporting people to be as independent as possible

   c helping people to do things

   d doing things for people that they cannot do

4 How do person-centred approaches **best** help active participation?

   a They look at what things the person needs help with.

   b They support the person to do what is important to them.

   c They encourage the person to do things they are able.

   d They ensure workers do things the person cannot do.

5 James is a child with cerebral palsy. The children in the setting are going to play games outside, but a care and support worker says James will not be able to take part in the group games and suggests he stays inside with another worker to play.
Which of these terms is demonstrated in the scenario?

   a equality

   b diversity

   c inclusion

   d discrimination

6 You see a worker talking in a derogatory way to another worker about people with a disability. What is the best way of responding to this?

   a Tell him firmly that you can't believe he would say that.

   b Report it straight to your manager.

   c Ignore it as he doesn't usually say things like this.

   d Tell him why you felt it was inappropriate and mention it to your manager.

7 What is a 'best interest' decision based on?

   a the total cost to the service

   b views and opinions of staff members

   c assessment of an individual's mental capacity

   d views and wishes of an individual's family

8 Which two of the following are benefits of encouraging and supporting acceptable levels of risk in play?

   a preventing slips and trips

   b building positive resilience

   c developing life skills

   d reducing conflict with peers

9 Which of the following is the most important for workers to consider when encouraging individuals, children or young people to participate in activities and take positive risks?

   a the experience level of the staff and gender ratio

   b the number of people in the group and their ages

   c the individual's/child's abilities, ages and stages of development

   d the number of trained staff available to support

10 Which of the following do you need to take into account when assessing teenager/adult risks related to road safety?

   a the individual's age

   b the individual's ability

   c their verbal communication skills

   d where the individual lives

LO6 UNDERSTAND HOW TO DEVELOP POSITIVE RELATIONSHIPS WITH INDIVIDUALS/CHILDREN AND YOUNG PEOPLE AND THEIR FAMILIES AND CARERS IN THE CONTEXT OF PROFESSIONAL BOUNDARIES

GETTING STARTED

Relationships are an important part of everybody's lives. In order to provide outcome focused, person-centred support, you need to build effective relationships with individuals, children and young people and the people important to them. You also need to know the boundaries to these relationships to ensure that people's needs are met and you don't step outside your job role.

Think about professionals you have come into contact with in your personal life, such as healthcare workers and tradespeople.

- How did they develop positive relationships with you?
- What boundaries were there in these relationships?

AC6.1 The term 'relationship-centred working'

'Relationship-centred working' ensures that you recognise the importance of working in partnership with the individual, family, carers and other professionals, with the individual at the centre of everything you do. It is a collaborative approach where you support each other to ensure the best outcomes for people.

When working in social care, you must adhere to professional boundaries in your relationships with individuals, children and young people. This will be looked at in more detail in Unit 005 and in AC6.3 in this unit.

Relationship-centred working recognises the importance of developing positive relationships with people you support. It is a relationship which must be built on mutual trust and respect. You must treat each other as equals where you respect diversity.

AC6.2 The importance of developing a positive relationship with individuals, children and young people and their families and carers

Positive relationships are really important when supporting people and their families and carers. Partnership working ensures the needs of the individual are met and creates a holistic approach to their well-being.

Positive relationships are built on trust. If people feel they can trust you, they will feel confident that they can talk to you. As a care and support worker you need to ensure you communicate effectively with people you support. This builds up trust and rapport, and gives individuals the chance to voice their concerns, needs, likes and dislikes.

When working with children and young people, positive relationships provide a role model. This is important for growth and development as some children and young people may not have had many good role models in their lives. This will help them learn how to develop relationships in their future lives.

REFLECT ON IT

- Use two pieces of paper. Draw a person in the middle of both pieces of paper, then draw a small circle around them, then another two circles, as shown in the diagram.
- In the inner circle, write the names of people who are very important to you, such as your family, spouse, partner, children.
- Write names of close friends in the middle circle, and in the outer circle write the names of acquaintances.
- Now do the same for somebody you support or an older person you know.

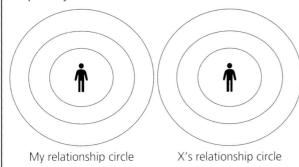

My relationship circle   X's relationship circle

Look at your relationship circles and consider these questions:

- Are there any differences in the two diagrams?
- Are there fewer professionals in your own diagram?
- What impact might any differences have?
- Is there anything you can do as a care worker?
- How can you do this?

Sometimes you will find that people who are receiving care and support have less people in their circle of relationships than you do. They often have a greater proportion of professionals and fewer friends.

This illustrates the importance of building positive relationships with individuals, children and young people and their families and carers. We all rely on people close to us for support at different times in our lives. People should be supported and encouraged to develop their own network of relationships within their local community.

REFLECT ON IT

Think about someone you have a very good relationship with or someone you can trust.

- What makes this a good relationship?
- Why do you feel you can trust them?
- How important is that relationship in your life?

We all need people we get on well with and can confide in, as it can often help to talk to someone when things get difficult. For people you support it is often other workers that fill that role. Developing positive relationships makes people feel safe enough to tell you what they want.

AC6.3 The term 'professional boundaries' and how to balance these with relationship-centred working

As we have seen from the activities above, people you support often have professionals as some of their closest relationships. This can create difficulties at times, as people can sometimes see you as friends, and it can be difficult to know where the boundaries of your relationship lie.

You must always remember you are not friends – you are a paid professional. Professionals have certain boundaries that they must adhere to when supporting people. Here is a list of some. See if you can think of any others:

- Ensure confidentiality – only pass information on when there is a need to know. Most times the individual should be told who you will be sharing information with. Some safeguarding cases would be an exception here. You must also remember not to discuss individuals, children and young people you support outside work.
- Do not give out personal information about yourself, such as your personal phone number, email address or where you live.

- Protect your privacy on social media. You should not accept friend requests from people you support.
- Establish clear physical boundaries – hugging, holding hands and other forms of touch may be seen as inappropriate. However, there are times when this is appropriate, for example, if a young person is upset or if someone is dying.

  Situations should be assessed individually. For example, a young person who is upset may just need a hug to make them feel better whereas hugging a different young person could make them feel embarrassed. If an individual or young person touches you inappropriately, you should explain why it is inappropriate. You should also report it in case of any complaints from the individual, and ensure other team members give the same response if it occurs again.

  An individual's care plan may say some form of touch is required, for example, you may need to link their arm to cross the road to ensure safety. This should be agreed with the individual and other professionals.
- Dress appropriately – remember that you are at work. Your clothes should portray a professional image while still remaining casual. Low-cut tops or cut-off jeans could make an individual feel uncomfortable or could portray the wrong image.
- Ensure you manage any conflicts of interest – you may know the individual from another setting, or you may know their family or friends. If you do, you should inform your manager so they can decide if it is appropriate that you support them. You should also not discuss or disclose this to the person as you are not there in that capacity.

  If you see an individual, child or young person outside or in a social setting, you should remain polite and professional but keep any interactions to a minimum. You should not agree to do favours for individuals you support out of work, such as picking something up from the shops for them, as this could be abused and could compromise professional boundaries.
- Use appropriate language – swearing, insulting languageand stereotyping are not acceptable. Even if the person you support uses language like this, you need to remain professional.

AC6.4 Types of unacceptable practices that may occur within relationships with individuals, children and young people and their families and carers

Section AC6.3 illustrates what constitutes professional practice. There are a number of practices which are classed as unacceptable and could be seen as abusive. Unacceptable practices include:

- sexual contact with an individual, child or young person using the service, for example, touching someone in an inappropriate way
- intimate relationships with people you support or former individuals you have supported: these relationships are unethical and could be seen as exploitative
- causing physical harm or injury to individuals, for example, hitting or bruising someone
- making aggressive or insulting comments, gestures or suggestions, even if they are only intended to be a joke
- seeking information on personal history where it is unnecessary or irrelevant
- watching an individual, child or young person undress where it is unnecessary – privacy should always be respected
- discussing your personal life – personal problems or your own religious/political views should never be discussed with people you support. You are there to support the individual, child or young person in their lives. Stories about your personal life are not required. It may also confuse the individual about the nature of your relationship
- inappropriate touching or hugging
- concealing information about individuals, children and young people from colleagues, for example, not completing daily records or not reporting errors in medication administration
- spreading rumours or hearsay about an individual, child or young person or others close to them, for example, sharing information about a child's family that you know from living in the same village as them

- accepting gifts or money from people you support – your organisation should have a policy on this. It may allow small gifts such as an occasional box of chocolates, but any other gifts not listed and frequent gifts would be seen as inappropriate. Never accept money from individuals.
- misusing an individual's money or property – if supporting individuals or young people when they are shopping, you should not use your own loyalty cards. The individual may have their own loyalty card. If they don't have one, you shouldn't use yours as this is an abuse of power: it could be seen that you are influencing the person about what to buy or what shops to buy from
- encouraging individuals, children and young people to become dependent or reliant for your own gain
- giving special privileges for 'favourite individuals' or children, for example, spending excessive time with someone, becoming over-involved or using influence to benefit one individual more than others
- providing forms of care that will not achieve the planned outcome – you should always follow the personal plans

- providing specialist advice or counselling where you are not qualified to do so
- failing to provide agreed care and support for or rejecting an individual, for example, due to negative feelings about them
- trying to impose your own religious, moral or political beliefs on an individual
- failing to promote dignity and respect or not respecting people's views
- any practices specifically prohibited in relevant legislation, statutory regulations, standards and guidance.

REFLECT ON IT

What might the consequences of poor practice be for the following:

- the individual, child or young person
- families and carers
- yourself
- the organisation you work for?

LO7 UNDERSTAND THE IMPORTANCE OF EFFECTIVE COMMUNICATION IN HEALTH AND SOCIAL CARE

GETTING STARTED

Communication is important in all aspects of our lives. We communicate with people regularly to build relationships, and share our thoughts and feelings for our well-being and to ensure our needs are met.

Workers in health and social care communicate with many different people including adults, children, young people, families, carers, colleagues and other professionals. You will need a range of communication skills to communicate with different groups of people and in different situations. You will also need to identify barriers to communication and how to overcome these.

Imagine you are living in a care home.

- How would you like workers to communicate with you?
- What skills do you think would be important for them to have?

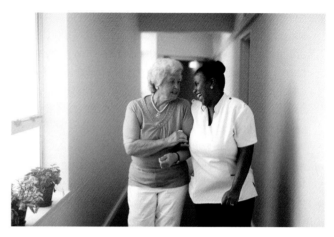

▲ Figure 1.11 Effective communication

AC7.1 The importance of 'effective communication' for the well-being of individuals, children and young people and development of positive relationships

Supporting well-being is about ensuring health and happiness in every part of a person's life. When supporting people's well-being you need to ensure that people have access to the services they need. Effective communication and the development of positive relationships is crucial here to enable services to provide person-centred support. This involves

finding out the individual's needs, likes and dislikes, and planning services with the individual in order to meet these needs.

Working in care involves making a positive impact on the lives of young people, adults, their families and carers. Good communication is essential for developing supportive relationships and working successfully as part of a team. The role of care and support workers involves interaction with a variety of people. You may need to use a range of **communication methods**, such as speaking, writing, on the telephone or by using computers.

You might need to liaise with other professionals in the development and delivery of support plans or on behalf of people you support.

KEY TERM

Communication methods: different ways of communicating, such as verbally, in writing, non-verbal communication, using digital technologies.

Reasons for communication

When we are with people, we are communicating all the time. Even if we are not talking, we are communicating just by the way we sit or our facial expression, gestures, body language and eye contact: this is **non-verbal communication**. Emojis are used in text messages to convey emotion as this is an important part of any interaction. When looking at an emoji, we can usually tell what the person is trying to convey.

How you communicate with the people you support will affect the quality of your relationships and the support you provide. People communicate for many different reasons, such as:

- to express likes and dislikes
- to express wants and needs – being hungry or thirsty, or choosing activities
- to tell others how they are feeling, such as being cold or in pain
- to develop relationships – to find out about the other person, and build trust and rapport
- to share thoughts – discussing opinions on a topic, or how activities can be improved
- to obtain and share information – with team members, individuals or families
- to discuss tasks and responsibilities – discussions in team meetings or supervision meetings with a manager
- to socialise – humans are naturally social, and most people don't like being lonely
- to offer choices
- to show compassion and **empathy**
- to give instructions
- to encourage, motivate and persuade.

In your role you will need to communicate well in order to build meaningful working relationships with your colleagues, as well as the individuals you support and the others involved in their lives.

You can do this by **building rapport**: being friendly and making sure people feel comfortable around you. Doing so will mean that they will trust you, feel positive and safe.

Good communication skills mean that you can encourage individuals to express how they are feeling, and building that trust means they may share information with you that will allow you to offer better, more informed care. For example, an individual may share with you their concerns about how to manage living at home. This means you can offer care and support that will be most helpful to them.

KEY TERMS

Non-verbal communication: communicating without talking, using body language, eye contact, gestures and facial expressions.

Empathy: being able to see things from another person's point of view in order to understand their situation and feelings.

Building rapport: establishing a connection with someone. This usually takes place at the start of a relationship. It is based on mutual trust and involves finding common ground. Showing you understand someone and listening to them establishes rapport.

CASE STUDY

How communication affects well-being

Jameel has developed health problems and become depressed.

Discussion points:

- How might effective communication help Jameel's well-being?
- Who might you need to communicate with if you were supporting Jameel?
- How might you communicate with Jameel?

AC7.2 Key features of effective communication

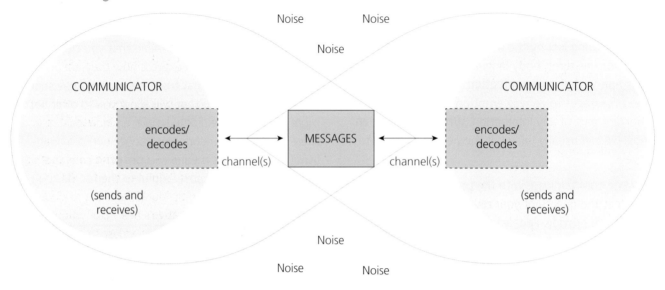

Person A   **Person B**

▲ Figure 1.12 Transactional model of communication

Effective communication involves a number of key elements:

- the person who sends the communication
- the person who receives the communication
- the communication.

A number of things affect communication, which means you are constantly interpreting or formatting the information you send and receive to what you think is suitable for the situation. This can affect how you understand a message. Things that affect communication include:

- external noise, which can make you lose concentration or make it difficult to hear
- your own abilities, such as your hearing or cognitive abilities
- your own values
- past experiences, such as attempts to communicate in similar situations
- how you are feeling at the time.

We will look at barriers to effective communication later in this unit.

REFLECT ON IT

- Can you think of examples of how the above factors have influenced your communication?
- Can you think of a time when you have communicated with someone and they have completely misinterpreted what you meant?

Misunderstandings often happen when text messaging as there is no body language or intonation of voice to help us understand what the message is trying to convey.

Imagine you were drawing up a list of features of effective communication for new staff. What would it include?

Effective communication

There are many ways of ensuring you communicate effectively:

- Listen to what the individual is saying. To show you are listening, you need to think about your body language, facial expression and eye contact. If you look bored or distracted, the other person will think you are not listening or don't care. How many times have you been speaking to someone and they continue to look at their phone? How did you feel? You need to give people your full attention in order for effective communication to take place.

- Show empathy and understanding. Look at things from the other person's point of view to help you understand them better. We naturally look at things from our own perspective. Looking at things from another person's perspective can open up whole new meanings.
- If the individual has any communication difficulties, you will need to be patient and not rush them or make them feel pressured. The individual may need aids such as glasses or a hearing aid to help them.
- Speak clearly so the individual can understand you. Remember that individuals can struggle with accents so you may need to talk slowly. Remember not to be patronising. For example, if we think someone can't understand us, we often talk louder even though they are not hearing-impaired.
- Show the individual that you are genuinely interested in them and what they have to say. Remember to have open body language and good eye contact.
- Be open and honest with people. This will help people feel they can trust you.
- Be aware of the individual's body language. This might help you understand their communication. For example, they may tell you they are okay but their face tells you something else. If you ask again, showing you genuinely care, they may then open up and tell you what is troubling them.
- Be aware of tone of voice. This can tell us a lot about a person. Messages can carry different meanings because the tone of voice might give out a different signal from what the message is trying to convey.
- Understand any communication difficulties the individual might have, such as hearing loss. You may need to adapt your way of communication to ensure they can understand.

To understand individuals and what they are communicating, you need to get to know them. When individuals understand you and what you are communicating, they will show you in their unique way; it is important you can spot the signs so that you can continue to communicate with them and provide them with high quality care and support. Encouraging others to trust you will also reflect your professionalism.

To communicate effectively, you will need to think about who you are communicating with and the reasons you are communicating with them. You can then change or adapt the way you communicate based on your observations. For example, using photographs alongside discussions when communicating with an individual about where they want to go on holiday can ensure that they are making their own choice about where they want to go.

Knowing how to adjust or change your communication to different situations that may arise at work can also mean that you are able to encourage participation from individuals, and show kindness and consideration in your working practices. You may need to do this, for example, when an individual's family is anxious or worried about their relative's health, or when an individual is finding it difficult to adjust to living in a care setting for the first time.

If you empathise with individuals, they will feel they can approach you with any concerns or difficulties. Listen carefully to what they say and pay attention to the feelings and emotions they express. You will then be able to respond appropriately, and the experience will be positive for both of you.

AC7.3 Skills that are needed to communicate effectively

To ensure people understand what you are communicating, you need to be aware of a number of skills. You may be communicating with people with communication or sensory difficulties, dementia or autism, so good communication skills are essential to build relationships and meet individual needs.

REFLECT ON IT

Think of a time when you had a really positive interaction with someone.

- What communication skills were you and the other person demonstrating?

If you find it easier, think of a time when your interaction wasn't so good.

- Why do you think this was the case?
- What could you both have done to make this a more positive interaction?

Reflecting on your interactions in this way can often help you to improve your communication skills. As you go about your day, reflect on the communication skills that you and the people you are interacting with are demonstrating. Think about how you can improve these interactions.

Skills for effective communication

- Active listening skills – you may have heard the saying, 'We have one mouth and two ears so we should listen twice as much as we should speak'. Active listening ensures we understand the other person. It also shows them we are engaged in the conversation. Using sounds like 'uum' and nodding your head demonstrates you are listening.
- Be able to adjust your communication to suit the situation; for example, you would need to use different language in a formal meeting from speaking to your friends on social media.
- Ask questions to help you understand the person better.
- Speak clearly and slowly – this helps people understand you. Mumbling and talking too fast or too quietly can create misunderstandings.
- Allow time for individuals to think and respond. Some may take longer to think about things than others.
- Clarify and summarise what has been said to check you understand it, and also to show the other person you understand what they are trying to convey.
- Effective body language and non-verbal communication – approximately 90 per cent of our communication is non-verbal. Smiling can make the other person feel happy, whereas frowning can make them feel there is something wrong. Posture can also express feeling. If you are facing the person or leaning forward, it looks like you are interested in them. If you have your arms folded, it could look like you are bored or angry.
- Ensure effective eye contact – this can be a way of building trust. Short or broken eye contact can show someone that you are nervous or shy. Not looking at the person can look like you are bored or uninterested. Long periods of eye contact can show you are actively listening, but if you never break eye contact it may be a little intimidating.
- Be clear and succinct – speak in a way which is easy to understand without using jargon or terms the listener may not know.
- Be empathetic – try to understand and share the feelings of others.

- Develop trust and rapport – build relationships on trust and integrity.
- Be confident – this shows colleagues that you believe in what you are saying and will follow through.
- Show respect – people will be more open to communicating with them if you show respect for them and their ideas. When sending emails and texts, check them before sending to ensure they are professional and respectful, and cannot be misinterpreted.
- Pick the right medium – sometimes picking up the phone is far better than sending an email or text. Some people find it easier to say things they are not confident with saying over email, although this can be misinterpreted. It is often better to hold difficult conversations face to face, and this might show more respect for the individual.
- Know how to keep a conversation going – ask **open questions** so that individuals are more likely to talk.
- Organise a conversation – don't keep going off at tangents so the other person finds it hard to follow. Depending on the conversation, it may be helpful to plan a beginning, a middle and an end. The beginning could be an outline of what you are doing to discuss and to check the other person is happy with that. The middle would be the main conversation, and the end could be a summary. This is useful in longer and more formal discussions.
- Understand cultural differences and how these might impact on communication.
- Understand how a person's sensory loss, health or disability might affect communication. For example, if an individual uses lip reading, you will need to ensure you are facing the person and they can see your mouth clearly.

KEY TERM

Open questions: starting a question off with 'Why ...?', 'What ...?' or 'How ...?' encourages the person to share facts, opinions, feelings and emotions. It encourages conversation as opposed to a closed question, such as 'Did you ...?' The answer here is likely to be 'yes' or 'no'.

AC7.4 How to find out an individual's, child's or young person's communication and language needs, wishes and preferences

As a social care worker it is important that you find out how people like to communicate. The easiest way to do this is to ask them, their families or your colleagues. You will need to understand what their responses mean because you will need to develop skills to meet their needs. You could also ask colleagues and look at care plans. Chatting with the person will also help you to understand how they communicate.

Not only do people have different communication and language needs and preferences, but these can also be affected by other factors such as illness and disability.

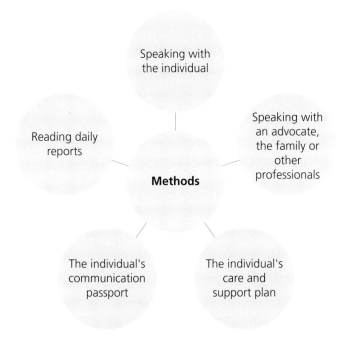

▲ Figure 1.13 How to find out about an individual's, child's or young person's communication needs, wishes and preferences

Different communication needs and preferences

There are many reasons why people you support might have different communication and language needs, wishes and preferences. Here are just a few of the reasons that you will need to think about:

- **Hearing impairment** – communication will be difficult for both of you if the individual has a hearing impairment. They may feel left out of group conversations or misunderstand what is being said to them.
- **Language** – individuals you support may have a different first language from you. If Welsh is their first language, speak to them in Welsh or get someone else who can to speak to them. When someone speaks a different language it can make it difficult for them to form relationships. People may also use sign language or have their own signs and language.
- **Cultural needs** – each culture has its own rules about acceptable behaviours when communicating verbally and non-verbally. For example, a handshake may be acceptable in some cultures but not in others.

RESEARCH IT

Research how disabilities and illnesses can affect the communication, language needs and preferences of the people you support.

- How might a physical disability affect an individual's communication needs?
- Find out about **aphasia** and **dysphasia**.
- How might having an **autistic spectrum disorder** affect an individual's needs and preferences?
- How might an illness such as dementia affect an individual's needs and preferences?

KEY TERMS

Hearing impairment: hearing loss, which could be in one or both ears. It may be a partial loss or a full loss.

Cultural needs: the particular traditions, customs and values shared by a group of people or society.

Aphasia: a condition that affects a person's speech, understanding and use of language. This condition can cause difficulties in putting words together to form sentences.

Dysphasia: a condition that affects how a person understands language. It is a less severe form of aphasia. For example, they may have difficulties listening to and understanding what another person is saying.

Autistic spectrum disorder: a lifelong condition that affects how a person perceives the world and interacts with others. For example, they may have difficulties interacting and socialising with others or expressing emotion.

Reactions to communication

Observing people's reactions to communication can help you understand their communication needs. You can usually tell from people's reactions whether or not they have understood you. If you are not sure if they have, you might need to check this or adapt your communication. This will give you a better understanding of how to communicate with them in the future.

Remember that individuals' needs are different and unique, and therefore different ways of communicating are needed for communications to be effective.

REFLECT ON IT

Reactions to communication

Reflect on an occasion when you observed an individual's reactions while communicating with them.

- What messages did their reactions convey or express to you?
- How did you adapt or change your communication?

If you have not done this yet, think of a time when you had a conversation with a friend.

- Did you observe or look at the way they reacted?
- What messages did you receive from their reactions?
- Were they interested in what you were saying?
- Did they look tired?
- How did you adapt or change the way you communicated?

CASE STUDY

Steve is deaf and blind, and has severe learning disabilities. He spends a lot of time sitting in his chair. When workers approach Steve to take him somewhere, for example, to the table for dinner or to put his coat on if they are going out, he often hits himself and screams.

Discussion points:

- What could Steve be communicating?
- How would it be best to communicate with Steve in this situation?

AC7.5 How the stage of development of a child or young person will impact upon their communication skills

Children learn to communicate by watching and listening to their parents and carers. Young children mimic words and actions. The more you communicate with children, the more they will develop their communication skills.

It is important to remember how stages of child development affect communication so that you don't expect too much from them. You should also remember that these stages can be affected by a number of factors such as education, disability, sensory impairment and environmental issues.

Table 1.7 is a guide to how children should develop their communication skills. They develop at different rates, and if a child has not met one of the milestones it doesn't necessarily mean they have a communication difficulty. However, it is worth talking to a health visitor or other professional if there are concerns that a child isn't developing at the expected rate.

Age	Milestone
	Children develop at different rates but usually they will:
0–6 months	• turn towards a sound • watch your face when you talk to them • be startled by loud noises • recognise a parent's voice • smile and laugh when others do • make baby sounds such as cooing and gurgling • have different cries for different meanings, for example, when tired, hungry or needing a nappy change

▲ Table 1.7 Communication milestones for children

Age	Milestone
6–12 months	• listen carefully to sounds in the room and turn towards sound • take turns in conversation by making pre-speech sounds, such as babbling • enjoy songs and rhymes, and become excited when they hear them • recognise familiar names, such as Mummy • get your attention by making noises, looking at you and pointing • start to understand words such as 'bye bye' or 'good girl'
12–18 months	• enjoy music and move their body or dance • say up to 20 single words such as Mummy, Daddy, cat, cup • enjoy looking at books with an adult and being read to • understand simple commands or questions, for example, 'Where is Daddy?' or 'Hug teddy' • understand a number of words, such as clothes and body parts
18–24 months	• sit and listen to simple stories with pictures • understand 200–500 words • copy sounds and words • concentrate on activities for longer • use 50 or more single words which others can understand over time • start to string a couple of words together, for example, 'Teddy gone' • use a more limited number of sounds in their words than adults. Some sounds are difficult, and young children might say 'pate' instead of 'plate'
2–3 years	• put 4 or 5 words together • understand longer instructions, for example, 'Where is Mummy's shoe?' • listen to and remember simple stories • ask lots of questions – they will be very inquisitive at this age • sometimes sound like they are stammering or stuttering – they want to speak before their language is developed enough • use action words as well as the names of objects, such as run, sleep
3–4 years	• listen to longer stories and are able to answer questions about stories they have just heard • use longer sentences and link sentences together • muddle up tenses, for example, 'I runned' instead of 'I ran' • understand colour, number and time related words • talk about past events • ask many questions, for example, 'Why?'
4–5 years	• understand more complicated language • understand sequences, such as 'First we are going to Grandma's house, then we are going to the park' • use sentences that are well formed although they may still struggle with some grammar; for example, say 'I comed' instead of 'I came' • be able to use most sounds effectively but struggle with some longer words
5–7 years	• rely less on pictures and objects to learn new words • learn to read, write and spell • use language in a range of social situations • share and discuss more complex ideas • learn that the same word can have two meanings • understand feelings and descriptive words
7–11 years	• understand comparative words, for example, 'It is colder than yesterday' • understand other's points of view and show they agree or disagree • use long and complex sentences • use language to predict and draw conclusions • keep a conversation going by giving reasons • start conversations with people they don't know
11–17 years	• use long sentences with conjunctions, for example, 'meanwhile' • follow complicated instructions • use subtle and witty humour • use slang words • use and understand sarcasm • tell long and complicated stories

▲ Table 1.7 Communication milestones for children *(continued)*

AC7.5 AC7.6 Potential barriers to effective communication and ways to address these

There are times when communications are not effective. Barriers to communication are problems that get in the way of you being able to communicate effectively with individuals, or them being able to communicate with you. It is important, therefore, that you think about what barriers could exist and learn what you can do to overcome them. Put yourself in the place of the individual and the difficulties they may have with communicating. What barriers are there for the individual? What barriers are there for you?

Environmental barriers

- Too much noise.
- Not enough time to communicate.
- Not enough space to communicate effectively.
- Too hot or too cold so people are uncomfortable.
- Poor lighting so people cannot see each other properly.

Personal barriers

- Language – an individual's first language could be Welsh and the other person might not speak Welsh.
- Sensory loss – hearing, sight loss.
- Attitudes – the individual's attitude towards the other person can affect the way they communicate with them.
- Previous experience – if you have had poor communication with someone in the past, this can form an ongoing barrier.
- Physical health – if someone is in pain they may not communicate effectively.
- Mental health – for example, an individual suffering with depression may not be able to communicate effectively.
- Cultural – differences in what is acceptable in different cultures.
- Emotional problems – for example, fear or mistrust.
- Terminology – using words or terminology the other person cannot understand.
- Communication skills – a lack of verbal communication or inability to use body language.

As a social care worker you must be aware of potential barriers in the environment or any barriers you might have. Perhaps you feel so busy that you don't have the time to give people. You could be feeling tired, or in a bad mood because of something that has happened earlier in the day. You might not have had training on communication, or **Makaton** for example, if that is how somebody communicates.

You must also be aware of barriers the individual may have, such as lack of confidence, cultural needs, illness such as dementia which affects communication, autism or sensory impairment.

REFLECT ON IT

This activity demonstrates how hard it can be to communicate, especially when you are only allowed to use words and cannot use non-verbal communication.

- Find a partner and sit back to back so that you cannot see each other.
- The partner will need a blank piece of paper and a pencil, and is not allowed to speak or see this book.
- Describe the diagram to your partner, who will draw it.

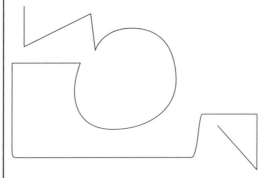

Look at your partner's drawing and discuss the following points:

- Did the drawing look like the diagram?
- What were the barriers for you when describing the picture to your partner? How did this make you feel?
- What were the barriers to your partner receiving the instructions? How did your partner feel?
- How can you apply this to people you may support now or in the future?

KEY TERM

Makaton: a method of communicating that uses symbols, signs and speech to help people with communication difficulties. It is often used with people with learning disabilities and children.

Communicating with somebody with dementia

There will be a number of potential barriers when communicating with somebody with dementia. There are a number of actions you can take to reduce these barriers.

- The individual may be confused about what has or hasn't happened; for example, they ask for their lunch when they have already had it. You will need to be tactful and use your judgement here as to how to respond, especially if they keep asking for lunch. Telling them they have already had it may cause them to be confused. Diversion tactics may be appropriate, such as suggesting you do something together so they forget about lunch.
- Avoid raising your voice or speaking abruptly as this could cause distress.
- Allow plenty of time for the person to process what you are saying.
- Don't shout and don't speak to them as if they were a child. Always show respect.
- Don't make things complicated. Ask questions one at a time.
- Using humour can help situations and save the individual becoming embarrassed, if they have got confused.
- Avoid asking direct questions. These can cause frustration if the individual becomes confused and can't find the answer.
- If the individual doesn't understand, use objects to help or increased non-verbal communication such as gestures.
- Don't keep challenging an individual. For example, if they are waiting for their husband to come home from work and you know the husband has died, use diversion or agree with them, as challenging them can cause upset.

Communicating with somebody with autism

Autism can affect people in different ways, and many people develop coping strategies. The list below gives some ways of overcoming barriers to communication in autism, although these may not be appropriate to everyone.

- Give precise instructions – people with autism often take language literally and do exactly as you say. For example, if you say 'Put some clean trousers on', they could put some on over the dirty trousers.
- Communicate clearly – people with autism may find it difficult to read social cues and body language so don't rely on them reading these. For example, if you are putting your coat on, ready to leave, and expect the individual to do the same, they might not do so. You might need to say 'Are you ready to leave?' and suggest that they wear a coat.
- Don't get frustrated if the person doesn't look interested or as if they are not listening. Sometimes people with autism find it hard to identify with their emotions so when you ask a question, they may say they don't know. This could come across as if they are uninterested, but this might not be true. They may find eye contact difficult and look like they are not listening, when in fact they are.
- People with autism often experience **anxiety** that they hide – keeping communication clear and to the point will help reduce their anxiety as they have a greater chance of understanding what you say.
- Sharing interests – when people with autism are interested in something, they often develop a real in-depth knowledge of the topic. Showing your interest in it or finding common interests will help build rapport.

KEY TERMS

Anxiety: a feeling of fear or worry that may be mild or serious and can lead to physical symptoms, such as shakiness.

Asperger's syndrome: a disability that affects how individuals interact with others. They may have difficulty understanding and relating to other people, and taking part in day-to-day activities.

CASE STUDY

Reducing communication barriers

Trefor has been providing one-to-one support to Michael, a young man who has **Asperger's syndrome**. This affects Michael's ability to communicate and interact with other people. Michael has difficulties understanding what others are saying and following conversations with other people. He finds it difficult to interpret other people's non-verbal communication such as their body language, including their sense of humour, feelings and emotions.

Michael has many interests and tends to tell people he meets what they are, but avoids interacting with them fully. In addition, Michael prefers to avoid eye contact with others. He becomes anxious when eye contact is maintained with him and when he is being asked questions about himself.

Michael has been invited to a family gathering as it is his nephew's birthday. He is anxious about attending this social occasion as he knows there will be lots of people there who know him.

Discussion points:
- How can Michael's communication needs make communications with others difficult?
- What strategies can Trefor use to reduce these barriers to communication?
- What are the benefits of effective communication when working with individuals?

LO8 UNDERSTAND THE IMPORTANCE OF WELSH LANGUAGE AND CULTURE FOR INDIVIDUALS, CHILDREN AND YOUNG PEOPLE

GETTING STARTED

The Welsh language is a key part of the country's culture and identity. It is the main language spoken in many communities and workplaces. The ability to speak Welsh is often seen as an essential requirement in many job roles.

Perhaps your first language is Welsh and you have lived all your life in an area where Welsh is the main language spoken. If you are not, imagine yourself in that situation. Now think about how you would feel if you moved into a care home where nobody spoke Welsh and there was no recognition of Welsh culture.

AC8.1 The importance of recognising and supporting Welsh language and culture

In order to support equality and respect people's individual needs, services must be provided in Welsh so that people whose first language is Welsh can communicate in the language they choose. Benefits of providing services in Welsh include:

- removing the risk of isolating individuals by failing to provide services in their first language
- assessing individual needs by communicating with people in their preferred language
- achieving quality standards
- preventing poor or deficient Welsh language provision
- promoting the reputation of the organisation as a bilingual service
- meeting the requirements of the Social Services and Well-Being (Wales) Act.

Services must ensure they have adequate staff who can speak Welsh. This should be taken into account at recruitment.

As a care worker, if you cannot speak Welsh then you should try to learn as much as possible. Even if you can only speak enough Welsh for basic conversation, for example, greetings and asking how people are, you are showing respect for people's individuality.

RESEARCH IT

If you can't speak Welsh, look up and learn some key Welsh words that will be helpful for communicating with Welsh speakers. Social Care Wales have a resources page on this link:

https://socialcare.wales/learning-and-development/using-welsh-at-work#section-30166-anchor

There are also a number of free apps to help you learn Welsh.

Sometimes when people have dementia, they might revert to Welsh if that is their first language, even though they may have spoken English in the past. It seems that they forget how to speak English.

AC8.2 Legislation and national strategies for Welsh language

As we saw in section AC2.2, there are a number of pieces of legislation which support the Welsh language.

1 The Social Services and Well-Being (Wales) Act says the industry must provide person-centred services. If someone's first language is Welsh then there would be an expectation that services would be available in Welsh.

2 The Welsh Language Act 1993 requires government funded and statutory organisations to offer services in Welsh. As care and support services are funded by the Government, they have a responsibility under this legislation to provide services in Welsh. Communication under the Act refers to verbal and written communication. Any documentation provided to individuals, children and young people must be available in both languages.

The law requires services to ensure that the provision of Welsh medium services are:

- of the same standard and as easily available as English medium services
- as wide-ranging and thorough
- available without being specifically requested.

3 The Welsh Language Measure 2011 and the Welsh Government Strategic Framework for the Welsh Language in Health and Social Care 2013 set standards for services to achieve in relation to Welsh language. The aim is:

- to ensure greater consistency in Welsh language services
- to improve the quality of services to Welsh-speaking individuals, children and young people
- to ensure the Welsh language needs of individuals are met.

The Strategic Framework details how health and social care services can achieve this through the principles of *Mwy Na Geiriau*.

AC8.3 Principles of *Mwy na Geiriau* / More than just words

Mwy na Geiriau is part of the Welsh Government Strategic Framework for the Welsh Language in Health and Social Care 2013. It requires organisations to:

- meet the language needs of Welsh speakers
- provide Welsh language services for those who need it
- demonstrate that Welsh language is an integral part of services and not just an 'add on'.

While it is the responsibility of everybody who provides health and social care services for people and their families across Wales, the Government have targeted a number of services as priority groups. These are:

- children
- older people
- people with learning disabilities
- people with mental health problems.

These priority groups are particularly vulnerable if they don't receive services in their chosen language.

AC8.4 The meaning of the 'active offer'

The 'active offer' is a term used in the 'Mwy na Geiriau' framework. It requires services to be provided in Welsh without a person having to ask for it. Workers who are Welsh speakers should be available as a matter of course.

Welsh newspapers and magazines should be available alongside English ones. Signage in services that help people to orientate should be in Welsh and English.

REFLECT ON IT

How does Welsh language legislation support person-centred approaches?

Check your understanding

1 How can effective communication affect an individual's well-being?

2 List three reasons why people communicate.

3 Who else might a social care worker need to communicate with in order to ensure an individual's well-being?

4 List four skills you need for effective communication.

5 Explain how body language can affect interactions.

6 Explain what adjustments you might need to make to your communication if someone has learning disabilities.

7 How can you help someone with a hearing impairment when communicating?

8 Outline three barriers to communication and describe how you can overcome them.

9 Jake's first language is Welsh. None of the staff who support him speak Welsh. How might this might affect Jake?

10 What is the aim of the Welsh Language Act?

11 Give two examples of how you can support the Welsh language and culture.

Question practice

1 Which of the following best describes relationship-centred working?

   a making friends with families and carers

   b going to regular meetings with other professionals

   c developing positive relationships with other workers across a range of care settings

   d working with individuals to form positive relationships when providing support

2 The parent of an individual you support asks for your personal telephone number so they can call you if they need help when you are off duty. What is the best course of action to take in this scenario?

   a Give the number but ask that it is not passed on to others.

   b Refuse, but provide a personal email address instead.

   c Give the number but state only to call at certain times.

   d Give a number of someone who can help.

3 When may it be suitable for a care and support worker to share personal information about themselves, in line with professional boundaries, when providing care to individuals?

   a to ensure person-centred care

   b to promote relationship-centred working

   c to increase the benefits of co-production

   d to meet data protection legislation

4 Which is the best method of communication for someone who is deaf?

   a eye contact with the individual

   b using professional language

   c using language that will be understood

   d using Makaton

5 Which of these is an environmental barrier to communication?

   a speaking a different language

   b using Makaton

   c hearing impairment

   d noise

6 Which of the following is a key principle of the *Mwy na Geiriau* initiative?

   a to provide Welsh language options before English ones

   b to ensure care services actively provide Welsh language options

   c to provide free Welsh translation services in all care settings

   d to ensure care services only use workers who speak both Welsh and English

7 What is the main reason for recognising the Welsh culture?

   a to meet government requirements

   b we should always recognise culture

   c it is part of Wales

   d to recognise individual diversity

LO9 KNOW HOW POSITIVE APPROACHES CAN BE USED TO REDUCE RESTRICTIVE PRACTICES IN SOCIAL CARE

> **GETTING STARTED**
>
> Think about an occasion or situation that arose that was perhaps difficult or challenging.
> - Why was it difficult or challenging?
> - How could a positive approach have been used?
> - Would this have made a difference? Why?

Positive approaches recognise people's individuality and support their well-being. They support people whose problem behaviours are barriers to reaching their goals. The main focus is understanding the behaviour so it can be predicted and diverted to a more positive response.

Can you think of some examples of positive approaches to behaviour?

AC9.1 The terms 'positive approaches' and 'restrictive practices'

Positive approaches

Positive approaches means working with an individual, child or young person in a person-centred way with an aim of supporting their well-being. This in turn will reduce or prevent challenging behaviour.

When using positive approaches, you should:

- get to know the individual and their likes and dislikes
- understand the individual's skills and abilities

- understand previous experiences the individual/child or young person has had
- respect the individual and their values
- understand the individual's support needs
- understand how someone is feeling and what makes them upset
- understand certain behaviours can be a way of expressing feelings
- understand the stages of development and how this applies to the individual, child or young person
- develop support plans so that you know how to support someone in a positive way when they are feeling upset
- understand how the environment impacts on the person
- implement care and support plans in a way which will ensure the individual's well-being
- ensure effective communication with individuals, children and young people.

If the above actions happen, this can reduce the amount of challenging behaviour. These actions can have a big impact on individuals, helping them to have more positive feelings and a sense of well-being.

> **KEY TERM**
>
> **Positive approaches:** these are based upon the principles of person-centred care. Their aim is to support the individual's well-being and prevent the need for more restrictive practices.

REFLECT ON IT

- Think about times when you are feeling stressed or anxious. What helps you in that situation?
- Imagine you were feeling really stressed and upset but you felt no one understood you or even cared. How would this make you feel?

Positive approaches ensure you give the support that is required when individuals, children and young people are feeling stressed, anxious, upset or scared. It prevents behaviour escalating and avoids the need for more restrictive interventions to be used.

Developing good relationships with people is crucial when using positive approaches. Individuals will feel listened to, and they will feel safe and secure when you are supporting them.

CASE STUDY

When Amy moved into a care home for people with dementia, she displayed some behaviours which challenged the team. She spent large parts of the day screaming, and she would often hit out at workers or the other people she lived with.

The workers decided to keep a record of when this happened. They found it happened much more when Amy wasn't doing anything, or when she was in a crowded, noisy situation.

In response to this, the workers put together an active support plan so that Amy could be more involved in activities in her own home, and supported in the community, doing quiet activities with only a few people.

Over time Amy's screaming had almost stopped, and she rarely hit out at people.

Discussion points:
- What positive approaches were used by the team?
- How did these positive approaches benefit Amy?
- How did these positive approaches benefit others?
- What would have been the potential consequences if the team had not used these positive approaches?

Restrictive practice

Restrictive practice includes actions that deliberately limit an individual's movement or freedom. They prevent people from doing the things they want to do. There may be times when a person needs a restrictive

intervention as this can be a useful way of helping individuals manage their behaviour.

There are a number of guidelines which must be followed to ensure that restrictive practices are in the best interests of the individual, child or young person.

Guidelines for restrictive interventions

Restrictive practices must:

- always be agreed as part of a multi-disciplinary decision and detailed in behaviour support plans
- be well considered, after alternative positive approaches have been considered or attempted
- only be used as the last resort when there are no other options
- be an immediate response to behaviours that challenge, or in an emergency situation to prevent danger and harm
- never be used for longer than necessary
- be appropriate and proportionate to the risk
- never be used as a punishment
- be legal, ethical and justifiable
- be made in a transparent manner with clear lines of accountability
- be reported following each intervention, and never hidden
- be regularly reviewed to ensure they are still required and appropriate
- be in line with training, policy and procedures.

When used inappropriately, restrictive interventions can:

- cause abuse, harm and neglect
- deny an individual their basic human right of freedom and movement
- have serious consequences including pain, harm, suffering and even fatalities if not used correctly
- inflict pain, suffering and humiliation to achieve compliance.

KEY TERM

Restrictive practice: a wide range of activities that stop individuals, children and young people from doing things that they want to do, or encourages them to do things that they don't want to do. They range from limiting an individual's choices, to physical interventions which restrict their movements in an emergency situation.

Examples of restrictive practice

There are many different types of restrictive practice:

- Physical restraint – this should not be used unless you have been specifically trained to do so. Physical restraint is defined by Welsh Government in the Framework for Restrictive Physical Intervention Policy and Practice: Welsh Assembly Government, 2005, as:

  direct physical contact between persons where reasonable force is positively applied against resistance, either to restrict movement or mobility or to disengage from harmful behaviour displayed by an individual.

- Medication used for the purpose of controlling or subduing behaviour.
- Mechanical restraint – an individual's movements are restricted by an object to ensure behaviour control; for example, straps in a chair, a table in front of a chair, or raised bed sides.
- Environmental interventions – making changes to the environment to prevent a behaviour occurring; for example, moving furniture from somebody's room if they throw the furniture in anger.
- Psychosocial restraint or sanctions – these are coercive social or material sanctions or threats of sanctions in order to control behaviour; for example, grounding somebody for a period of time if they act in a way which puts them at risk.
- Seclusion – this is against regulations and should not be used in any social care setting.
- Time out or giving a person space away from a situation – this is not the same as seclusion or isolation. The person should be supported to discuss their feelings, and have space and time to calm down and think about what has happened.

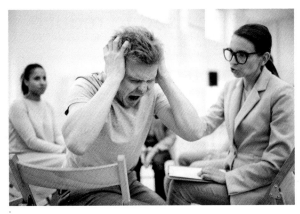

▲ Figure 1.14 Restrictive practices must be appropriate and justifiable

When restrictive practices may be used

Restrictive practices may be appropriate in these situations:

- when a person is self-harming
- to calm somebody down if they need life-saving treatment and are being physically aggressive
- to protect somebody else; for example, if somebody is under the influence of drugs or alcohol, they may need to be physically restrained if they are attacking another person
- keeping knives in a locked drawer if there is a risk of them being used inappropriately to cause harm
- only giving somebody a choice of two items because giving them more choice will cause confusion. This can then be increased so the individual has an increased range of choices when they can cope with this
- when they have been agreed as part of someone's behaviour plan
- when there is a DoLS (soon to be LPS) in place
- when staff have received appropriate training.

> ### REFLECT ON IT
> Restrictive practice
> For each situation below:
> - Think about whether the restrictive practice is appropriate and justifiable, or inappropriate.
> - Think of a positive intervention which might be used as an alternative.
> 1 Mr Walker lives in a care home for people with dementia. The exit doors are locked because he tends to wander out and down the street.
> 2 Ben has learning disabilities and urgently needs an intravenous drip when in hospital. When the doctors try to come near him with the drip and needle, he gets very upset and tries to hit them. They give him some mild sedation to relax him.
> 3 Phillipa is known to bite other people when she is angry. When this happens, workers carry Phillipa to her bedroom and keep the door locked until she has calmed down.
> 4 Hakim has his phone taken from him for a week every time he absconds.
> 5 Callum is given £5 a day if he keeps his room tidy and does the washing up.
> 6 Rosie has learning disabilities. She has sides on her bed at night as she tries to get up and wander round. Staff are scared she might fall downstairs.

AC9.2 Underlying causes that may impact upon behaviour of individuals, children and young people

All behaviour has a meaning and a reason. People's behaviour is in response to a situation, experience or interaction. It is important for workers to understand the meaning behind any behaviour they might find challenging.

If you can understand the meaning, then you might be able to take action to prevent the situation from escalating. There are many things that cause people to behave in the way they do. You need to keep an open mind when supporting people so that you can identify the reason. Often it is because something is happening that the person doesn't feel they can control. Stages of development can have an impact on behaviour as children often use behaviour to test out situations and boundaries.

Sometimes people who have limited communication skills might display their frustrations with a situation in a way which might challenge you, such as aggression, violence, self-harm or screaming. This might be because they have no other way to voice their pain, fear or upset. Even when people can communicate, they still may have difficulty expressing their feelings in a more appropriate way. This can often be due to past experiences; for example, they might feel they are never listened to so their behaviour escalates to become more challenging.

The list below includes some of the reasons people may display behaviour that challenges:

- chronic or acute pain
- infection or other physical pain
- sensory loss
- an acquired brain injury or other neurological condition
- communication difficulties which means the person cannot express their wishes
- noisy environment
- fear and anxiety
- unhappiness
- boredom
- loneliness
- unmet needs
- demands placed on a person, for example, a child may be asked to tidy their bedroom
- change and transitions such as moving house
- recent significant events, such as death of a family member
- past events or experiences
- abuse or trauma
- bullying
- over-controlling care
- being ignored.

> **REFLECT ON IT**
>
> Causes of behaviour
> Think about when you are stressed or upset.
>
> - How do you respond?
> - Does your behaviour change?
> - Does this cause any problems for you or those close to you?
> - Are you able to change the situation so that you feel better?
> - What if you didn't have control — how would you feel?

> **CASE STUDY**
>
> Ianto has limited verbal communication following a stroke and mainly communicates through body language and facial expression. Over the last year or so Ianto has started becoming increasingly withdrawn.
>
> **Discussion points**:
>
> - What might be the cause of this?
> - What should social care workers do in this situation?

Sometimes it can be difficult to find out the cause of somebody's change in behaviour. Adopting positive approaches and trying different strategies will help people feel better and their behaviour might change as a result.

AC9.3 Positive approaches that can be used to reduce restrictive practices and promote positive behaviour

Restrictive practices should only be used as a last resort, with positive approaches always tried first. Being a positive role model for individuals is a positive approach that can have a big influence on individuals' behaviour.

When thinking about what positive approaches can be used, the principles from the Social Services and Well-Being (Wales) Act provide a useful framework for improving support and delivering positive interventions. This is shown in Table 1.8.

Principle	Questions raised by the Social Services and Well-Being (Wales) Act
Voice and control	• Does the individual, child or young person have a voice? Are you listening to them? • Have you found out their likes and dislikes, and what is important to them? • Does the individual have an advocate if they need one? • Have you supported the individual to find alternative methods of communication if they have difficulties communicating their wishes? • Are you communicating with the individual in a way which they understand? • Are you speaking to others to find out past experiences, for example, family and carers? • Are you respecting individuals' rights? • Have you got detailed personal plans in place so that everyone knows the best way to enable voice, control and effective communication? • Do you need to provide any accessible information about services to the individual? • Do individuals know how to complain if they are not happy? • Are you providing support in Welsh if the person needs it? • What else can you do to support voice and control?
Prevention and early intervention	• Can you develop any prevention strategies to help individuals, children and young people deal with situations they struggle with? • What are the trigger points for an individual's behaviour? Is everybody aware of these? Can you prevent these? • Can you support the individual to develop coping strategies? • Does the individual receive the help they need when they need it? • Does the individual have any health problems that need to be addressed? • Can you provide additional support if you know the individual will be facing a stressful situation? • Do you need to make any changes to the environment to prevent the individual from becoming distressed? • Can you support individuals in more or different activities to prevent them from becoming bored and ensure positive outcomes? • Can you support individuals, children and young people to develop their resilience?
Well-being	• Does the individual have any unmet physical, mental or emotional needs? • Is there anything more you can do to support the individual's social and economic well-being? • Is the individual protected from danger, harm and abuse? • Does the individual have access to work, education and leisure activities as appropriate? • Does the individual have suitable and safe living accommodation? • Does the individual have support for domestic and family relationships and friends? • Is the individual's uniqueness recognised and their individual needs met? • Are the individual's beliefs, culture, gender and race respected? • Is the individual an active participant in decisions affecting them? • Is the individual, child or young person involved in meaningful activities? • Does the individual feel in control of their life? • Is the individual supported with positive risk taking?
Co-production	• Are there equal partnerships between individuals, children and young people, families, carers and professionals? • Are key issues discussed between everyone so a solution can be agreed which suits everyone? • Does everyone in the partnership have mutual respect and understanding of each other? • Do you establish what individuals, children and young people want and need, and base services around that? • Do you ensure individuals, children and young people have valid ways of giving feedback and participating?
Multi-agency working	• Do professionals and multi-agency partnerships work together to provide person-centred services? • Do professionals understand each other's roles and have trusting relationships? • Do individuals, children and young people understand how information will be shared? • Is support co-ordinated with clear communication channels? • Is consistent support provided between professionals?

▲ Table 1.8 Questions raised by the Social Services and Well-Being (Wales) Act

Positive Behaviour Support

Positive Behaviour Support (PBS) is a framework that can be used to support positive behaviour. It is person-centred and supports people to make improvements to their quality of life, thus changing behaviour that can cause difficulties and reducing the need for restrictive interventions.

Through using the PBS framework, an understanding is developed of why an individual has behaviours that challenge. It also looks at whether any changes are required to the environment to support the individual to reduce their challenging behaviour. It then looks at alternative communication strategies the individual can use to communicate their needs, and also looks at how services can respond to behaviour in a way which values and respects the individual, child or young person.

The framework has three different stages:

1 **Primary stage** – this is the most important stage as it looks at what triggers behaviour and then identifies actions that can be taken to reduce or eliminate the behaviour. It is therefore proactive in reducing the behaviour.
2 **Secondary stage** – this stage supports the individual when they are becoming upset and distressed, looking at ways of preventing this.
3 **Reactive strategies** – the final phase is used when the first two stages haven't been successful. Safe responses are noted that can be used after the behaviour has occurred to protect the person and others, and defuse the situation. This stage should be carried out within the above guidelines on restrictive interventions.

LO10 UNDERSTAND HOW CHANGE AND TRANSITIONS IMPACT UPON INDIVIDUALS, CHILDREN AND YOUNG PEOPLE

GETTING STARTED

A transition is a period of change from one significant stage to another. These changes happen to everyone throughout life. They can happen suddenly or gradually, and can last for different periods of time. This LO will look at the types of change people may face, factors that affect these changes and how you can support people with change and transitions.

List the key transitions you have faced in your own life and what effects these had on you.

AC10.1 Types of change that may occur in the course of an individual's life as a result of significant life events or transitions

We all face significant life events at certain times during our lives. These are a natural part of the ageing process. These can include:

- having new siblings
- leaving home
- getting married
- moving house

- starting a new school or job
- having children and grandchildren
- retirement
- death of parents or other close family member.

In addition, some people may face additional transitions such as:

- parents getting divorced
- a member of the family developing an addiction
- a member of the family going to prison
- going into care
- becoming a carer
- ill-health
- becoming disabled
- dementia.

Some of these changes have a positive effect on our lives, while others can have a negative effect.

We can experience a whole host of emotions when facing significant changes. These can range from happiness, excitement and thankfulness to apprehension, fear, anger and **depression**. The changes may cause disruption to routines. People might wonder if they will cope, become worried about the future and develop a feeling of hopelessness.

Changes may occur to our daily lives as a result of these transitions or life events.

KEY TERM

Depression: a medical condition causing low mood that affects your thoughts and feelings. It can range from mild to severe, but usually lasts for a long time and affects day-to-day living.

REFLECT ON IT

Think about the transitions and life events listed below. What changes may occur as a result?

- a young child's parent getting divorced
- starting a new school
- having children
- a child's father going to prison
- going into care
- becoming disabled
- death of a spouse.

AC10.2 Factors that make these changes either positive or negative

REFLECT ON IT

Thinking about the changes in your own life above:

- What made you respond in the way you did?
- What positive and negative emotions and feelings did you experience?

Everybody responds to situations differently. Some people are able to deal with stress and challenges better than others. Other people, particularly people with autism, can find change extremely stressful, and it can be a period of heightened anxiety.

How you deal with change can be based on past experiences, your personality, coping mechanisms, resilience and support networks. It is natural for people to resist change but there are positive outcomes from change and transitions as you learn to become more flexible. Change can be an opportunity, and a way of developing new relationships. For most people, having control in their lives is important to them. When faced with change and transitions, they can feel out of control.

How to support people with change and transitions

There are many ways you can support people with change and transitions. An individual may need time to accept change or time to grieve. People can experience grief in many different situations such as death of a loved one, a change of home or loss of health.

There are a number of stages people go through when experiencing grief, which, as we have seen, can occur during significant life changes. These stages are:

- denial – people pretend the change isn't happening
- anger – they might blame others
- bargaining – they try to control the change by suggesting alternatives
- depression – they can get depressed when they realise the change is going to happen
- acceptance – they finally accept the change and work out how to deal with it.

Time might help a person work through these changes on their own. There are also ways your support can turn what might have been a negative experience into a positive one.

- Planning and decision making should be done in a person-centred way – individuals should have voice, choice and control with access to advocacy where required.
- You can help individuals to think about the positive aspects of the change. If you talk about it positively, it may help the individual to look at it from another viewpoint.
- You could encourage the individual to think about what they want to achieve, and what is important to them, both now and in the future.
- You could support the individual to identify ways that they can reduce their stress levels. This could be going to the gym, sitting in a garden or park,

talking over their concerns or just thinking about the positive benefits of the transition.

- Support is very important when facing change. Being able to talk things through with people you trust often helps you deal with things better. Having strong support networks can help your well-being, give you a sense of identity and build self-esteem.
- You can support people to plan for change as early as possible so they feel in control of the situation.
- Ensure that individuals have access to the information they need and that they understand it.
- Support should be co-ordinated across all services.
- Families and carers may also need support – consideration should also be given to this.
- You might be able to sensitively support people to move from one stage of grief to another, for example, by helping them to accept the change if it is inevitable. There is no point in fighting against it if it is definitely going to happen.

AC10.3 How to support young people to develop the skills, confidence and knowledge that will prepare them for adult life

Helping young people to prepare for adulthood will give them a sense of control and readiness which will help them feel more able to cope. Some people may be looking forward to it as it can give them a sense of freedom. Others may be filled with dread as it might mean they will move from services for children and young people into adult services. They may feel they won't have the same support as they will be expected to cope with adulthood.

Feedback from young people shows that the earlier they start preparing for adulthood, the better. Young people themselves need to take the lead role in this planning. Education, children's and adult services need to work together to ensure positive outcomes.

As we saw in LO1, the Social Services and Well-Being (Wales) Act requires people transitioning from children's services to adulthood to have a pathway plan which identifies how they will be supported with this change.

> **REFLECT ON IT**
>
> Imagine a teenager needs to change his living situation when he turns 18. Explain the approaches that can be used to make this transition a positive one.

There are many ways you can help young people to prepare for transitions:

- Develop practical skills – this can include budgeting and opening bank accounts, cooking and other household tasks such as cleaning.
- Build resilience – this will help them to face future challenges. Exposing young people to challenges will help them face future challenges. It will give them self-confidence and a sense of achievement, as well as develop their coping mechanisms and problem solving skills.
- Ensure young people have information about what support is available in their local communities.
- Support young people to think about what they would like to do for leisure, career, education. They might like to try some volunteering work, which will help to prepare them for the world of work.
- Develop goal plans with them. This can include what they would like to do in the short, medium and long term.
- Support young people to understand the benefits system and apply for any benefits they may need.
- If young people have spent most of their time with their families or carers, support them to do things independently.
- Support young people to put emergency and contingency plans in place.
- Support young people to weigh up risks and benefits of things that they do, and to realise that making mistakes is a natural part of growing up.
- Ensure that young people know what will happen before, during and after the transition, and what support will be available to them.

LO11 UNDERSTAND HOW OWN BELIEFS, VALUES AND LIFE EXPERIENCES CAN AFFECT ATTITUDE AND BEHAVIOUR TOWARDS INDIVIDUALS, CHILDREN, YOUNG PEOPLE AND CARERS

GETTING STARTED

Our beliefs reflect what we think is true. Our values are usually based on these beliefs, and tell us what is right and wrong and how we should live our life. These beliefs and values affect everything we do, including our relationships, quality of life and work. They form an essential part of our identity.

Think about your own beliefs and values.

- What are they?
- How have they developed?

AC11.1 The impact of own attitude and behaviour on individuals, children and young people and carers

Throughout your life your attitudes and values develop. These make up the person you are today. They define what is important to you and influence your decision making. Your beliefs and values are formed because of a number of different influences in your lives. These could include:

- Your parents – you may do things because your parents did, or you may purposely do things differently from your parents.
- Role models – these can be famous people or people you know that you admire and try to imitate.
- Peer groups – these can have a big influence, especially for children and young people. Peer groups can influence how you dress, what activities you take part in, your use of language, the activities you get involved in and what you regard as important.
- Education – school, further education and any other form of learning has an impact on our values and beliefs.

- The media – radio, television and social media have been proven to affect people's values. For example, media messaging and advertising influence what society sees as beautiful or attractive. They have a powerful effect on self-esteem and body image.
- Culture and religious beliefs – people may choose to observe customs and practices related to their culture or religion.

REFLECT ON IT

How your beliefs affect your interactions
Look at this list of beliefs that some people may have:

- All human beings are equal and should be treated fairly.
- People with disabilities cannot do a job as well as people who do not have a disability.
- Refugees should not be allowed into Britain.
- People should not have to retire by the age of 67, and should work while they feel they are able to.

If you have or were to have these beliefs, how could they affect the way you interact with the individuals you support?

When working in health and social care, you must ensure that your own beliefs, attitudes and values do not influence the people we support. This ensures you provide person-centred support which values the person as an individual with their own needs and aspirations. It respects other people's cultures and any religious beliefs they may hold.

Respecting other people's attitudes and values can increase opportunities for you to think about and develop an understanding of other beliefs, traditions and cultures.

Sometimes you might not agree with the attitudes and behaviours of individuals, children and young people we support. However, remember that all people have:

- the right to freedom of thought and religion
- the right to freedom to express their beliefs as they wish
- the right to freedom of conscience (personal values and a sense of right and wrong).

Oppressing people's values and trying to influence them with your own is discriminatory, denies them their freedom and is a form of abuse.

REFLECT ON IT

Give examples of when workers' attitudes, values and beliefs may inadvertently influence the people they support.

Check your understanding

1 Define the term 'positive approaches'.

2 List some restrictive practices and think of positive alternatives.

3 Give some examples of what might cause behaviours that challenge.

4 Describe three potential outcomes if team members have a negative attitude towards young people who misuse substances.

5 Describe how to make sure that your own beliefs and values do not affect people you support.

Question practice

1 Linda displays behaviours that challenge. On a few occasions, restrictive interventions have been used to ensure her safety and that of others. Workers in the setting are anxious to reduce the need to use restrictive interventions. Which of these will best support this aim?

   a Plan activities to meet Linda's individual needs.

   b Exclude Linda from activities when she becomes angry.

   c Treat Linda the same as the others at all times.

   d Look at what makes other people angry.

2 Which of the following actions is most likely to reduce the need for restrictive practice?

   a Treat all individuals the same.

   b Request feedback on a monthly basis.

   c Control the range of resources available to individuals.

   d Support individuals to engage in activities that are important to them.

3 Gillian has a terminal illness. She tells her care and support worker Jim that she is struggling to come to terms with her own death as she has no religious belief. What is an unacceptable way for Jim to respond to Gillian in this scenario?

   a Arrange pastoral support for Gillian with her permission.

   b Ask Gillian if she would like to speak to a palliative nurse or advocate.

   c Express his beliefs around dying and contact Gillian's family to support her.

   d Listen with empathy to Gillian's concerns and report the incident to a manager.

FURTHER READING AND RESEARCH

Weblinks

Information about the Social Services and Well-Being (Wales) Act 2014:
https://socialcare.wales/hub/resources

Information about the Codes of Practice:
https://socialcare.wales/dealing-with-concerns/codes-of-practice-and-guidance

Information on the Code of Conduct for Healthcare Support Workers in Wales and the Code of Practice for NHS Wales Employers:
www.wales.nhs.uk/nhswalescodeofconductandcodeofpractice

Outlines all the rights contained in the Human Rights Act:
www.equalityhumanrights.com/en/human-rights/human-rights-act

An outline of *Mwy na Geiriau* (More than just words):
https://careinspectorate.wales/more-just-words-follow-strategic-framework-welsh-language-health-social-services-and-social-care

Mwy na Geiriau (More than just words) action plan:
https://gov.wales/welsh-language-healthcare-more-just-words-action-plan-2019-2020

Summary of the Mental Health Act:
www.nhs.uk/using-the-nhs/nhs-services/mental-health-services/mental-health-act/

Summary of the Mental Capacity Act; discusses consent and how to support people to make decisions:
www.nhs.uk/conditions/social-care-and-support-guide/making-decisions-for-someone-else/mental-capacity-act/

Outlines the seven aims adopted by Welsh Government:
https://gov.wales/sites/default/files/publications/2019-06/seven-core-aims-for-children-and-young-people.pdf

Information on Shared Lives:
https://sharedlivesplus.org.uk/

Further information on PBS:
www.challengingbehaviour.org.uk/understanding-behaviour/keymessagespbs.html

A resource on positive approaches and reducing restrictive practices in social care:
https://socialcare.wales/cms_assets/file-uploads/Positive-Approaches-Final-English-June-2016.pdf

Useful information about transitions from childhood to adulthood, including a downloadable guide:
www.nice.org.uk/guidance/ng43

Links to Say Something in Welsh (an app with 25 free Welsh lessons):
https://socialcare.wales/resources

HEALTH AND WELL-BEING (ADULTS)

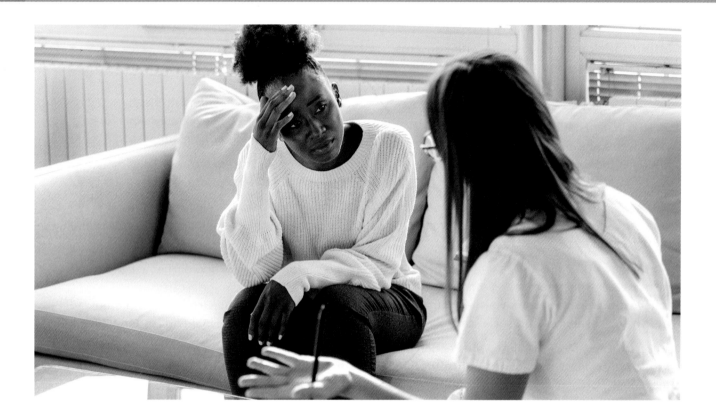

ABOUT THIS UNIT

Guided learning hours: 80

In this unit you will learn what well-being means and develop an understanding of well-being in the context of health and social care. You will look at:

- how you can support the well-being of individuals and the factors that impact upon the health and well-being of individuals
- the roles and responsibilities related to the administration of medication in health and social care settings by learning about the legislation and national guidance
- the links between misadministration of medication and safeguarding
- the factors that affect end of life care
- how supportive technology can be used to support active participation
- how individuals with a sensory impairment can be supported
- dementia – what it is, the signs and indicators and how person-centred approaches can be used to support individuals living with dementia
- how mental ill-health can affect health and well-being, factors that contribute or lead to mental ill-health, and the signs and potential indicators of mental illness
- substance misuse and the impact this can have upon health and well-being.

Learning outcomes

LO1: Know what well-being means in the context of health and social care

LO2: Know the factors that impact upon the health and well-being of individuals

LO3: Know how to support individuals with their personal care and continence management

LO4: Know what is meant by good practice in relation to pressure area care

LO5: Know how to support good oral health care and mouth care for individuals

LO6: Know the importance of foot care and the health and well-being of individuals

LO7: Understand the roles and responsibilities related to the administration of medication in health and social care settings

LO8: Understand the importance of nutrition and hydration for the health and well-being of individuals

LO9: Know how to support falls prevention

LO10: Know the factors that affect end of life care

LO11: Know how assistive technology can be used to support the health and well-being of individuals

LO12: Know how sensory loss can impact upon the health and well-being of individuals

LO13: Know how living with dementia can impact on the health and well-being of individuals

LO14: Know how mental ill-health can impact upon the health and well-being of individuals

LO15: Know how substance misuse can impact upon the health and well-being of individuals

LO1 KNOW WHAT WELL-BEING MEANS IN THE CONTEXT OF HEALTH AND SOCIAL CARE

GETTING STARTED

Think about what well-being means you to you. What contributes to your well-being? It might be your family and loved ones, your friends, your hobbies, your networks, your childhood experiences, the environment you live in.

- Why is well-being important?
- Think about what it would mean to you if you didn't have these contributing factors around you. How would you maintain your well-being?

AC1.1 The term 'well-being' and its importance

We explored well-being in Units 001/002, AC1.1. Look back at this section for a definition of the term. Good well-being will have a positive effect on many aspects of individuals' lives, such as:

- good physical and mental health
- the development of resilience

- positive self-esteem
- encouraging positive behaviour
- encouraging social interactions and positive relationships
- combating loneliness
- helping to support mental health.

The Social Services and Well-Being (Wales) Act 2014 provides definitions of well-being and is applicable to people who need care and support in Wales. The Welsh Government has published a 'Well-being statement for people who need care and support and carers who need support'. The Welsh Government's definition of well-being includes:

- being physically, mentally and emotionally happy
- securing rights and entitlements
- having education, training and recreation
- protection from abuse, harm and neglect
- positive relationships with family and friends
- social and economic well-being
- suitable living accommodation.

AC1.2 Factors that affect the well-being of individuals and carers

It is important to understand the background of the individual or carer in order to understand how this may have affected their health and well-being. There are a variety of factors that affect the well-being of individuals and their carers. These may be social, cultural, economic, emotional, spiritual or physical factors such as:

- healthy relationships, which support emotional well-being
- enjoyable and fulfilling career, which supports self-esteem
- regular exercise, which supports physical and mental health
- enough sleep and rest, which supports physical and mental health
- access to healthcare services
- health conditions which can affect an individual's physical and mental well-being, for example, diabetes, cardiovascular disease, multiple sclerosis
- healthy self-esteem, which promotes well-being
- healthy diet, which supports good physical health
- a sense of belonging, which supports emotional well-being and good mental health
- being able to explore your spiritual beliefs and access suitable places of worship
- having your cultural needs recognised
- being able to communicate in your language of choice
- resilience and ability to adapt to change
- enough money
- placement breakdowns when being looked after
- physical disabilities
- learning disabilities
- secure attachment.

Table 2.1 presents some factors that may impact negatively on well-being.

Factor	Negative impact of the factor on well-being
Adverse Childhood Experiences (ACEs)	Negative childhood experiences such as abuse, neglect, domestic violence in the home, substance misuse and parental separation, can impact on the individual's well-being throughout their lives. *'Evidence shows children who experience stressful and poor quality childhoods are more likely to develop health-harming and anti-social behaviours, more likely to perform poorly in school, more likely to be involved in crime and ultimately less likely to be a productive member of society.'* (NHS Wales, www.wales.nhs.uk/sitesplus/888/page/88524)
Emotional factors	Emotional factors such as loneliness or mental ill-health can have a negative impact on well-being. Everyone deals with situations differently and emotional needs should always be addressed when an individual is going through change, a transition or a challenging experience.
Social deprivation	Not having the opportunities to mix and meet other people can lead to isolation and affect well-being.
Disabilities and physical ill-health	This could impact on an individual's ability to exercise and socialise, leading to isolation.
Economic factors	If an individual experiences poverty, poor diet, financial stress and limited opportunity, this can impact on their well-being.
Cultural factors	Individuals from different cultural backgrounds may struggle to access services due to language barriers, religion or gender.
Spiritual factors	Spirituality is personal and unique to the individual and support should be person-led when considering these factors. It is important to note that spirituality may not always link to religion and an individual may express their spirituality in a variety of ways.
Environment	Individuals living in cramped conditions, with inadequate facilities, pollution and hazards will experience a poorer level of well-being than those who are living in stimulating, safe, caring and supportive environments.
Stress	Chronic stress can affect the body, thoughts and feelings of an individual. It can hinder brain development, impact on the ability to concentrate and learn. This in turn will impact on well-being. If left untreated, it can contribute to health problems such as high blood pressure and heart disease.

▲ Table 2.1 Factors which negatively affect well-being

CASE STUDY

Ian is a 25-year-old man who lives in support housing. Ian has a history of drug and alcohol abuse; he is currently unemployed and struggles to hold down a job.

Ian was taken into care when he was seven, and was a looked-after child in foster homes and residential children's homes before ending up in a secure unit at the age of 18. This was due to his residential placements breaking down because of concerning behaviour. Ian would go missing from care for days, he would often return back to the home with stolen items he claimed to have 'found' or been given by 'friends', and he would often have aggressive outbursts and break property in the home.

Ian struggled to develop attachment to any foster parents or support staff, always appearing to push them away. Ian had a difficult relationship with his mother, who was a recovering drug addict and had severely neglected him as a young child. His education was very limited due to long absences from school, and as a result he still struggles to read and write.

Discussion point: What factors have affected Ian's health and well-being?

AC1.3 The importance of families, friends and community networks on the well-being of individuals and carers

Families, friends and community networks are important for the support of well-being on individuals and carers. As humans, we desire a sense of belonging and this can be nurtured by our families, friends and networks.

Your early childhood experiences will impact on your experiences as adults. Friendships with people who share your interests can help you to feel you belong. Family, friends and communities can help to build foundations for good health and well-being through positive relationships, social participation and community connection.

REFLECT ON IT

Think about how you support others – not just your friends and families, but the wider community too. How does this help you to feel a sense of belonging?

AC1.4 Ways of working that support well-being

There are many ways you can support individuals' well-being as a health and social care worker:

- Spend time with someone, with no distractions.
- Treat individuals with respect.
- Find out what their beliefs, religion, spiritual needs and culture are and talk openly about these.
- Encourage independence; allow individuals to make choices and decisions.
- Help individuals to follow their chosen routines – these give structure and support security.
- Support individuals to set realistic goal and gain new skills.
- Create a culture of trust so individuals open up to you and feel they can talk freely.
- Support physical and mental health.
- Encourage healthy eating and hydration.
- Support individuals to have social interaction and maintain friendships.
- Support individuals to keep safe.
- Raise concerns about health and well-being with the appropriate service.
- Be a positive role model.

LO2 KNOW THE FACTORS THAT IMPACT UPON THE HEALTH AND WELL-BEING OF INDIVIDUALS

GETTING STARTED

Think about some of the factors that might affect your well-being: where you live, who you live with, where you work or study, your hobbies, your physical health.

Now think about a time when you may have been unwell.

- How did that make you feel?
- Did it affect your mental well-being?
- Did you feel alone, isolated, frustrated that you could not do the things you enjoy?

AC2.1 Factors that can affect human development

We explored some of the factors that can affect well-being earlier in the unit. We will now look at factors that can affect human development.

Physical factors	Social and emotional factors	Economic factors	Environmental factors
Exercise – promotes physical development	Family – an individual's family structure can impact on their emotional development	Debt – living in debt can cause huge stress and anxiety, and have a large impact on mental well-being	Barriers to accessing services – individuals living in remote locations, or being members of cultures that prevent individuals from accessing services, can impact on their development and well-being
Disabilities – can impact on physical and intellectual development	ACEs – negative childhood experiences that individuals experience can impact on them throughout childhood and into adulthood	Poverty – living in poverty can mean that an individual's development suffers through lack of nutritious food, inadequate housing and limited access to social opportunities	Air pollution – this can severely impact on physical twell-being and development
Diet and nutrition – can impact negatively on physical development if not balanced	Relationships – positive relationships can have a good impact on emotional development, but unhealthy relationships can hugely affect how an individual sees themselves, and severely impact on their self-esteem and mental well-being	Wages – low wages and income can impact on development through low self-esteem, poor mental and physical health	Housing – poor housing can impact on physical well-being and also mental and intellectual well-being. Is there enough space to learn? Is there adequate heating and lighting?
Genetic inheritance – can impact on physical and intellectual development	Gender – we still have gender stereotypes and pay gaps: boys and girls learn differently and can often be treated differently		

▲ Table 2.2 Factors that can affect human development

REFLECT ON IT

Pick one factor from each column in Table 2.2 and discuss why you think this might impact on human development.

CASE STUDY

Owen, who is 21 years old, spent his childhood in care. His partner Faye, 19, had their first baby when she was 17 years old. They now have two small children. Owen left school with few qualifications and is currently working night shifts at a local factory. Owen and Faye struggle on his low income and on occasion have been late with their rent.

They argue a lot as Owen spends all night working and then sleeps during the day. This means Faye gets little help with their small children. She is frustrated and feels overwhelmed.

One day Owen is told that the factory is going to be making redundancies and he will hear in due course whether he will lose his job. Owen worries but does not tell Faye as he is worried that she will leave him.

Discussion points:

- What factors are impacting on Owen and Faye's well-being?
- How might their background affect their ability to cope in these circumstances?
- What support might be available for Owen and Faye?

AC2.2 Factors that may affect the health, well-being and development of individuals and the impact this may have on them

There are many factors that may affect the health, well-being and development of individuals, and the impact on individuals can vary. We will look at these factors in the four categories of physical, social and emotional, economic and environmental.

Factors that may affect the health, well-being and development of individuals may include:

- adverse circumstances or trauma before or during birth
- autistic spectrum conditions
- dementia
- family circumstances

- frailty
- harm or abuse
- injury
- learning disability
- medical conditions (chronic/acute)
- mental health or physical disability
- physical ill-health
- poverty
- profound or complex needs
- sensory needs
- social deprivation
- substances misuse.

Physical factors that can affect health, well-being and development

Disabilities

Individuals may be born with their disability or they can acquire it at any stage in life. This could be due to an accident, illness or related to their age, such as dementia.

Genetic or inherited disorders

Individuals may be born with a genetic disorder caused by an abnormal gene in their genetic make-up. Some examples of this are:

- cystic fibrosis
- haemophilia
- Huntington's disease
- sickle cell anaemia
- muscular dystrophy
- thalassaemia
- fragile X syndrome
- Hunter's syndrome.

Sensory disabilities

Some individuals may have a disability of the senses which affects their sight, and their sense of hearing, taste and smell. Some examples of this are:

- autism
- blindness or poor vision
- deafness or hearing loss
- **anosmia**
- somatosensory impairment.

KEY TERM

Anosmia: loss of smell.

Physical disability

A physical disability can reduce the individual's opportunities to develop friendships, and may affect their physical development which then impacts on their health. Some examples of physical disabilities are:

- **cerebral palsy**
- **spina bifida**
- multiple sclerosis
- muscular dystrophy
- **dwarfism**.

Learning disabilities

Learning disabilities can be mild, moderate or profound, and will affect how an individual learns new things throughout their life. Some examples of learning disabilities are:

- **Down's syndrome**
- **Williams syndrome**
- autism (this is not a learning disability but some individuals with autism will have some level of learning disability).

For further information on these disorders, see Unit 004.

KEY TERMS

Cerebral palsy: a condition that causes lifelong conditions affecting movement. It is caused by a problem with the brain before, after or during birth.

Spina bifida: a birth defect caused when the spine and spinal cord do not form properly.

Dwarfism: a medical or genetic condition causing short stature.

Down's syndrome: a genetic condition that causes physical and mental development delays.

Williams syndrome: a rare genetic disorder causing mild learning or developmental challenges.

RESEARCH IT

Research the different physical disabilities and factors listed above. These videos might help you to understand what it can be like to live with a sensory, physical or learning disability:

Sensory disability awareness

https://youtu.be/LU0dQXJ-YQM

Physical disability awareness

https://youtu.be/CL8GMxRW_5Y

What is a learning disability?

https://youtu.be/tfkVA2BKIyY

Diet and nutrition

Having a healthy diet and good hydration can have lasting benefits on the health of individuals. They will have more energy, maintain a healthy weight, an improved mood, good sleep, better oral health, healthy muscles and kidneys, and a lower risk of developing chronic health conditions, such as cancer, heart disease and stroke.

See Unit 004, AC2.2 for more information on the benefits of breastfeeding, for the child and the mother.

Physical activity

Staying physically activity can affect health, development and well-being in many positive ways. Physical activity will:

- keep the body healthy and reduce the risk of disease, such as cardiovascular disease
- help support mobility and maintain a healthy weight
- support mental health by improving self-esteem and reducing stress, depression and anxiety.

For older individuals, it can:

- help to maintain cognitive function
- reduce the risk of falls by maintaining mobility and independence.

CASE STUDY

Dylan is a 40-year-old man with learning disabilities, and lives at home with his elderly parents. Dylan played football in a local team for adults with learning disabilities every week, but has recently sprained his ankle and is now too frightened to return to the team.

Discussion point: What are the factors that might impact on Dylan?

Experience of illness and disease

Some illnesses can affect an individual's health and well-being. For example:

- asthma
- Crohn's disease
- kidney disease
- cystic fibrosis
- stroke
- appendicitis
- respiratory infections.

These illnesses can:

- cause pain and discomfort
- require regular visits to hospital
- stop individuals partaking in activities
- affect their emotional well-being
- cause depression and low moods due to living with an illness
- affect their physical well-being if mobility is affected.

Individuals could be affected either by the illness or the medication. Their quality of life may be reduced if the illness is not managed correctly. They may need to be in hospital for longer, they may need to give up activities that were important to them and make other changes to their lives. The illness or disease could also affect other areas: the individual may have to give up their job, which may lead to financial problems and could affect their self-esteem and the way that they see themselves, and the family dynamic can also be affected when one individual needs to be cared for.

Social and emotional factors that can affect health, well-being and development

Gender

Issues around gender stereotypes, inequality and transgender discrimination can all have an impact on health, well-being and development. Men, women and children are still often expected to conform to gender roles. Inequality, discrimination and harassment can directly impact on health and well-being.

> ### REFLECT ON IT
>
> *One of the reasons for differences in the gender pay gap between age groups is that women over 40 years are more likely to work in lower-paid occupations and, compared with younger women, are less likely to work as managers, directors or senior officials.*
>
> (www.ons.gov.uk/employmentandlabourmarket/ peopleinwork/earningsandworkinghours/bulletins/ genderpaygapintheuk/2019#the-gender-pay-gap)
>
> - Why does the gender pay gap still exist?
> - What are the reasons behind the above statement?
> - How can the pay gap affect well-being?

Relationships

An individual will have many relationships throughout their life, starting with the relationship they have with their parents and siblings through to friendships, sexual relationships and working relationships.

Feeling connected to their parents gives children a healthy start in life. If they feel safe and secure and know their parents are there for them, children are less likely to be influenced by external relationships in their teens. Mutual respect and attachment will allow them to grow into secure adults.

Sibling relationships will vary dependent on age and gender, and not all siblings remain close in adulthood. Some sibling relationships remain strong and are placed above all other relationships. Many will maintain a close friendship, but this will be secondary to their partner and children, and some will grow to feel no connection or even hostility towards their siblings.

Friendships can support health and well-being if the friendship is positive. However, some friendships can be negative and dysfunctional, leaving the individual with poor self-esteem and feeling pressured.

Intimate relationships can have a positive or negative impact on health and well-being. This will depend on honesty and trust: is there a healthy sexual relationship, or does one person feel pressured?

An individual working relationship can be positive if the individual feels valued, respected and part of a community. It helps to give them a sense of purpose, which has been discussed under LO1, AC1.3.

ACEs

ACEs occur before the age of 18 and will have a lasting traumatic effect on the child. They can include:

- physical abuse – intentionally causing physical injury or trauma
- sexual abuse – abusive and/or inappropriate sexual behaviour towards an individual
- emotional abuse – also called psychological abuse; this can be any type of mistreatment, such as bullying, humiliation, verbal abuse, isolation, belittling or scaring
- domestic violence – any kind of abuse between current or former partners, this can include physical, sexual, emotional, financial abuse

- neglect – failure to meet an individual's basic needs, including their physical and psychological needs
- parent separation – parents separating/divorcing and living apart.

RESEARCH IT

Research the way ACEs can have an impact on an adult's health and well-being. You might like to look at the following websites:

ACEs and their association with chronic disease
https://bit.ly/ACEs-chronic-disease-report-pdf

The Early Action Together ACEs learning network
www.rsph.org.uk/our-work/resources/early-action-together-learning-network.html

ACEs and their impact on health-harming behaviours
https://bit.ly/ACEs-health-harming-behaviours-pdf

ACE Aware Wales
www.aceawarewales.com/welcome

Employment

Employment supports health and well-being as it:

- provides individuals with purpose and routine
- supports them financially
- promotes feelings of security
- can help with self-esteem
- stimulates individuals mentally and physically, depending on the job.

Unemployment can consistently impact negatively on individuals, as it:

- increases poverty, stress, unhealthy behaviours
- can affect future employment
- can increase mental ill-health, causing anxiety and depression.

Cultural and racial diversity

Cultural beliefs, customs and behaviours can impact on health and well-being.

- They can impact on how groups approach topics of health, illness and death; for example, in the Jewish faith, after death there is a washing ritual, and the body must not be left alone until burial.
- Seeking medical help and receiving treatment can be affected; for example, Jehovah's Witnesses do not accept blood transfusions of blood products, based on biblical readings.

Likewise, race can impact on health:

- Some races have a higher chance of certain diseases; for example, people of African, African American or Mediterranean heritage are more prone to sickle cell disease, although sickle cell disease can occur in any ethnic group.
- Other issues that can affect different racial groups could come from racism which can impact on well-being. People subjected to racism may find they have lower self-esteem, suffer with anxiety and depression, or will even be too scared to go to work or school, which could impact on their development.

Economic factors that can affect health, well-being and development

Wages, benefits, bills and debt

Studies have shown that earning a low income can link to unhealthy lifestyles, and virtually all **domains of health** potentially have a worse outcome. With a greater income, individuals can purchase items and services that can improve their health, such as gym memberships. The stress of managing on a low income can affect the individual's physical and mental health.

KEY TERM

Domains of health: physical, emotional, occupational, spiritual, social, environmental and intellectual areas of health.

Being the sole earner can be very stressful, especially if you are a low earner and have to rely on benefits to earn a living. Living with low wages or receiving welfare benefits can also have a negative impact on health, well-being and development.

- There can be a stigma attached to families who live on benefits, which can impact on their self-esteem and mental well-being.
- Low wages mean an individual may not be able to provide for their family in the way they want, or keep up with all the additional cost such as activity clubs and school equipment.

High levels of debt can also have a negative impact on well-being:

- It can cause stress, depression and a feeling of hopelessness.
- Families could break down.
- Access to healthy food and exercise opportunities can be impacted, leaving to health risks.

Poverty

Poverty can affect the health of individuals at all ages. The causes of poverty could include economic and social factors such as:

- unemployment
- low income
- inadequate benefit entitlements
- lack of affordable housing
- having a disability
- being a full-time carer
- being a lone parent or from a large family
- being an older adult living alone.

Studies show that:

- Children living in poverty are more likely to have chronic diseases and diet-related problems.
- Childhood poverty can have a long-term effect on their life chances and their health as adults.
- Mental health problems are much more prevalent in those individuals living in poverty.

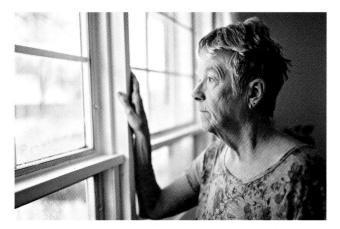

▲ Figure 2.1 Economic factors can affect individuals at all ages

Environmental factors that can affect health, well-being and development

Housing conditions

Housing conditions can have a huge impact on health and well-being. Where we live is important for giving us a sense of security and safety: Is it free from damp? Is it warm? Is there is enough space for everyone living there?

Poor quality housing can impact on health conditions but can also lead to poor mental health or even domestic violence in the home.

Homelessness impacts on an individual's physical and mental well-being. They may not have a regular abode, they may be living in hostels or sleeping rough. Homeless individuals are often also suffering from poverty and struggling to find employment. All this means it is very difficult for that individual to access the means to look after their well-being.

Availability of services and barriers to accessing them

Health and social care services are there to support individuals from conception to the end of their lives. If individuals are healthy then resources can be used for those most in need. But even healthy individuals need to access services from time to time:

- Health services are there to help keep individuals healthy. They can help with choosing healthy lifestyles, recovering from illness and preventing further health problems.
- Social care services will assist in improving quality of life, and offering help and support for those who are struggling with aspects of day-to-day living. They will identify those at risk and put plans in place to support them.

If there is a lack of availability of services in an area, this could affect the health and well-being of individuals, and might mean they miss out on crucial services.

There are also many other barriers that individuals may face:

- physical – individuals living in a rural location may struggle to get to services, while individuals with mobility issues may also have problems
- financial – whilst prescriptions are free in Wales, there may be financial implications for travel or access
- psychological – individuals may have had a negative experience of services in the past and are reluctant to access them again, they may have a fear of going to the doctor or dentist or are worried about the potential outcome

- cultural and language – there may be cultural and language barriers, for example, in some cultures an individual may require a chaperone, or information may not be provided in their first language
- resources – sometimes the demand for a service is high or there are not enough staff for the service and this can mean increased waiting times.

Air pollution

According to the **World Health Organization (WHO)**, outdoor air pollution is a major cause of death and disease. It is linked to heart disease, stroke, pulmonary disease, lung cancer and acute respiratory infections.

Air pollution can also cause less severe effects such as fatigue, headaches, anxiety, irritation of eyes, nose and throats. It can affect children's growth of lung function that can go on to have an impact throughout their life.

RESEARCH IT

Find out what the Welsh Government think we need in order to live healthy and happy lives, by researching the Well-Being of Future Generations (Wales) Act 2015.

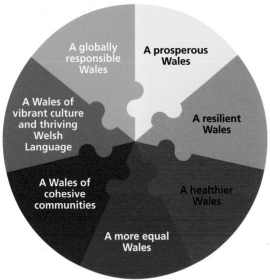

For more details, see:

www.futuregenerations.wales/about-us/future-generations-act/

You may find these videos useful:

https://youtu.be/rFeOYlxJbmw

https://youtu.be/5erVqthMd4c

AC2.3 Differences between the medical and social models of disabilities

The **medical model of disability** focuses on the disability as the focus of the problem. For example, if an individual using a wheelchair cannot access a building because the only way of accessing the building is to climb some steps, it would be because of the wheelchair and not because of the lack of access. This model focuses on what is wrong with the individual rather than what the individual needs.

By contrast, the **social model of disability** would see the steps as a disabling factor. This is a problem that can be overcome. The social model of disability believes that society needs to support a disabled person's rights. The social model is proactive and has an inclusive approach.

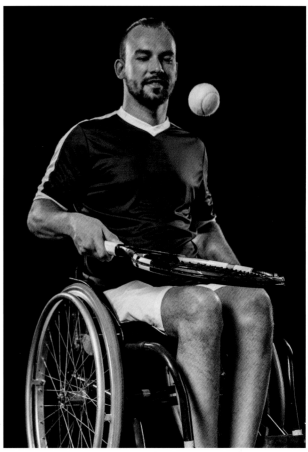

▲ Figure 2.2 There are different models of disabilities

KEY TERMS

World Health Organization (WHO): an organisation that promotes health across the world by promoting access to health services and medicines and responding to emergencies, such as the COVID-19 pandemic.

Medical model of disability: a way of providing care and support that focuses on the medical condition

Social model of disability: a way of providing care and support that focuses on the individual

REFLECT ON IT

Think about your learning environment.

- What impact might this have on an individual with a physical disability?
- What could be done differently?

AC2.4 The terms 'good physical health' and 'good mental health', and how these are interdependent

In the past, physical and mental health were viewed as separate issues. We now know that taking care of physical health has a positive effect on mental health.

Think about how your physical health impacts on your mental health.

- Do you feel good after exercise?
- Do you feel low when you are ill or not able to do the things you enjoy?

Physical health

Individuals need to look after their physical health in order to remain fit and healthy, and do the things they enjoy. Alongside this, getting enough rest and having a healthy, balanced diet will support physical health.

Mental health

Having good mental health is important for our moods, thinking and behaviour. Many things can affect our mental health, and having poor mental health does not always mean you have a mental health problem.

For example, nerves and anxiety before an interview could impact on your mental health, affecting your sleep and increasing your stress levels. Once the interview is over, it is likely these feelings will subside. Signs of a mental health problem are when these feelings stay for longer and are a part of your everyday life.

Taking care of mental health helps to develop resilience and the ability to cope with stressful situations.

How does physical health impact on mental health?

There are many interconnections between physical and mental health. Having good self-image and good self-esteem are indicators of good mental health, so having good physical health can help to promote this. Feeling healthy and fit can help you feel good about yourself.

Suffering from anxiety or depression can hugely impact on your health and well-being. Exercise is known to release endorphins which help to create a positive chemical balance and alleviate low moods.

The routine of exercise can also help with mental health. Having something to focus on, and small, achievable goals, can create positive changes.

Physical activity also links to enhanced cognition – the ability to think – by reducing insulin resistance and inflammation and stimulating the growth of new blood vessels.

Sedentary behaviour can have negative impacts on the health and well-being of individuals and can lead to long-term illnesses such as cardiovascular diseases, obesity and diabetes, as well as affecting mental well-being and mood. We all know that sitting on a computer all day can make us feel tired, and after a short break and some movement we feel refreshed. Children often have better concentration after breaktime.

REFLECT ON IT

Think about how much time you spend sitting, and on screens. Sedentary behaviour can have a large impact on health and well-being. It can affect your physical health and reduce your energy levels. It can also impact on your mental health, especially if you are isolated.

- What can you do to get more movement in your day?
- How could you motivate yourself to be more physically active?
- What stops you from doing more physical activity? How could you overcome this?

AC2.5 The impact of prolonged inactivity on physical and mental well-being

Inactivity and a sedentary lifestyle mean we are not keeping our bodies healthy, are at more risk of mobility problems and weight gain and can be a contributing risk factor for cardiovascular disease and other conditions such as high blood pressure, type 2 diabetes and certain cancers. Physical activity can help reduce this risk, especially in later life. Physical inactivity can hinder an older person's ability to stay mobile. Over time, their muscles may weaken, making it harder for them to stay physically fit and healthy, which can have an impact on their weight and cause them to become overweight or obese.

Lack of activity can also add to feelings of depression and anxiety, as well as increase feelings of isolation. As mentioned above, exercise releases endorphins which relieve stress and pain.

RESEARCH IT

You may wish to carry out some further research on the impact of physical activity on well-being. Try the following links:

www.mentalhealth.org.uk/sites/default/files/lets-get-physical-report.pdf

www.mind.org.uk/information-support/tips-for-everyday-living/physical-activity-and-your-mental-health/about-physical-activity/

Think about the impact of inactivity on both physical and mental well-being.

AC2.6 Social, mental and physical benefits of engagement in activity and experiences

We have explored the impact that physical activity can have on the mental and physical well-being of individuals. But there are other benefits to meaningful activities, whether these are physical, intellectual, emotional or social.

Physical benefits

As well as the health and mental well-being benefits described above, physical activities can also:

- help with **gross motor skill** and **fine motor skill** development
- improve strength, stamina and muscle tone.

REFLECT ON IT

- Can you think of some activities that require gross motor skills, and others that require fine motor skills?
- What are the other benefits to these activities you have chosen?

Intellectual benefits

Meaningful activities help to develop the brain. For example, puzzles, crosswords and number games help to improve memory, problem solving and concentration. These activities are often described as 'brain trainers'.

Reading can help to develop an understanding about something new. It can increase an individual's understanding of language, which will help them to develop literacy skills.

Emotional benefits

Meaningful activities, such as physical, social or leisure activities, can boost self-esteem and confidence. They can help individuals relax and find a sense of belonging or a sense of pride.

Individuals tend to choose activities they enjoy and bring them pleasure. They might be able to express themselves through their chosen activity, such as writing or painting.

KEY TERMS

Gross motor skills: skills that require the large muscles in the body.

Fine motor skills: skills that require the smaller muscles in the body, especially the hands and fingers.

Social benefits

Many activities can be done as groups and therefore there is a social interaction, which can help individuals to make friends and feel a sense of belonging. Group activities can help to teach co-operation and teamwork, and develop communication, for example, sports teams, fundraising groups, crafting circles or book clubs.

AC2.7 Ways that people can engage in a range of personal activities, including the use of social media and technology

Individuals can participate in a range of activities. These could be recreational, creative or therapeutic; they can be carried out individually, or as part of a group.

Some activities can also have more than one of the benefits discussed in the previous section.

REFLECT ON IT

Think about an activity from the list below and discuss with your group the type of activity it is – physical, creative, intellectual, emotional or social. Could it fit into more than one category?

Then discuss the benefits of this activity to an individual. Remember, there could be more than one benefit:

- cooking
- playing football
- running in a club
- creative writing class
- knitting
- attending a book club
- gardening
- choir
- online gaming
- reading
- board games.

Social media and technology can play a part in engagement of meaningful activities. Online forums can be a place to meet people who share your interests and help to develop your skills, such as gardening or mechanics forums. However, they can also pose a risk. Playing computer games online can be enjoyable and social, but:

- There is a risk of online bullying.
- Computer games are highly addictive, and individuals can develop what is known as gaming disorder. This affects a small portion of gamers, around 1–9 per cent, and tends to affect males more than females. The WHO added 'gaming disorder' to its 2018 medical reference book, *International Classification of Diseases*. You can read more about gaming addiction here:

https://hampshirecamhs.nhs.uk/issue/gaming-addiction/

There are also the benefits that come with using technology and social media, such as finding out about clubs and groups, reaching out to like-minded people and being able to contact friends and family who may live far away. This can help an individual to feel less isolated.

However, there are risks to using social media:

- It can be addictive: individuals become addicted to 'likes' and this can have a negative impact on their self-esteem.
- There is also the risk of bullying, identity theft and data security breaches.

Individuals should be educated on the danger of using social media and online forums so they can use them safely.

CASE STUDY

Wendy is 50 years old and suffers with mental ill-health. She has anxiety and depression, and sometimes has to spend long periods of time on her own. Sue is a mental health worker who is assigned to work with Wendy.

On her first visit, Sue questions Wendy about her likes and dislikes as well as her history. Wendy mentions that when she was younger, she used to enjoy art and excelled at this in school.

Sue suggests they look into an adult art class. Wendy is unsure as she feels anxious about meeting new people. Sue suggests they use the internet to do some research first, to see if they can find something that might interest Wendy.

Sue and Wendy find a local club that runs art classes and has an active social media page. Wendy is able to contact them through social media and the teacher gets in touch. Wendy and the teacher strike up a conversation over the following weeks, and slowly Wendy feels more confident and interested in attending. Sue agrees to attend the first few classes with Wendy until she feels confident to go alone.

Discussion points:
- How did technology and social media help Wendy?
- What could be the benefits of attending an art class for Wendy?

AC2.8 How engagement in the arts can support health and well-being

We have looked at the benefits that activities can have on health and well-being, and touched on creative activities. This section will explore the benefits of engagement in the **arts** and the impact this can have on health and well-being.

KEY TERM

Arts: music, dance, drama, painting, drawing, sculpture, photography and crafts.

Creative expression gives an individual the freedom to express their thoughts and feelings, which in turn supports emotional health. Think about Wendy from the previous case study – being able to express herself through art may give her an outlet for her anxious thoughts and feelings, and in turn can help her to work through those feelings. Art therapy would be something to explore.

Engagement in the arts can help with mental growth, as they encourage problem solving skills and trying out new ways of thinking.

There is a clear link between creative activities and well-being, as detailed in the Creative Health Inquiry Report 2017:

> The arts can help keep us well, aid our recovery and support longer lives lived better.

(www.culturehealthandwellbeing.org.uk/appg-inquiry/Publications/Creative_Health_The_Short_Report.pdf)

AC2.9 The term 'attachment' and the impact that this can have on individuals in adulthood

Attachment is the term given to the relationship between child and care giver that makes that child safe, secure and protected. However, it can also apply to older individuals, especially when you take into account their experience of early childhood attachment.

- If there is healthy attachment, the individual is confident their needs will be met, and feels secure to explore the world around them, knowing they have a safe space to return to. An attached child will probably feel safe and secure, and receive comfort and protection.
- Where there is poor attachment, the individual does not feel confident in the care givers around them. They will often present as anxious and insecure with low self-esteem. Early attachment experiences can impact on them in later life and will influence all their relationships. There might be a lack of trust in those giving care, which can impact on behaviour if the individual has never learnt how to manage their feelings.

John Bowlby is the theorist who explored attachment between child and care giver, and considered how poor attachment in the early years can impact on the individual as an adult.

See Unit 003, LO2 for more information on John Bowlby and his attachment theory.

AC2.10 The importance of self-identifying, self-worth and sense of security and belonging for the health and well-being of individuals

Knowing what you identify as helps you to understand yourself. Feelings of self-worth and security will help you to support your own health and well-being. Without these feelings, you have a higher risk of physical or mental ill-health.

Having a healthy self-image, self-worth and a sense of security and belonging supports individuals' resilience – the ability to cope with change and manage emotions.

Self-identity

The Oxford English Dictionary defines self-identity as

> the perception or recognition of one's characteristics as a particular individual, especially in relation to social context.

Self-identity can also be referred to as self-concept, and includes physical, psychological and social attributes.

Self-identity begins to develop very early in infancy. When a baby smiles at his caregiver, the caregiver smiles back. He therefore starts to recognise himself as separate individual. As he grows older, he will begin to categorise himself and this builds on his self-identity; for example, 'I am two and half. I am a big boy now.'

We all have beliefs about ourselves, and we split these into our **personal** and **social identity**.

KEY TERMS

Personal identity: the concept we develop about ourselves over time; for example, I am smart/funny/kind.

Social identity: the self-concept we have of ourselves based on social groups; for example, I am a teacher/Muslim/parent.

There are a range of factors that influence our self-identity:

- sexual orientation
- appearance
- age and gender
- relationships
- social roles
- labels that others ascribe to us
- skills and attributes
- value and cultural beliefs
- personal preferences
- personality traits.

REFLECT ON IT

Using the listed factors above, think of words to describe yourself under these factors. For example:

- Cultural beliefs – I am vegan.
- Relationships – I am single.

How many words do you have for each factor? Reflect on how long your lists are, and think about how these may grow in time due to changes in your life.

Self-image

Your self-image also affects your self-identity. Self-image is how you see yourself when you look in the mirror and the opinions you have of yourself, which can be influenced by many factors.

Self-image can make it very difficult for people to work outside their comfort zones. We give ourselves descriptions, such as:

- physical descriptions – I am tall
- social roles – I am a student/parent
- personality traits – I am kind
- existential statements – I am a human being.

When we are younger, we often focus more on our personality characteristics, but later in life we may focus more on our social roles. This may be because we give more value to these at certain stages of life.

REFLECT ON IT

- Think about some of the characteristics/descriptions you would use to describe your self-image.
- Could this limit you in some way? For example, 'I am not sporty, therefore I do not try new sports or avoid sporting events'. This could limit your friendship groups and your access to meaningful exercise. Could this impact on your health and well-being?

Self-worth

Self-worth can be referred to as self-esteem, and is the value an individual places on themselves. Over time this can change – you can have positive or negative evaluations of yourself.

The Oxford English Dictionary defines self-esteem as

confidence in one's own worth or abilities; self-respect.

Low self-esteem can have a serious impact on well-being:

- An individual with low self-esteem will have a negative view of themselves which can contribute to feelings of anxiety and depression.
- They might feel they cannot achieve well in life and therefore avoid new situations and approach challenges negatively.

Someone with high self-esteem who gets constructive feedback at work may see this as a way to improve – 'I know I can do better'. On the other hand, someone with low self-esteem who received the same feedback might think – 'I can't do anything right'.

CASE STUDY

Stacey is 20 years old and lives in supported housing following a move from children's services to adult services. Stacey had a difficult childhood and was the victim of sexual abuse and neglect. Stacey has periods of depression when she will remember her childhood and experience feelings of self-loathing and worthlessness.

The staff in the supported housing are trying to help Stacey to access employment. Stacey is interested in animals and, when she was younger, had some animal therapy sessions which had positive results for her. She now has a pet cat which she is very attached to. The staff suggest she does some volunteering at the local animal sanctuary and investigate an apprenticeship for animal care.

Stacey is excited by this and the staff support Stacey to enquire with the local sanctuary. Stacey sends the sanctuary an email and waits to hear back. When she has not heard after two days, Stacey becomes very low, telling the staff she is 'useless and no one would want her anyway'.

Discussion points:

- What is Stacey experiencing here?
- Why might she react in this way and how can the staff support her through this?

Sense of security and belonging

Having a sense of security and belonging is important for developing the confidence and resilience to explore your surrounding environment and build a place for yourself in the world. A sense of security and belonging is often developed in early childhood through attachment. A child who is securely attached will have a safe base from which to explore, knowing that if something frightening happens they have a safe space to come back to. This, in turn, helps them to develop resilience and to learn about themselves.

However, we continue to need a sense of security and belonging throughout our lives. We will seek this in our families, relationships and working environment. It allows us to take chances and positive risks and explore new possibilities, safe in the knowledge that we are accepted and that we belong.

AC2.11 How the way that individuals are supported will impact how they feel about themselves

> **REFLECT ON IT**
>
> Think about a time when a decision was made for you without your opinion being asked.
>
> How did that make you feel?

Person-centred care is about thinking and doing things that sees the individual as a partner in planning, developing and reviewing their care so that it meets their needs. It is putting the person at the centre of all you do. For more on person-centred care, see Units 001/002, LO3.

To support well-being, individuals need to be involved in their own care and support. They must have a voice. One of the principles of the Social Services and Well-Being (Wales) Act 2014 is 'voice and control' which means 'putting the individual and their needs at the centre of their care, and giving them a voice in, and control over reaching the outcomes that help them achieve well-being'. This is supported by the Code of Professional Practice for Social Care which states that workers should:

> *promote the well-being, voice and control of individuals and carers while supporting them to stay safe.*

Working in a person-centred way will help support the individual to have an input into their care and this supports their well-being. The individual will look at themselves as an equal partner which in turn supports them to feel more empowered and independent. A confident individual who is independent is more likely to seek the care and support they need and ask for help when needed.

RESEARCH IT

Further reading can be found here:

https://socialcare.wales/hub/sswbact

https://socialcare.wales/dealing-with-concerns/codes-of-practice-and-guidance#section-29491-anchor

AC2.12 Health checks that individuals need to support their health and well-being

There are many health checks available to support individual health and well-being in Wales. Examples include:

- bowel cancer screening – screening to look for early signs of bowel cancer
- cervical screening – screening carried out to look for cell changes that can lead to cancer if left untreated
- cholesterol tests – helps to determine if cholesterol levels are high as a result of age, weight or other conditions such as high blood pressure
- blood pressure tests – a simple test to determine if your blood pressure is too high, too low or normal
- breast screening – screening to look for breast cancer before symptoms show
- abdominal aortic aneurysm screening – screening to determine if there is a bulge or swelling in the main blood vessel that runs from your heart down through your tummy
- dental health checks – these determine any issues with teeth, gums or dental hygiene; supports good oral health
- newborn screening – the newborn bloodspot test screens for nine rare but serious health conditions and the newborn hearing test helps to spot any problems with babies' hearing
- antenatal screening – screening to help to determine some conditions that may affect mother or baby. It is the pregnant mother's choice which, if any, tests she has.

Health check programmes also run in Wales for people aged over 50. The programmes include physical checks, checking current health problems, health advice and preventative advice and making sure families receive the support they need and discussing medication.

AC2.13 Services and information that support health promotion

There are many services and sources of information that support health promotion, from the NHS to voluntary services and charities. Regular health promotion campaigns are run, for example, to promote the Eatwell Guide and 'stop smoking' campaigns. Information is often available in bilingual posters and leaflets and is also made available online.

Public Health Wales is part of the NHS, and offers advice and services about many issues such as:

- healthy eating
- oral health
- substance use
- sexual health
- mental health and well-being.

GPs, nurses and other primary care professionals operate social prescribing schemes such as gardening, cooking, group learning and arts activities to combat anxiety and depression.

Local authorities are required to tackle causes of ill-health as well as reduce health inequalities in the community. They must take a leading role in improving health and well-being. One way they can do this is through schools.

- Topics that schools cover include healthy eating, mental health, well-being and sexual health.
- In Wales, schools follow anti-bullying programmes and can encourage children to work on projects that improve well-being.

RESEARCH IT
There are a number of national and local charities that promote health.
- Research some national charities and what they do.
- Can you find more local charities in your area?

AC2.14 Types of changes in an individual that would give cause for concern for their health and well-being

When supporting individuals, it is important to notice any changes that give cause for concern. These could include the following:

- **Signs of a heart attack** – this could include chest pain, when the chest feels like it is being pressed or squeezed, shortness of breath, feeling weak, lightheaded, an overwhelming feeling of anxiety.

- **Breathing difficulties** – shortness of breath, difficulties catching breath, feeling breathless, wheezing, rapid breathing.
- **Signs of stroke** – sudden numbness or weakness in face, arms or legs (especially if just on one side of the body), sudden confusion, trouble speaking, or difficulties understanding speech, slurred speech, sudden difficulties with vision in one or both eyes, dizziness, loss of balance, trouble walking, lack of co-ordination. These signs will all suddenly present. Severe headaches can also be a sign, especially if there is no known cause.
- **Any pain** – especially new and sudden pain.
- **Skin changes** – rashes, bruises, wounds, moles, red scaly skin, wart-like growths.
- **Diabetes** – increased thirst, frequent urination, extreme hunger, unexplained weight loss, fatigue, irritability, blurred vision.
- **Sepsis** – fever and chills, low body temperature, urinating less, fast heartbeat, diarrhoea, fatigue, weakness, blotchy skin.

It is important to note that women might have additional symptoms of stroke, such as general weakness, confusion or memory problems, fatigue and nausea or vomiting.

- **Mood changes** – sudden mood swings, irritable, irrational, aggressive, weepy.
- **Expressing suicidal thoughts** – suicidal thoughts should always be taken seriously, with immediate support provided.
- **Changes in behaviour** – changes in normal behaviour, inactive when previously active, staying in bed for longer, not motivated, forgetful or confused, eating less or more, withdrawing from people, hyperactivity. Anything that would be unusual behaviour for that individual should be treated as a cause for concern.
- **Memory loss** – forgetfulness, confusion, sudden memory loss, severe memory loss, such as not remembering where you are or who you are.
- **Self-neglect** – not attending to personal care, not eating well or refusing meals, looking unkempt, dirty clothes, soiling themselves.

- **Social isolation** – withdrawing from social engagements, spending more time alone, showing signs of anxiety, not enjoying their usual favourite activities, withdrawing from friendship groups.
- **Changes in sleeping patterns** – wakefulness in the night, sleepwalking, rising early when previously slept later, sleeping later when previously woke early, nightmares, disturbed sleep, difficulty falling asleep.
- **Mobility loss** – trouble walking, stumbling, foot problems, stiffness.
- **Incontinence issues** – having accidents, soiling, not recognising the need to go to the toilet, not asking for help to go to the toilet, not recognising when they have been incontinent.
- **Weight gain/loss** – whether this is sudden or slow.
- **Aggressive or irritable** – sudden aggressive behaviour or irritability that is not considered normal for that individual.

REFLECT ON IT

From the list above, note down which could impact on physical or mental well-being.

AC2.15 The importance of observing, monitoring and recording the health and well-being of individuals affected by particular health conditions

It is important, and our duty of care, to observe and monitor individuals with a health condition. This can help you to:

- determine the level of care they need
- note any changes in behaviour
- identify whether changes indicate any mental health issues or deterioration in their health condition
- see whether their medication is working or needs to be reviewed.

Changes in behaviour and mood can often be an indication that something isn't right, and therefore it is important to observe and record all changes to an individual's behaviour.

Clear recording is vital to ensure consistent and safe care. Record keeping also enables you to see any trends or patterns, and helps to work towards a decision. It also supports health professionals to obtain a clear picture of the problem.

AC2.16 The importance of reporting any concerns or any changes in the health and well-being of individuals

It is important to report concerns or any changes in health and well-being for a number of reasons:

- Individuals may require a change in their treatment or their care plan.
- There may be concerns around neglect or abuse which will need to be investigated.
- The families may need to be updated regarding these changes, so accurate records will help.
- Accurate records can also help to highlight any mistakes, and settings can learn from these.
- It is a legal requirement to keep accurate records and report concerns.
- The information could be required in a court of law.
- Accurate reporting helps to identify any trends with behaviours or health.
- Accurate reporting is important for accurate handovers and continuity of care.

AC2.17 Links between health and well-being and safeguarding

We will explore safeguarding in Unit 006, but it is important to recognise how safeguarding links to health and well-being. Everyone has the right to live free from harm, abuse and neglect. Safeguarding is about protecting people from harm, abuse and neglect, and therefore naturally promotes health and well-being. If an individual suffers a safeguarding concern, this can have a lasting impact on their physical and mental well-being.

In practice, safeguarding means:

- being proactive and reactive: putting preventative measures in place to stop harm, abuse and neglect from happening but also stepping in if it does
- addressing the cause of the abuse and neglect, learning from this and ensuring it is not repeated.

By working in a person-centred way under the Social Services and Well-Being (Wales) Act 2014, you can ensure that individuals have control over their lives and are involved in making decisions. This in turn promotes safeguarding – individuals know their rights and are supported to make choices.

> **REFLECT ON IT**
>
> Write down as many types of abuse as you can think of. You will explore these more in Unit 006.

AC2.18 Links between health and well-being and the Mental Capacity Act

As we saw in Units 001/002, the Mental Capacity Act applies to everyone over the age of 16, and protects individuals who may lack the mental capacity to make their own decisions. It covers a range of decisions, from day-to-day thinking such as what to buy at the shop, to life-changing decisions such as whether the individual should move into a care home.

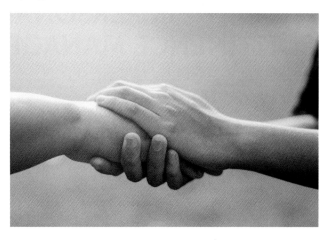

▲ Figure 2.3 A helping hand

Table 2.3 shows the five principles of the Mental Capacity Act.

Principle number	The principle
1: A presumption of capacity	Every adult has the right to make their own decisions and it must be assumed they have the capacity to do so unless proved otherwise.
2: Individuals being supported to make their own decisions	All practicable help must be given to the individual to make their own decisions. If lack of capacity is established, the individual should still be involved in making decisions where possible.
3: Unwise decisions	Even if others may think a decision is unwise or eccentric, the individual still has the right to make this decision.
4: Best interests	Any decisions made on behalf of an individual must be done in their best interests.
5: Less restrictive option	Anyone making a decision on behalf of an individual must take the least restrictive option. This is the option which would interfere least with the person's rights and freedom of action.

▲ Table 2.3 The five principles of the Mental Capacity Act

There may be a number of reasons why an individual may lack capacity:

- dementia
- a severe learning disability
- a brain injury
- a mental health illness
- a stroke.

However, just because a person has one of these conditions does not mean they lack capacity. Also, they may lack capacity for some decisions but not all. The Mental Capacity Act says you must assume a person has capacity to make their own decisions unless it can be proved otherwise, so you should help people to make their own decisions if possible. Even if a decision appears unwise, you should not assume this is due to lack of capacity.

An individual being able to make as many choices for themselves supports their well-being. They are more likely to have positive outcomes when able to make their own choices about things that matter to them. They are also more likely to engage in activities if the choices are theirs. This in turn promotes good self-esteem and independence.

RESEARCH IT

Read more about the principles of the Mental Capacity Act here:

www.nhs.uk/conditions/social-care-and-support-guide/making-decisions-for-someone-else/mental-capacity-act/

www.scie.org.uk/mca/introduction/mental-capacity-act-2005-at-a-glance

LO3 KNOW HOW TO SUPPORT INDIVIDUALS WITH THEIR PERSONAL CARE AND CONTINENCE MANAGEMENT

GETTING STARTED

Think about a routine you like doing, such as styling your hair or having a soak in the bath.

Now consider how it would feel if you couldn't do this for yourself and someone had to do this for you. How would you like to be treated?

AC3.1 The term 'personal care'

Personal care is the act of helping individuals in a number of daily tasks:

- using toilet facilities
- showering/bathing
- dressing/undressing
- applying creams/make-up
- oral hygiene
- continence care
- foot care
- shaving

- changing stoma or catheter bag
- maintaining nutrition
- support with eating and drinking
- hair care
- avoiding pressure sores.

You may need to support an individual with some or all their personal care, depending on their needs. This could be a short-term or long-term need, depending on their circumstances and the reason they need support; for example, an individual recovering from an operation may need short-term support with their personal care.

Personal care supports health and well-being in many ways:

- It promotes good hygiene, which in turn improves health as it reduces the risk of catching infections and illness caused by bacteria.
- It also helps an individual to feel good about themselves, therefore promoting a sense of well-being.
- It supports self-esteem and a sense of identity.

AC3.2 Ways to establish with an individual their preferences in relation to how they are supported with their personal care

It is important to treat individuals with dignity and respect, and to consider their preferences and choices. Here is a guide to how you can achieve this:

- Speak to the individual about their preferences for personal care.
- Check with the individual after personal care to find out if their needs were met or if they would like you to change anything.
- Involve family or other carers – they may know more about the individual.
- Follow the care plan and take into consideration what has previously worked well.
- Find ways to communicate if the individual does not understand verbal communication.
- Involve an occupational therapist if speciality equipment is needed.
- Work with an advocate if needed.

> **CASE STUDY**
>
> Mabel recently moved into a care home as she has dementia and was struggling to look after herself at home. Mabel will often forget to carry out her personal hygiene and has had incidences of incontinence at night when she will forget where the bathroom is.
>
> **Discussion points:**
> - How might the staff in the care home support Mabel with her personal care in a person-centred way?
> - Who should they involve in putting this support plan together?

AC3.3 Ways to protect the privacy and dignity of an individual when they are being supported with their personal care

It is also important to remember that personal care can be intimate, and it are therefore essential the privacy and dignity of the individual are considered and respected at all times. For example:

- Always gain consent for any activity.
- Ensure you follow all policies and procedures.
- Ensure you work in line with confidentiality policy.
- Ensure you have had training before you carry out any task.
- Respect privacy and ask permission to enter a personal space.
- Support dignity – for example, ensure that the individual is covered during a bed wash.
- Ensure the individual has choice and options.
- Ensure that en-suite toilets or same-sex toilets are available.
- Consider whether the individual wishes to have a male or female worker to carry out tasks.
- Be respectful in communication with colleagues, for example, do not shout out to colleagues for help – plan ahead for any difficult issues.
- Offer a choice of toiletries and clothes.
- Ensure privacy by drawing curtains and windows.
- Respect individuals' personal belongings.

REFLECT ON IT

Think about how you would support an individual to get dressed for the day.

- How would you support dignity and treat the individual with respect?
- How might it feel for the individual to have personal care carried out?
- How would you feel if someone had to help you with personal care?

AC3.4 The term 'continence'

KEY TERM

Continence: the ability to control movements of the bowels and bladder. A continent individual knows when they need the toilet and uses it.

AC3.5 Factors that may contribute to difficulties with continence

There are many factors that affect **continence** through all stages of life, shown in Table 2.4.

Factor	Explanation
Following a stroke	It is common for an individual to experience continence issues following a stroke. • The stroke may have damaged part of the brain that controls the bowel and/or bladder, and it may take time to recover. • An individual may be less mobile after a stroke and not able to get to the toilet in time. • Communication difficulties can also contribute to continence issues if people cannot understand what the individual is asking.
Following childbirth	Pelvic floor muscles can be weakened following childbirth. Some women may also experience a prolapse, which can affect continence.
Being overweight	Being overweight can weaken pelvic floor muscles due to the pressure of fatty tissue on the bladder.
Certain medications	Some medications such as diuretics and opioids can disrupt how the body stores and passes urine.
Crohn's disease	Individuals with Crohn's disease can experience incontinence due to having an overactive bowel, inflammation of the rectum, and damage to the muscles or nerves.
Constipation	Straining during bowel movements can weaken the pelvic floor muscle. A full bowel can cause the bowel to press on the bladder, creating the need to urinate frequently.
Substance misuse	If the substance the individual is misusing is an opioid, this could affect their body's ability to deal with urine storage. • Substance misuse can hinder an individual's ability to recognise signs or urges to use the toilet. • Ketamine has been found to cause shrinkage of the bladder if used in large or repeated doses.
Diabetes	Individuals with diabetes can experience incontinence caused by a neurogenic bladder. This is caused by nerve damage that can happen when blood sugar levels are not brought under control.
Urinary tract infection (UTI)	UTIs develop when the urinary tract is infected by bacteria. Most symptoms tend to be mild, and UTIs are more common in women than in men.
Neurological disorders	Conditions such as Parkinson's disease or multiple sclerosis can affect the nerve signals involved in bladder control.
Spinal cord injury	Injury to the spinal cord can interrupt communication between the nerves that control bladder and bowel function.
Mobility issues	The individual knows they need the toilet but cannot get there quickly enough.
Dementia or memory problems	• The individual may not be able to react quickly enough to the urge to use the toilet. • They may forget that they need to use the toilet or fail to get there quickly enough. • Confusion can mean they do not recognise the right area to use for their toileting needs.
Family history	Genetic factors can play a role in continence problems.

▲ Table 2.4 Factors that affect continence

AC3.6 Ways in which difficulties with continence can affect an individual's self-esteem, health, well-being and day-to-day activities

Incontinence can be very upsetting for both the individual and those around them. The impact on the individual's well-being can be huge as it affects their day-to-day life.

- It can have an impact on them socially. This can lead to isolation, and feelings of anxiety and depression.
- It can impact on their ability to work, to exercise and to carry out daily routines.
- It can affect the individual's self-esteem if they are left feeling dirty and smelly. For example, they may need to wear continence pads which may worry them and may affect how they can dress, thus impacting on their self-image.
- It can affect their health by causing infections and problems with skincare.

AC3.7 How an individual's beliefs, sexual preference and values may affect the management of their continence

You must understand an individual's beliefs, sexual preference and values. They may affect how you support them to manage their continence, as they may impact on their personal wishes when it comes to personal care. For example, in some religions cleanliness is linked to prayer and individuals may feel worried that they cannot fulfill religious obligations, which can contribute to worry and stress.

People from all backgrounds are likely to be embarrassed talking about continence and may find it easier to talk to a professional of the same gender.

Other barriers such as communication and language could be present. Without a translator, an individual may not seek help, as they do not want the embarrassment of admitting to someone they have continence issues.

Urinary incontinence can affect sexual intercourse, and the odour and fear of incontinence during sexual intercourse can have an impact on an individual's confidence and sexual function.

> **REFLECT ON IT**
>
> Think of other reasons that a person's gender, sexual preference, religion, beliefs and culture may impact on the management of their continence.

RESEARCH IT

Research the impact that incontinence has on Muslim women, taking into account the cleaning ritual they have to perform before prayer. Incontinence would leave them 'unclean', meaning that prayer could not take place. Think about the impact this would have on these women's lives.

AC3.8 Aids and equipment that can support the management of continence

There is support available to help an individual manage continence. Aids and equipment include:

- enuresis pads (technical name for incontinence pads)
- absorbent bed pads and waterproof mattress protectors
- chair protectors
- pull-up pants with built-in pad
- male continence sheath – a silicone condom which drains into a bag attached to the leg
- protective duvet covers and pillowcases
- catheters which drain urine directly from the bladder into a bag
- bedpans and commodes
- male urinal bottles
- raised toilet seats for those with mobility issues.

AC3.9 Professionals that may help with continence management

The GP should always be the first point of contact when seeking help. It can be very difficult for people to admit if they have a problem with continence and seek help. The GP will be able to review if there are any underlying health conditions or urinary tract infections and make an assessment.

The GP could then refer the individual to a continence adviser/nurse. They will carry out an assessment and see how the incontinence affects the person's quality of life. It is likely the individual would need to keep toileting charts to see if there is any pattern. The adviser/nurse will then develop a plan with the individual, and their carer if necessary. In some cases the individual may need to be referred to a specialist such as a geriatrician, urologist or gynaecologist.

Other professionals that may be able to help include:

- **A community nurse** can help individuals to access NHS products and advise individuals on the management of their problems, including how to maintain hygiene and protect their skin.
- **An occupational therapist** will give advice on which adaptations and equipment can be helpful.
- **A physiotherapist** could help if the individual has problems with co-ordination or movement.
- **Community mental health team** could help to detect whether an individual's mental health is impacting on their continence, if it is linked to a change in behaviour.

AC3.10 Ways to support individuals with their personal care and/or continence management in a way that protects both the individual and the worker supporting them

It is of vital importance to protect you and the individual during personal care routines, which could include personal hygiene, bathing, cleaning teeth, continence care and menstruation:

- Wear personal protective clothing (PPE) – this could include aprons and gloves.
- Wash hands before and after contact.
- Support individuals to wash hands, for example, after using the toilet or before meals.
- Ensure areas are clean and ready for use.
- Use safe, appropriate equipment and materials – and ensure you are trained to use these.
- Safely dispose of waste and soiled materials (for more details of safe disposal of materials, see Unit 007).
- Ensure any concerns or physical marks are recorded and reported.

RESEARCH IT

Read the following scenarios and research the support and aids that would be available for these individuals.

1 Harry has had his prostate removed and now has no bladder control.
2 Megan has suffered a pelvic organ prolapse and as a result has stress incontinence.
3 George has recently been diagnosed with dementia. He is repeatedly forgetting to go to the toilet.

Check your understanding

1 Why are families, friends and communities important in relation to well-being?
2 What is meant by a sensory disability?
3 What barriers might there be for accessing health and social care services?
4 Public Health Wales is part of what service?
5 Name the theorist who explored attachment.

6 What is another term to describe self-worth?
7 What does the term 'continence' mean?
8 Who should be the first point of contact for continence problems?
9 Why are women more likely to experience incontinence following childbirth?

Question practice

1 There are many factors that can impact on well-being. Which of the following is an example of a physical factor?

   a healthy eating

   b a sense of belonging

   c an enjoyable job

   d healthy relationships

2 What type of disabilities could be caused by autism (there could be more than one)?

   a physical disability

   b learning disability

   c sensory disability

   d intellectual disability

3 What type of disabilities could be caused by multiple sclerosis (there could be more than one)?

   a physical disability

   b learning disability

   c sensory disability

   d intellectual disability

4 Which of the following is classed as an adverse childhood experience (ACE)?

   a cyber bullying

   b neglect

   c poverty

   d parent separation

5 What does the following statement define?

   'The value an individual places on themselves'

   a self-image

   b self-worth

   c self-identity

   d self-esteem

6 Which **three** of the following are essential when record keeping?

   a fact

   b opinion

   c accuracy

   d date

7 Which two of the following are benefits to meaningful activities?

   a social

   b financial

   c emotional

   d employability

8 'A presumption of capacity' is which principle of the Mental Capacity Act?

   a Principle 2

   b Principle 4

   c Principle 1

   d Principle 5

9 Which of the following statements links to Principle 4 of the Mental Capacity Act?

   a best interests

   b unwise decisions

   c less restrictive option

   d a presumption of capacity

10 Which of the following is an aid to assist with continence problems?

   a hoist

   b PPE

   c incontinence pads

   d adjustable bed

11 Why is it important that the individual is given choice about their personal care?

   a It makes it easier for the carer.

   b It ensures the individual has a voice.

   c It helps treat individuals the same.

   d It means the family don't have to do it.

12 What is the community nurse's role in supporting individuals with continence problems?

   a They can give advice on equipment.

   b They can give a diagnosis.

   c They can help access NHS products.

   d They can refer the individual to a specialist.

LO4 KNOW WHAT IS MEANT BY GOOD PRACTICE IN RELATION TO PRESSURE AREA CARE

GETTING STARTED

Pressure ulcers and sores can be a common problem but can be avoided with the right care. This section will explore how to provide pressure area care, the risk factors and the legislation that underpins this care.

Think about an older individual who has poor mobility and has gone into hospital for a short period of treatment. Why might this individual be at risk of developing pressure ulcers and sores?

AC4.1 The terms 'pressure area care', 'pressure damage' and 'pressure ulcers'

Pressure area care

Pressure area care is the term used for the care given to the areas that are prone to pressure damage on individuals.

With good pressure area care, most pressure ulcers/sores can be avoided. Risk assessments help to determine the care needed and help reduce the occurrence (see Unit 007 for more on risk assessments). Pressure area care can include:

- changing positions when in bed or sitting for long periods of time
- keeping the skin clean and dry and checking the skin for signs of ulcers
- using pressure-relieving equipment correctly
- avoiding shearing forces
- keeping a healthy balanced diet
- changing soiled incontinence pads
- making sure bedsheets are not creased
- not smoking.

Pressure damage

This refers to the damage caused by pressure to the skin. Examples of different pressure:

- Low pressure: sitting or lying in bed for prolonged periods.
- High pressure: damage to the skin caused in relatively short periods of time, such as rough handling or lying on the floor after a sudden fall.
- Pressure from equipment: for example, catheter, oxygen tubing, heart monitors.

Pressure ulcers

This is the area of the skin and underlying tissue that is damaged by the pressure. Pressure ulcers can range from redness to open wounds and develop when:

- pressure is applied to the skin and underlying soft tissue
- damage occurs to local capillary, venous and lymphatic networks. The cells around the vessels die and, if the pressure is not removed, the damage will spread.

RESEARCH IT

Research the most common types of pressure ulcers and their causes. You may find the following web links useful:

https://nhs.stopthepressure.co.uk/

www.oxfordhealth.nhs.uk/wp-content/uploads/2015/08/OP-014.14-Pressure-area-care.pdf

---

REFLECT ON IT

We all at times experience a 'numb bum'. What do you do when this happens?

Now think about an individual with mobility issues. If they cannot just stand up, what support will they need and what needs to be considered?

AC4.2 Legislation and national guidelines in relation to pressure damage

There are pieces of legislation and guidance to support pressure area care. These are in place to support individuals and those involved in the care of vulnerable adults and children. They will help to guide you to minimise the risk of pressure damage and to understand how to treat the damage if it does occur.

Social Services and Well-Being (Wales) Act 2014

As we saw in Units 001/002, there are five principles to the Social Services and Well-Being (Wales) Act 2014, and we can apply these principles to every aspect of care and support. Table 2.5 relates these principles to pressure area care.

Principle	How the principle relates to pressure area care
Voice and control	*'putting an individual and their needs at the centre of their care and support, with individuals having voice and control over the outcomes that will help them achieve well-being'* • Does the individual wish to be at home or in the hospital? • How can you support pressure area care in line with their wishes?
Prevention and early intervention	*'increasing preventative services within the community to minimise the escalation of critical need'* Being proactive in pressure area care can limit the need for more serious care if ulcers appear.
Well-being	*'supporting people to achieve their own well-being and measuring the success of care and support'* Well-being is at the heart of all care and support, including pressure area care.
Multi-agency	*'working together and co-operating'* The GP may need to work with the community nurses and occupational health to support pressure area care.
Co-production	*'encouraging individuals to become more involved in the design and delivery of services'* This would mean working with the individual to support them how they wish to be supported and encouraging independence whenever possible.

▲ Table 2.5 Applying the five principles of the Social Services and Well-Being (Wales) Act 2014 to pressure area care

CASE STUDY

John lives alone. He has children living nearby. He is 86 and until recently has still been very active. He enjoys gardening and usually spends a few hours each day outside in his garden and vegetable patch. John recently had to go into hospital for an operation and needs a period of recovery, which he can do at home if he has support.

John's mobility will be reduced during this recovery period and he will have to spend a period of time on bed rest. There is a risk that John could develop pressure sores from prolonged periods of bed rest.

John is also feeling upset about the amount of time he will be away from his garden.

Discussion point: Thinking about the principles of the Social Services and Well-Being (Wales) Act, how can John be supported during this recovery period?

Pressure Ulcer Reporting and Investigation (All Wales Guidance) 2018

This document promotes consistency and Welsh Government targets for zero tolerance to pressure damage. It also:

• provides guidance on when pressure damage should be referred into safeguarding processes
• aims to reduce the risk of pressure area damage by facilitating effective learning and standardised approaches to reporting.

NICE guidelines

These guidelines cover risk assessment, prevention and treatment in children, young people and adults at risk of, or already suffering, a pressure ulcer/sore. It aims to reduce the number of pressure ulcers in people receiving NHS care.

NHS Wales guidelines

The NHS Wales guidelines on pressure care are covered in the NHS Wales Health and Care Standards under Standard 2.2 Preventing Pressure and Tissue Damage. It focuses on minimising the risk of individuals developing avoidable pressure ulcers through an assessment of factors.

European Pressure Ulcer Advisory Panel (EPUAP)

This panel educates the public and influences pressure ulcer policy in Europe, with an aim towards patient centred and cost-effective pressure ulcer care.

aSSKINg

aSSKINg is a guide for carers and patients in the management of pressure area care. It gives guidance on the following areas:

- **a** – assess risk
- **S** – Skin inspection
- **S** – Surface selection
- **K** – Keep moving
- **I** – Incontinence and increased moisture
- **N** – Nutrition and hydration
- **g** – give information

RESEARCH IT

You can find more on the above legislation and guidance here:

Stop the Pressure

https://nhs.stopthepressure.co.uk

Pressure ulcer reporting guidance

https://bit.ly/pressure-ulcer-reporting-investigation-pdf

Pressure ulcers: prevention and management guidance

www.nice.org.uk/guidance/cg179

European Pressure Ulcer Advisory Panel

www.epuap.org/

AC4.3 Factors that cause skin breakdown and pressure damage

There are many factors that cause skin breakdown and pressure damage:

- problems with mobility; for example, using a wheelchair, difficulty standing and walking for periods of time
- poor circulation, which could cause muscles to cramp and is often made worse by lack of movement
- moist skin; for example, due to incontinence
- inadequate diet and poor fluid intake
- previous tissue damage, such as scar tissue
- pressure against the skin, for example, from sitting and lying for periods of time
- lack of sensitivity to pain or discomfort; for example, following a stroke or from conditions such as diabetes, nerve or muscle disorders
- pain, such as a reluctance to move
- individuals who are overweight may experience more pressure on their skin from the body weight pressure
- being underweight could mean the individual has poor nutrition and fluid intake; this can mean they are at more risk of pressure ulcers
- shear – when two surfaces move in opposite directions; for example, while supporting an individual to move on their bed, the ankle bone moves in one direction and the skin in the other, causing friction.

AC4.4 Stages of pressure ulcer development

Stage 1 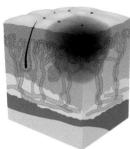   Stage 2 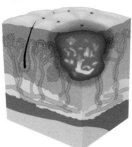   Stage 3 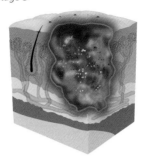   Stage 4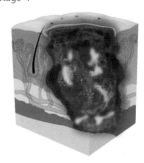

▲ Figure 2.4 The four stages of pressure ulcer development

Table 2.6 details the four main stages of pressure ulcer development.

Stage 1	Stage 2	Stage 3	Stage 4
• Closed wound • Skin is painful • No breaks or tears • Reddened skin • Warmer skin temperature • May go away in 2–3 days	• Skin breaks and forms an ulcer • Sore expands • Deeper layers of the skin are affected • Looks like a crater, abrasion or blister • Some skin may damage beyond repair • Can heal within 1–6 weeks	• Sore becomes worse • Extends to tissue beneath the skins • Forms a small crater • Fat may be visible but not muscle, bone or tendon • May take several months to heal • May never heal, especially for those with ongoing health problems	• Wound is so deep it reaches to muscle and bone • Damage to deeper tissues, tendons and joints • Dead tissue may need to be removed to minimise further infection • May take several months to heal • May never heal, especially for those with ongoing health problems

▲ Table 2.6 Stages of pressure ulcer development

AC4.5 Parts of the body that are commonly affected by pressure damage

There are parts of the body that are more commonly affected by pressure damage. These tend to be the more bony parts of the body:

- elbows
- heels
- hips
- base of spine
- tips of toes
- shoulder blades
- back of the head.

LO5 KNOW HOW TO SUPPORT GOOD ORAL HEALTH CARE AND MOUTH CARE FOR INDIVIDUALS

AC5.1 The terms 'oral health care' and 'mouth care'

It is important that oral health care is covered in the individual's personal plan.

When supporting an individual with **mouth care**, this could include activities such as:

- removing and cleaning dentures
- tooth brushing
- mouth rinsing
- tongue moistening for those not able to drink
- checking for sores and treating mouth ulcers
- ensuring dentures are fixed correctly
- the use of fluoride toothpaste
- gum cleaning
- applying water-based lip balms
- regular visits to the dentist for oral checks.

Good mouth care, including the care of teeth and dentures, contributes to good oral health and supports the general health and well-being of individuals.

KEY TERM

Mouth care: oral hygiene and maintaining good oral health through different oral health techniques.

AC5.2 National policy and practice on oral health care

There is national policy and practice to follow for oral health care.

Social Services and Well-Being (Wales) Act 2014

As detailed in LO4, the Social Services and Well-Being (Wales) Act underpins every element of care and support given to an individual. For example, it ensures that the individual has access to the correct oral health support. Supporting oral health care supports an individual's well-being and prevents more serious problems occurring.

REFLECT ON IT

Using the five principles of the Social Services and Well-Being (Wales) Act 2014, think about how these contribute to the care and support of an individual's oral health care.

NICE guidelines

There are a number of NICE guidelines on oral health, including:

- oral health for adults in care homes
- oral health promotion: general dental practice
- oral health: local authorities and partners.

See further details at their website:

www.nice.org.uk/guidance/conditions-and-diseases/oral-and-dental-health

The All Wales Dental Public Health Team (AWDPHT)

This team provides advice and support for the health boards, NHS Shared Services Partnership, Healthcare Inspectorate Wales, the Welsh Government and dental teams. See further details at their website:

www.wales.nhs.uk/sitesplus/888/page/43708

AC5.3 Common oral and dental problems in older people and other individuals who need care and support

There are some common oral and dental problems in older people and individuals who need care and support. They include the following:

- **Teeth** – staining, brittle, loss of enamel, discolouring following nerve damage or root canal treatment.

- **Dental caries and tooth loss** – dental caries (decay) is caused by the acid generated by bacterial plaque present in every mouth. Older people can be more susceptible to root caries because of gum recession.
- **Gum disease** – gingivitis and periodontitis. Gum disease is a major cause of tooth loss in adults.
- **Receding gums** – a condition where the gums gradually shrink away from the teeth. It can be caused by gum diseases, poor dental hygiene and smoothing.
- **Badly fitting dentures** – can cause the denture to rub and cause trauma to the bone.
- **Mouth sores and ulcers** – a small, painful patch or lump inside the mouth that can cause pain and discomfort.
- **Badly fitting dentures** – can cause the denture to rub and cause trauma to the bone.
- **Mouth sores and ulcers** – a small, painful patch or lump inside the mouth that can cause pain and discomfort.
- **Dry mouth (xerostomia)** – decreased saliva production, which can be caused by age or a side effect of medication.
- **Oral cancer** – the chance of oral cancer increases with age and there is an increased risk for individuals who smoke or drink alcohol.

AC5.4 Reasons why oral health and mouth care are important

There are many benefits to good oral health and mouth care which support the overall health and well-being of individuals. Good care enables good nutrition and hydration and prevents:

- infection, which could lead to more serious problems such as cardiovascular disease, respiratory infections or sepsis
- decay and gum disease, and keeps teeth and gums healthy – missing teeth can affect speech and self-esteem
- bad breath, which can impact on social interactions and relationships.

AC5.5 Potential impacts of poor oral health and mouth care on health, well-being, self-esteem and dignity

Poor oral health and mouth care can have an impact on physical health. There are many diseases linked to poor oral health as detailed in AC5.4. Individuals who are suffering from poor oral health and mouth care may feel self-conscious, it could affect their self-esteem and put them in a low mood. It could cause a great deal of worry and anxiety. Their dignity may be affected through factors such as bad breath, not being able to feed themselves or problems with chewing and swallowing.

CASE STUDY

Carys is moving into a residential home after becoming unable to look after herself. Carys used to take great pride in her appearance, but lately has been forgetting basic care routines, including brushing her teeth. Carys has seen a dentist and is showing signs of receding gums.

The staff at the residential home have a meeting with Carys to discuss her arrival and put her personal plan together.

Discussion points:
- Why is it important that the team include oral health care on Carys's personal plan?
- What is the impact on Carys if they do not support her oral health?

AC5.6 Links between oral health and mouth care and nutrition

Good nutrition plays a vital role in good oral health. Poor diet can make it harder for individuals to fight infection, and this can lead to gum disease and tooth decay.

Foods that contribute to the production of plaque include those high in carbohydrates, sugars and starch. Eating foods with no acid helps avoid the breakdown of tooth enamel and keeps the mouth healthy.

Also important are:

- Vitamin D – it allows calcium to be absorbed.
- Vitamin C – a diet low in Vitamin C could lead to bleeding gums and loss of teeth.

Good nutrition and oral health support each other. Poor oral health can reduce the ability to consume and enjoy healthy food; for example, it can be difficult to enjoy foods that need to be chewed, such as fruit and vegetables, if you don't have healthy teeth.

AC5.7 Professionals that may help with oral health care

There are a number of professionals that may help with oral health care, as shown in Table 2.7.

Professional	Role
Dentist	Diagnoses, manages and treats general oral care needs.
Endodontist	Carries out specialised procedures.
Dental hygienist	Cleans teeth and advises on hygiene issues.
Orthodontist	Specialises in the prevention, diagnosis and treatment of problems affecting the teeth and jaw.
Periodontist	Specialises in prevention and treatment of diseases affecting soft tissues in the mouth.
Prosthodontist	Provides oral prostheses to replace damaged, decayed or missing teeth.
Dental technician	Creates braces, dentures and crowns.

▲ Table 2.7 Professionals who help with oral health care

LO6 KNOW THE IMPORTANCE OF FOOT CARE AND THE HEALTH AND WELL-BEING OF INDIVIDUALS

> **GETTING STARTED**
>
> People can face foot problems at any age but these tend to increase as they get older. Foot problems can have a big impact on individuals' health and well-being. Think about how foot pain and problems could affect your day-to-day routine.

AC6.1 The importance of foot care for individuals

There are many benefits to good foot care:

- **Mobility and increased physical activity** – problems with the feet can reduce mobility and stop physical activity, due to pain, discomfort or problems with standing and balance.
- **Reducing pain** – foot problems can cause varying levels of pain from minor discomfort, as blisters, to severe pain caused by diabetic neuropathy.
- **Reducing trips and falls** – foot problems can cause the individual to change the way they walk to compensate for the pain it causes. They can also reduce mobility, and both of these factors can increase the risk of trips and falls.
- **Self-esteem, confidence and independence** – foot problems can affect mobility or cause pain, which can stop an individual doing some of the things they have always done. Good foot care helps to maintain independence, increase self-esteem and confidence.
- **Supporting social interaction and exercise** – being able to get out and about can be vitally important to individuals. Foot problems can limit this.
- **Reducing the risk of infections** – this is particularly important for people who have diabetes.

AC6.2 Common conditions that can cause problems with feet

Table 2.8 shows some of the most common conditions that cause problems with the feet.

Condition	How this causes problems with feet
Athlete's foot	This is a fungal infection of the skin, usually found between the toes. It can spread and cause significant discomfort, itching and sometimes even pain.
Bunions	Abnormalities of the feet that cause a bump to develop on the large toe joint, causing the big toe to turn slightly inward.
Diabetic neuropathy	Caused by fluctuations in blood sugar. This is not just one condition but a group of conditions that causes damage to the feet.
Ingrown toenails	A condition where the toenail starts to grow into the nail groove, which can cause pain and discomfort.
Plantar fasciitis	The most common cause of heel pain and occurs when the plantar fascia (the ligament responsible for supporting the foot's arch) on the bottom of the foot becomes inflamed.
Blisters	Blisters are extremely common and are likely to appear after walking or running for long periods of time, especially if the feet have become moist from sweat or from wearing ill-fitting shoes. Blisters are fluid-filled sacs that usually heal on their own and are not generally a serious concern.
Corns	These usually occur on the sole of the feet or toes and are patches of thickened skin. They sometimes form to protect the skin and stop the body from developing blisters. However, over time they can become painful and need treatment.
Heel spur	An outgrowth of calcium between the heel bone and the arch of the foot. It can be painful and cause inflammation but for many there are no symptoms at all. They are caused by long-term strain on muscles and ligaments, arthritis, excess body weight and badly fitting shoes.
Claw toe	Also known as claw foot. It occurs when the first toe joint points up and the second toe joint points down. • It can be present at birth or appear suddenly. • It can be painless but for others very painful. Claw toe can be a sign of a more serious condition such as rheumatoid arthritis, diabetes and cerebral palsy.
Stone bruises (metatarsalgia)	Stone bruises cause a numbness with sharp pains between the toes and the arch of the foot. It can feel as if there is a stone in your shoe. Causes include high-impact exercises or poor-fitting shoes, though it can be a sign of an underlying condition.
Gout	A type of arthritis where crystals form inside and around joints causing pain. It can be caused by too much uric acid.
Raynaud's disease	This can cause numbness and cold toes. It is a vascular disorder that causes interruptions to blood flow.

▲ Table 2.8 Common conditions affecting the feet

AC6.3 Signs of foot and toenail abnormalities

Individuals should have their feet checked regularly for signs of any abnormalities, and seek advice to rule out any other underlying causes and prevent any long-term disability.

Some of the signs to look out for are:

- inflammation
- swelling of foot or around nails
- pain
- skin discolouration on feet
- signs of pressure damage
- fluid build-up
- change in walking
- bumps on foot
- itching
- stinging or burning
- numbness or coldness
- bleeding around nails
- changes in nail shape
- brittle or pitted nails
- changes to nail thickness
- changing in nail colour or discolouration.

AC6.4 The potential impact of foot conditions or abnormalities on the health and well-being of individuals

Foot care is extremely important for supporting an individual's health and well-being. Foot problems can impact on mobility. With reduced mobility comes a reduction in quality of life. An individual may find that:

- they struggle with walking, driving, shopping, working, socialising and exercising

- they lose their independence and miss out on social interactions
- their mental well-being suffers as a result, leading to depression and loneliness.

We have already learnt about the importance of physical activity for both physical and mental health. Foot problems can hinder exercise, resulting in the loss of muscle and strength. This could lead to weight problems and a higher risk of diseases such as diabetes and heart disease.

For individuals with diabetes, foot care is particularly important as high blood sugar can cause poor circulation and nerve damage.

CASE STUDY

Derek is 60 years old and has always been very active. He is a keen rambler and a member of a local walking group. Derek recently suffered with plantar fasciitis. His GP told him to rest and referred him to physiotherapy. Derek has missed the last three weeks of his walking group and has been struggling to walk around his garden without any pain. He is on the waiting list for physiotherapy but has been told it can take up to a month.

Discussion point: What impact might this have on Derek's well-being?

AC6.5 Professionals that may help with foot care

There are a number of professionals who can help with foot care. For details see Table 2.9.

Professional	Role
GP	A GP is usually the first point of contact for identifying and diagnosing any foot problems.
Podiatrist or chiropodist	These professionals treat ingrown toenails, fallen arches, heel spurs, calluses and some common foot and ankle injuries.
	They can also provide treatment for foot problems relating to diabetes and other systemic illnesses.
Orthopaedic surgeon	A surgeon who performs surgeries to correct foot problems.
Foot clinics / chiropody clinics	These clinics provide care and services such as nail cutting, dealing with corns, hard skin and cracked heels.
Diabetes speciality nurse	The diabetes nurse will always check the feet of their patients and refer to the chiropodist or podiatrist if there is something that requires support.
Sports injury clinics	These clinics will assess and deal with foot problems caused by sports injuries.

▲ Table 2.9 Professionals who help with foot care

Check your understanding

1 How many stages are there to a pressure ulcer?

2 How many principles are there in the Social Services and Well-Being (Wales) Act 2014?

3 What can cause low pressure damage?

4 What can cause high pressure damage?

5 What can increase your risk of oral cancer?

6 Why are older people more at risk of tooth decay?

7 What kind of infection causes athlete's foot?

8 Why are individuals with diabetes more prone to foot problems?

Question practice

1 Which stage of pressure ulcers usually goes away in two to three days?

   a Stage 3   c Stage 4

   b Stage 1   d Stage 2

2 Which of the following two factors can contribute to pressure ulcers?

   a smoking   c poor diet

   b drinking alcohol d sight impairment

3 What is an example of good mouth care?

   a tooth brushing

   b wearing dentures

   c using non-fluoride toothpaste

   d eating foods high in carbohydrates

4 Tooth decay is caused by:

   a bacterial plague   c dry mouth

   b irregular brushing d oral cancer

5 What is the role of an orthodontist?

   a creates braces, dentures and crowns

   b specialises in problems affecting the teeth and jaw

   c cleans teeth and advises on hygiene issues

   d carries out specialist procedures

6 Which of these is a heel spur?

   a fluid-filled sac

   b fungal infection

   c outgrowth of calcium

   d bump on toe joint

7 What could numbness and cold toes could be a sign of?

   a stone bruises

   b Raynaud's disease

   c plantar fasciitis

   d ingrown toenails

LO7 UNDERSTAND THE ROLES AND RESPONSIBILITIES RELATED TO THE ADMINISTRATION OF MEDICATION IN HEALTH AND SOCIAL CARE SETTINGS

GETTING STARTED

Think about an occasion when you or someone you know was unwell and required medication.

- What medication was administered and by whom?
- Why was this necessary?
- What were the potential side effects of this medication?
- Were any experienced?

AC7.1 Legislation and national guidance related to the administration of medication

There are a number of laws and national guidance documents to ensure that medications are safely administered.

- **Social Services and Well-Being (Wales) Act 2014** – the principles of this Act underpin the correct procedures for administering medication. If mistakes are made, and legislation and guidance are not followed, this can have a severely negative effect on an individual's health and well-being.
- **Misuse of Drugs Act 1971 (regulations 1972 and 2001)** – this Act's main purpose is to prevent the misuse of controlled drugs. It imposes a ban on the possession, supply, manufacture, import and export of controlled drugs.
- **Health Act 2006 (Controlled Medication)** – this Act deals with the management of controlled drugs, and sets out provision of pharmacy and ophthalmic services.
- **Control of Substances Hazardous to Health (COSHH) 1999** – this Act requires employers to control substances that are hazardous to health; for example, many cleaning products in care settings must be controlled, as well as bodily waste.
- **Hazardous Waste Regulations 2005** – these set out the regimes for the control and tracking of the movement of hazardous waste in England and Wales.
- **Mental Health Act 2007** – this is the main legislation that covers the assessment, treatment and rights of people with a mental health disorder. This legislation has to be followed when issuing medication to someone with a mental health disorder.
- **Mental Capacity Act 2005** – this legislation is very important when administering medication. Health and social care practitioners must not administer medication to individuals without their knowledge and consent, if that individual has the capacity to make decisions about their treatment and care.
- **All Wales Guidance for Health Boards / Trusts in Respect of Medicines and Health Care Support Workers 2015** – this guidance is intended for nurses and midwives who delegate duties to health care support workers.

AC7.2 Roles and responsibilities of those involved in prescribing, dispensing and supporting the use of medication

There are a number of roles in which people take responsibility for prescribing, dispensing and supporting the use of medication. See Table 2.10 for details.

Person involved	Role in prescribing, dispensing and supporting the use of medication
Doctor	Their role is to prescribe medication, indicating the dose, type and amount to be given.
Chemist/pharmacist	Their role is to dispense the medication, checking that the medication matches the prescription. They must label it with the name of the individual, making sure these details and instructions are clearly stated: • the dose • the date • the expiry date • how the medication is to be taken.
Manager of the setting	The manager must ensure that policies and procedures for the administration of medication are in place and all staff are regularly trained and updated. They should ensure that care plans are updated and record keeping systems are in place.
Care worker	The worker must ensure that the individual receives their medication, and that it is the correct dose at the correct time. They must: • always maintain the respect and dignity of the individual. • record the administration of medication with date, time and dose. • never administer medication without the correct training first.

▲ Table 2.10 Professionals responsible for prescribing, dispensing and supporting the use of medication

AC7.3 Remits of responsibility for the use of 'over the counter' remedies and supplements in health and social care settings

When buying **over the counter medication**, the following individuals have certain responsibilities:

- **The pharmacist** must ensure the medication is suitable to the individual and the condition they want the medication for. The pharmacist should also check any other medications that are being taken to ensure the medication is safe to take.
- **The manager** is responsible for confirming with the individual's GP that this will not affect prescribed medication. The manager is also responsible for ensuring there is a policy in place and that all staff have received training.
- **The care worker** must be aware that over the counter medication could impact on prescribed medication and should always confirm first.

KEY TERM

Over the counter medication: usually refers to non-prescription medication that you can buy in a pharmacy.

AC7.4 Links between misadministration of medication and safeguarding

While mistakes can happen at any stage of the medication process, for example, incorrect recording or a missed administration, this is often down to procedures not being followed correctly.

However, the misadministration of medication will be considered a safeguarding issue when there are the following concerns:

- deliberate act of harm using medication, such as giving an intentional overdose
- use of medicine for reasons another than for the benefit of an individual, such as to control the individual
- medication withheld without a valid reason, such as refusing to give medication as a form of punishment
- accidental harm caused by an administration of medication error
- deliberate falsification of records
- misuse or over-reliance on sedatives to control behaviour.

Social care staff have a duty of care to report any concerns regarding the administration of medication.

CASE STUDY

Moira is 75 years old and has recently moved to a residential setting following the onset of dementia. Moira has not adapted well and is having problems with her sleep. She spends all night howling and crying to 'go home'.

Katie is a new member of staff who usually works the day shift but agreed to cover a couple of night shifts when a colleague was on holiday. Katie hears Moira and tries to calm her down by chatting with her, offering her something to eat or drink, reading to her. After an hour another worker comes in and issues Moira with a sedative, stating 'Now we can all get some peace'.

Katie feels uncomfortable with this but does not challenge the staff member who is more experienced than her.

Discussion points:

- What are the potential safeguarding issues here?
- What should Katie do in this situation?

LO8 UNDERSTAND THE IMPORTANCE OF NUTRITION AND HYDRATION FOR THE HEALTH AND WELL-BEING OF INDIVIDUALS

GETTING STARTED

Good nutrition and hydration are crucial for the health and well-being of individuals who have care or support needs.

- Have you ever had a busy day where you didn't have time to eat or drink properly?
- Do you remember how this made you feel?
- Were you tired, irritable, low in mood?

Imagine being an individual with care or support needs feeling the same way but being unable to express how they feel.

REFLECT ON IT

Imagine you are an individual with care or support needs who has just moved in to a care setting and you are unable to eat and drink without support from an adult care worker.

- What might your concerns be about the support you will receive with your eating and drinking?
- Why?

AC8.1 The terms 'nutrition' and 'hydration'

Good **nutrition** means eating healthily and in a balanced way:

- eating sufficient for your needs – eating too much can make you put on weight, while not eating enough can make you will lose weight

- eating as wide a range of foods as possible – the body will be provided with all the nutrients it needs to work well
- eating lots of fruit and vegetables – they are a very good source of vitamins
- eating plenty of fish – they contain many vitamins and minerals essential for the body
- cutting down on eating salty and fatty foods – to avoid putting on weight and developing conditions such as heart disease
- cutting down on sugary foods – to avoid putting on weight, and prevent low and high mood swings and tooth decay
- support – individuals require the correct level of care or support to meet their nutritional needs, such as eating aids (adapted cutlery, plates) and diet sheets (diabetic, gluten free, vegetarian).

Good **hydration** means drinking healthily and in a balanced way. Consider:

- drinking fluids such as water and milk – avoid drinking too many sugary and fizzy drinks that can lead to tooth decay, and caffeine based drinks that can lead to putting on weight and sleep disturbances
- drinking enough and regularly (the UK Government recommends drinking 6–8 glasses of water every day)

- what will happen if someone drinks too much before meals – this can make you feel bloated and can reduce your appetite
- the use of drinking aids – some individuals will require the correct level of care or support to meet their hydration needs, such as adapted cups, a straw and fluid sheets (to record the amount and types of fluids they are drinking).

KEY TERMS

Nutrition: a healthy and balanced diet with the correct nutrients.

Hydration: ensuring the body absorbs enough water to keep hydrated.

AC8.2 Principles of a balanced diet and good hydration, and government recommendations for a balanced diet and hydration

It is important to have a balanced diet as no single food group contains all the essential nutrients the body needs to be healthy and function well. A balanced diet, therefore, should include a large variety of foods for adequate intakes of all the nutrients.

The Eatwell Guide in Figure 2.5 sets out guidance on all the food groups and how best to balance these.

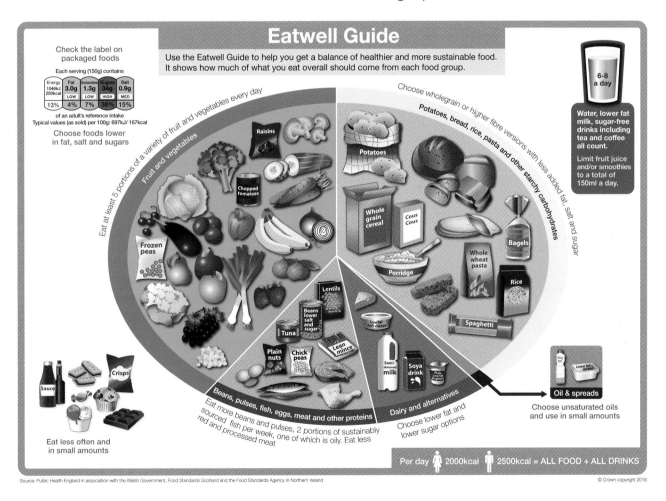

▲ Figure 2.5 The Eatwell Guide

Having a healthy diet is all about achieving the right balance and variety of food. The Eatwell Guide aims to reduce confusion about what makes a healthy diet. It is divided into five food groups:

- fruit and vegetables
- carbohydrates (potatoes, bread, rice, pasta and other starchy foods)
- proteins (beans, pulses, fish, eggs, meat)
- dairy and alternatives
- oils and spreads.

Foods from the largest groups should be eaten more often than the foods from the smallest groups.

It is equally important to keep hydrated. Fluid intake is essential for health. Individuals who do not drink enough fluids are at risk of repeated infections, confusion or falling over.

RESEARCH IT

Research more about the Eatwell Guide and the different food groups through this resource:
www.nhs.uk/live-well/eat-well/the-eatwell-guide/

AC8.3 National and local initiatives that support nutrition and hydration

As well as the Eatwell Guide, other initiatives include:

- NHS Live Well – provides advice, tips and tools to support individuals to improve their health and well-being:
https://www.nhs.uk/live-well/eat-well/

- Change4Life – supporting families to eat well and move more:
www.nhs.uk/change4life/

- Nutrition Skills for Life – available through your local Public Health Dietetics Department to support nutrition.
- Corporate Health standard – working to promote health, work and well-being:
www.healthyworkingwales.wales.nhs.uk/corporate-health-standard

- Nutrition in Community Settings – provides a pathway and resource pack for professionals working in the health and social care sector:
www.wales.nhs.uk/sitesplus/documents/862/FOI%20193j%2015.pdf

RESEARCH IT

See if you can find any other local initiatives in your local area.

AC8.4 The importance of a balanced diet for the optimum health and well-being of individuals

We need energy to live. A balance of carbohydrates, fat and protein must be achieved in order for us to remain healthy. Too little or too much of one element of the five food groups could have a negative impact. For example:

- Too little protein can interfere with growth and other body functions.
- Too much protein can be stored as fat and can lead to weight gain over time.
- Too much fat can lead to obesity and heart disease.
- Too little fat can cause issues such as dry rashes, hair loss and a weaker immune system.
- Too many carbohydrates can lead to an increase in blood sugar levels, which encourages the body to make more insulin and save up the glucose as fat.
- Too little carbohydrates can mean blood sugars drop too low and cause hypoglycaemia.

Vitamins, minerals and dietary fibre are all important for health. There is evidence that a number of bioactive plant substances (termed phytochemicals) found in fruit and vegetables are also important in promoting good health.

A varied and balanced diet should give you all the nutrients you need but some people need to take vitamin supplements:

- Vitamin A – can be found in cheese, eggs, oily fish, milk and yoghurt. It helps the body's natural defence against illness and keeps skin healthy.
- Vitamin C – can be found in citrus fruits, peppers, broccoli and potatoes. It helps maintain healthy skin

and blood vessels and protects cells, keeping them healthy.

- Vitamin D – direct sunlight on the skin can help the body create vitamin D, which can also be found in oily fish, red meat and fortified foods. Vitamin D helps to keep bones, teeth and muscles healthy.
- Iron – important for making red blood cells that carry oxygen around the body. Too little iron can cause iron deficiency, which can cause fatigue. Good sources of iron include red meat, beans, nuts, dried fruit and fortified breakfast cereals.

Diet can affect the following areas of health and well-being:

- balance of nutrients
- bone health
- immune function
- dental health
- bowel health
- blood
- skin
- cognition (thinking)
- maintaining a healthy weight
- can cause chronic diseases (such as heart disease and stroke)
- reproductive health
- mental health and well-being.

AC8.5 Factors that can affect nutrition and hydration

There are many factors that can affect the nutrition and hydration of individuals. These can include health, environmental, financial, cultural and social factors, as shown in Table 2.11. This table also covers Unit 004, AC10.5, Factors that affect nutrition and hydration for children and young people.

Factor	How this affects nutrition and hydration
Culture and religion	Culture affects the choice of foods, and how they are cooked and eaten.
	Some religious groups may avoid certain foods or require food to be cooked in a certain way. Children and young people who grow up in these families will usually follow these cultures too.
Individual preferences and habits	Understanding an individual's food preferences and requirements can help to understand their dietary needs. In health and social care settings it is important to discuss this with the individual regularly and to encourage a wide variety of food and drink options.
	Children may be resistant to trying new things, but can be encouraged through education and learning about food.
Physical factors	Health conditions can cause pain or difficulty when eating.
	People with disabilities may need additional support to ensure adequate intake. There may be an issue with swallowing, and the speech and language therapist may need to carry out an assessment.
	An individual may require assistance with feeding, using adapted cutlery and plate guards. Sitting in an upright position will aid individuals with eating and drinking.
Psychological factors	Stress, depression and anxiety can all impact on appetite. Eating disorders are most common in young women between the ages of 12 and 20, but can affect older women and men of all ages.
Income, lifestyle and social convention	Low income families struggle to be able to afford a balanced diet and are more at risk of having a poorer quality diet (for example, fast food). This will impact on the children and young people in those families.
Family and peer influences	It is important that individuals have positive role models when it comes to diet. Eating as a social experience can have more positive effects on an individual than eating alone.
	Introducing children and young people to new foods, having themed nights or going out to different restaurants can support a healthy attitude to food.
Neglect	Individuals suffering from neglect are likely to have a poor diet. It is important as a social care worker to recognise and report the signs of abuse and neglect.
Advertising and fads	Individuals may be influenced by advertising, meaning they may be inclined to choose foods and drinks that are widely advertised, but these are often high in fat, sugar and salt.
	Fad diets can be misleading and make false claims. Diets are often not supported by medical fact and can be unhealthy and dangerous.
Ethics, morals and political beliefs	Vegans and vegetarians base their diet on ethical choices and they must ensure that they replace the nutrients from food they do not eat with alternatives. More information can be found online through the NHS, the Vegan Society and Vegetarian Society.
	Other beliefs and preferences may be due to wanting to eat organic, making food choices based on environmental factors or wanting to shop and buy local.

▲ Table 2.11 How nutrition and hydration are affected by different factors

LO9 KNOW HOW TO SUPPORT FALLS PREVENTION

GETTING STARTED

Older individuals who are looked after can be more prone to trips and falls for a number of reasons. But is it just age that is a contributing factor?

Think about your current environment: can you highlight any obvious fall risks?

AC9.1 Factors that contribute to falls

There are many factors that could contribute to falls. They include:

- Physical factors, such as:
  - balance problems (can be caused by conditions such as stroke or Parkinson's disease)
  - muscle weakness (particularly if in the legs)
  - foot problems (think back to LO7 on foot care)
  - poor vision, including glaucoma, cataracts and sight deterioration caused by age.
- Memory loss or confusion, particularly with individuals with dementia.
- Substance misuse, too much alcohol or side effects from drug taking.
- Certain medications which make you feel dizzy or drowsy. It is important to know the side effects of any medication taken.
- Individuals who require mobility aids could be more at risk of falls if the aid is inappropriate or has not been fitted correctly.
- Some long-term health conditions (such as heart disease or low blood pressure) can lead to dizziness, fainting or brief loss of consciousness.
- Environmental factors such as:
  - wet floors
  - unsecure carpets or rugs
  - clutter
  - obscured doorways and corridors
  - dim lighting
  - stairs, going up or down
  - rushing to get somewhere
  - reaching for something too high.

AC9.2 Ways in which falls can be prevented

Reducing the risk of falls is an important element of health and social care. There are several ways to do this, and it is important, first and foremost, to follow your health and safety policies.

As a support worker you can do the following:

- Check that rugs and carpets are secure.
- Mop up spillages promptly.
- Ensure doorways and corridors are clear.
- Remove clutter and keep areas clear.
- Report any issues immediately.
- Support individuals to maintain good foot care.

The setting can also act to prevent falls by doing the following:

- Carry out regular inspections.
- Replace worn carpets and rugs.
- Use non-slip mats and rugs.
- Ensure the environment has good lighting.
- Install grip rails and handrails.
- Carry out assessment on individuals' needs.
- Carry out medication reviews.
- Provide training to staff.

An individual can also help to prevent falls by doing the following:

- Wear suitable footwear.
- Wear clothing that does not trail.
- Exercise that improves balance and muscle strength, such as pilates.
- Avoid alcohol.
- Have a regular sight test.
- Maintain good foot care.

CASE STUDY

Vera works in a care home. During her morning rounds, she notices that one of the handrails in the bathroom has come loose. Vera makes a mental note to mention it to the shift leader at handover but then forgets.

Discussion points:
- What are the potential risks of Vera not reporting this?
- What could Vera have done differently?

Check your understanding

1 What is the main purpose of the Misuse of Drugs Act 1971?

2 What is the manager's responsibility around prescribed drugs?

3 What is the government guidance on keeping a balanced diet called?

4 How many food groups are there?

5 Why can taking medication contribute to falls?

6 Explain why the following individuals might be more prone to falls:

   a individual with substance misuse problem

   b individual with dementia.

Question practice

1 When should the recording of administration of medication take place?

   a by the end of your shift

   b within 24 hours

   c when the manager is there

   d straight away

2 Which of these is an example of a psychological factor impacting on healthy nutrition?

   a low income

   b neglect

   c anorexia

   d vegetarianism

3 Which of the following is linked to a diet high in fat?

   a diabetes

   b cancer

   c heart disease

   d high blood pressure

4 Which of the following **two** environmental factors could contribute to falls?

   a poor lighting

   b fire doors

   c wet floors

   d exit signs

5 Which of the following is an example of how a worker can minimise the risk of falls to individuals?

   a drink less alcohol

   b install handrails

   c remove clutter

   d provide training

LO10 KNOW THE FACTORS THAT AFFECT END OF LIFE CARE

GETTING STARTED

There are many factors that surround individuals, their families and carers during end of life care.

You may have had experience of someone you knew dying. Spend some time thinking about how this made you feel and how it affected others around you, as well as the person who died. It is important as a support worker to understand these factors and get support to work effectively with end of life care.

AC10.1 Ways in which death and dying, grief and mourning may impact on individuals and key people in their lives

Death, dying, grief and mourning will affect individuals and key people in their lives in many different ways. There are no rules to follow and everyone will be on their own journey through the process.

The most well-known theory on grief is Kubler-Ross's five stages of grief, shown in Figure 2.6. This states that there are stages in the grief cycle that will eventually lead to acceptance, but that the time will vary, depending on the person who is grieving and, perhaps, the circumstances surrounding the individual's death.

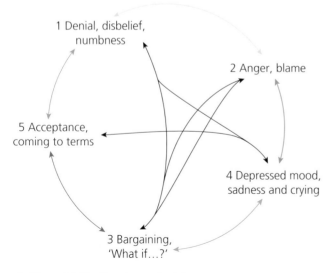

1 Denial, disbelief, numbness

2 Anger, blame

5 Acceptance, coming to terms

4 Depressed mood, sadness and crying

3 Bargaining, 'What if...?'

▲ Figure 2.6 The five stages of grief

Death, dying, grief and mourning can be displayed through a range of emotions and reactions.

- They can impact on individuals' sleep, cause changes in appetite, and affect their memory and ability to concentrate.
- Individuals may want to withdraw and isolate from others or they could become angry.
- They may feel an overwhelming sadness and despair.
- They could even become ill or develop physical problems.

It is important to understand these factors and how to support individuals during this process.

RESEARCH IT

Kubler-Ross's five stages of grief is not the only theory on grief. You may wish to research some other theories that argue that grief cannot be categorised into stages and is about multiple trajectories:

- Resilience to loss and chronic grief, Bonanno et al. (2002)
- Dual-process model, Stoebe and Schut (1999)
- Task-based model, Worden (2008).

AC10.2 Ways in which culture, religion and personal beliefs will impact upon approach to death and dying

It is extremely important to understand an individual's culture, religion and personal beliefs. These can have a significant impact upon their approach to death and dying. Every culture and religion has rituals related to death and dying as well as grief.

The individual's religion will affect the type of care they will receive during end of life care. For example:

- Catholics do not believe in cremation, and the Greek Orthodox church does not permit it.

- Catholics have the last rites read to them before they die.
- Muslims will have their bodies washed by family and friends after death.
- Prior to death, Muslims will often gather to recite the Qur'an and you should aim to turn the individual towards Mecca.
- Jewish people believe that the dying person should not be left alone until the funeral and burial should take place as soon as possible after death.
- Hindus prefer to die at home with support.

As well as culture and religion, it is also important to consider a non-religious individual's personal beliefs on how they wish to be cared for and their personal wishes for after death. Many people will plan their funeral and state their wishes for their end of life and after death.

It is important to understand how different cultures express grief. For example, Eastern Orthodox Christian widows will mourn for 40 days and wear black, Catholics will carry out a mass one month after the death, Jewish people will often wear a black ribbon following the death and the first anniversary is marked by the unveiling of a tombstone.

AC10.3 The terms 'advance care planning' and 'advance directives', and why these are important

Advance care planning allows the individual to plan for how they wish to be cared for during their end of life. It allows them to talk about their wishes and have their preferences written down. Advance care planning also allows individuals to make plans for who should care for them, as well as who should make decisions for them if they become too unwell to make them.

Advance care planning helps the family and carers ensure that the individual's wishes and needs are being met. Advance care plans can be updated as needed.

An **advanced directive** is a legal document in which an individual with mental capacity states the actions they wish to be taken if ill-health or lack of capacity results in them not being able to decide. It will detail issues such as refusing treatment that could sustain life, for example, a 'Do not resuscitate' order. The document

might also name an individual to make decisions on the individual's behalf.

These decisions must be written down and must be signed by a witness. This document is then legally binding if it complies with the Mental Capacity Act. It is only valid if:

- The individual is over 18 and has mental capacity.
- It is signed and witnessed.
- It is made without pressure.
- The individual has not said anything contradicting the directive.

Both these documents help to reduce the stress of making decisions for relatives and support effective end of life care. They support the Social Services and Well-Being (Wales) Act by giving individuals voice, choice and autonomy over decisions affecting their lives.

KEY TERMS

Advance care planning: the plan an individual will create stating the care they wish to receive at the end stage of life.

Advance directive: also referred to as a living will, this is a legal document detailing the actions to take at the end stage of life.

AC10.4 Support available to support individuals with end of life care

Individuals can be supported in many ways during end of life care. They may not have to go into a hospital and could choose other options more suitable for them, such as:

- community nurses – who provide end of life care in the home (including the Macmillan and Marie Curie nurses)
- care homes – can provide round the clock care
- hospices – providing care for terminally ill individuals until their death
- GP – prescribing medication and liaising with community nurses and hospices
- social services – ensure that the individual has help with equipment, respite services and other support such as personal care or meal delivery
- specialist social workers – can provide support for children, counselling, and so on.

AC10.5 Assistance that is available for workers when supporting individuals with end of life care

Supporting individuals and their families through end of life care can be very difficult, upsetting and stressful. It is important that support workers receive the right support and assistance to carry out this challenging role.

Building resilience is very important. You will need strategies to cope with this challenging role and to balance providing end of life care with your own self-care. It is important that you look after yourself, physically and mentally. This can include eating well, sleeping well, exercising and taking time for yourself outside work.

You need to be able to reflect on your own views and beliefs about death and dying, as well as being able to reflect on the way you supported individuals and their families through end of life care. Being a reflective practitioner is crucial in all aspects of health and social care, but it is very important in helping you to process the death of an individual you have supported.

You should seek to continue your professional development around end of life care, so that your practice remains up to date. This could be through:

- having a mentor who is more experienced
- attending training sessions on coping strategies and how to deal with difficult situations (such as angry family members).

All workers should learn how to handle relationships with family as they play such a large part of the end of life process.

It is also important to seek support and advice when needed. Struggling with end of life care is normal. It is very sad and can be very challenging. To be the best worker for the individual and their families, you need to look after yourself and ask for help with you need it. Without the right support, you could be at risk of 'burn out' or 'compassion fatigue'.

Getting support can take the following forms:

- Work colleagues – this informal support can be invaluable as you are all going through the same challenges.

- Debriefing session following death, particularly if it was sudden or distressing.
- Speaking to a religious leader – a worker may seek guidance in their own faith.
- Support from line managers – feedback and guidance are crucial, either informal or through formal supervision.
- Regular team meetings – it is important to work as a team and to be supportive of each other. Team meetings can be a safe space to discuss work-related feelings and stresses.
- Some workplaces offer counselling services.

CASE STUDY

Kate is 21 years old and has just started working at a care home. Kate has no prior experience of working in care, but she loves her new job and her mentor feeds back to the manager that Kate is doing really well. After three weeks, one of the individuals in the home dies suddenly from a heart attack while Kate is on shift.

Discussion points:
- How might this affect Kate?
- What support could be offered to her?

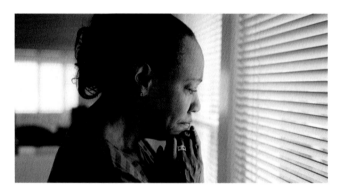

▲ Figure 2.7 Taking time to reflect on your practice

REFLECT ON IT

- Think about some of the emotions that might be experienced by staff supporting individuals with end of life care.
- What are the possible consequences of not receiving support?

A helpful video can be found here:

End of life care: Supporting staff in care homes

https://youtu.be/SBVZLaC3Ns8

LO11 KNOW HOW ASSISTIVE TECHNOLOGY CAN BE USED TO SUPPORT THE HEALTH AND WELL-BEING OF INDIVIDUALS

GETTING STARTED

Assistive technology can improve an individual's functioning and independence. They can enable individuals to actively participate in their lives, therefore improving their well-being.

Think about some of the technology you live with: how does it improve your way of life?

AC11.1 The terms 'assistive technology' and 'electronic assistive technology'

Assistive technology and **electronic assistive technology** can support individuals to live the way they want to and to access the care and support they need to do this.

KEY TERMS

Assistive technology: aids, devices and equipment that can support an individual with disabilities to actively participate in their lives.

Electronic assistive technology: equipment that can be used to overcome difficulties for accessing and using computer technology. It also refers to environmental control systems to operate equipment in an individual's environment (such as heating or lighting) using alternative technology.

AC11.2 Types and ranges of technological aids that can be used to support an individual's independence and how these can be accessed

There are many different technological aids that can be used to support individuals' independence, such as:

- Text readers – electronic system that reads text and can support an individual with visual impairment.
- Touch screen display – can be easier to use than a keyboard to support an individual with sensory loss.

- Hearing aids – to support hearing for individuals with hearing loss.
- Screen magnifiers – can increase the images and text on a screen to support individuals with visual impairment.
- Larger key keyboards – to support individuals with visual impairment or poor gross motor skills.
- Mobility devices such as scooters – a scooter designed to support individuals with mobility loss.
- Adapted cars – adapted to support access for individuals with mobility loss, or support wheelchair access.
- Automatic house lights and doors – to support individuals with sensory loss or mobility loss.
- Electronically operated beds and chairs – in order to support individuals with mobility loss, beds and chairs can be electronically moved to assist individuals getting in and out.
- Speech recognition programmes – individuals who have mobility loss can use their voice to turn items such as lights on or off.
- Adapted telephones – adapted to support hearing loss by flashing when someone is calling, or larger buttons for someone with visual impairment.
- Stairlifts – support individuals with mobility issues to get up and down stairs.

Technological aids can be accessed through the NHS, charities and voluntary organisations, or purchased privately. There are some grants available for those with a long-term illness. Occupational therapists can advise on suitable aids; there are also various organisations providing advice and support such as the Disabled Living Foundation and AbilityNet. See their websites:

www.dlf.org.uk/

https://abilitynet.org.uk/

AC11.3 Ways in which technological aids can be used to support active participation

We explored the term 'active participation' in Units 001/002. Individuals should be regarded as active partners in their own care and support. Active participation recognises the individual's right to participate in activities and relationships and live as independently as possible.

With technological aids, individuals can be independent and participate in everyday life. With the right aid and assistance, they can be more in control of their own life, promoting their self-esteem and boosting their well-being.

Technological aids can support active participation in the following ways:

- increase the individual's ability to stay in their own home
- assist in daily tasks such as personal care
- assist participation in social activities
- reduce isolation
- less reliance on others – promotes independence
- reduces accidents
- increases choice – individuals should not be limited by disabilities.

AC11.4 Support available for use of assistive technology

Individuals should be able to access support through the council or their GP. They may also be able to access support through the reablement team, occupational health, the district nurse or community physiotherapist, as well as the manufacturers and organisations that specialise in specific conditions..

LO12 KNOW HOW SENSORY LOSS CAN IMPACT UPON THE HEALTH AND WELL-BEING OF INDIVIDUALS

GETTING STARTED

Individuals with sensory impairment can experience many challenges that can impact on their health and well-being.

- Consider how important your sight and hearing are to your day-to-day tasks.
- Consider your other senses – smell, touch and taste – and think about how this would affect your well-being if these were impaired.

AC12.1 The term 'sensory loss'

KEY TERM

Sensory loss: mostly used to describe sight loss, hearing loss and deafblindness, but can also relate to a loss or impairment of any of the senses including sight, hearing, taste, smell and touch.

AC12.2 Causes and conditions of sensory loss

Some causes of **sensory loss** can be congenital (the individual is born with them) and some can be acquired (these occur during life due to accident or illness). Examples of conditions that could cause sensory loss include:

- glaucoma
- head trauma
- macular degeneration
- viral causes such as meningitis
- cataracts
- industrial/noise-induced deafness
- hereditary conditions such as otosclerosis
- premature birth
- viruses during pregnancy
- genetic conditions
- Ménière's disease
- cerebral palsy.

REFLECT ON IT

Ageing is the largest cause of sensory loss but it is not the only contributing factor.

- Research the conditions listed above to learn about their causes.
- Think about how this could impact on an individual in your care.

AC12.3 Potential indicators and signs of sensory loss

There are many signs and indicators of sensory loss. Some are more obvious than others. You might notice small changes over time, or a big change might happen quickly.

Sensory loss will be experienced by individuals differently, and it is important to know what the signs are so you can ensure the right care and support are offered: see Table 2.12.

Indicators of sight loss	Indicators of hearing loss	Indicators of other sensory loss
• Bumping into things • Not reacting to visual clues • Squinting in bright or dark lights • Holding reading material away or moving it closer than usual • Irises changing colour • White areas on the pupil • Difficulty with peripheral vision • Slower movements	• Speaking louder than normal • Not reacting to voices from behind • Apparent inattention • Difficulty following conversation • Stress or tiredness after conversations • Not hearing the doorbell or telephone • Turning the volume up on the radio, television or other device	• Experiencing tingling/shooting pains • Experiencing warm and cold sensations • Not feeling warm, cold or extreme heat • Inability to smell • Inability to taste • Stuffy nose • Congestion • Headaches • Weight loss • Nose bleeds • Sneezing and persistent running nose

▲ Table 2.12 Indicators of sight, hearing and other sensory loss

---

CASE STUDY

Mrs Jones lives alone and has carers visiting each day. Lately the carers have noticed some bruising to her arms and hips. When they question her about this, she says she keeps bumping into the table. They have also noticed her squinting when they turn the main lights on.

Discussion point: What could this be an indicator of?

AC12.4 Factors that impact upon an individual with sensory loss

There are a range of factors that can affect an individual with sensory loss.

- One of the biggest impacts can be communication. Individuals may not be able to follow conversation, which could lead to feeling lonely and isolated. They may become frustrated that they cannot join in.

- Sight loss may mean they struggle to recognise people and places. This can affect their ability to access information if they cannot read timetables and signs clearly.
- Sensory loss can also affect individuals' routines as they may not feel confident in doing things they usually do.
- Sensory loss can also put individuals at risk of accidents in the community if there are unexpected hazards, such as blocked pathways or no dipped curb.

AC12.5 Considerations when communicating with an individual with sight loss, hearing loss, deafblindness

Table 2.13 shows what you need to consider when communicating with an individual with sensory loss.

Sight loss	Hearing loss	Deafblindness
Stand where you can be seen.	Face the individual and speak clearly – stay in their field of vision.	Allow extra time.
Identify yourself and speak clearly.	Do not shout. Speak slowly.	Use good lighting.
Use non-verbal communication.	Use alternative communication methods, such as sign language.	Stand before a clear, plain background.
When writing, use large printed words.	Make sure hearing aids are switched on and working.	Stand in front of the individual.
Use different formats for information, for example, braille, large fonts and audio tapes.	Ask the individual to repeat what has been said.	Tactile communication – use touch with objects.
Allow for extra time.	Write things down.	Tactual communication – use touch with individuals.
	Use a loop system.	Use clear speech.
	Allow extra time.	Use the **deafblind manual alphabet**.
	Reduce background noise	

▲ Table 2.13 What you need to consider when communicating with an individual with sensory loss

KEY TERMS

Deafblindness: a combination of hearing and sight loss which affects the individual's ability to communicate, impacts on their mobility and reduces their access to information.

Deafblind manual alphabet: a method of spelling out words on an individual's hand by using signs and certain places on the hand.

AC12.6 The importance of supporting individuals to use aids such as hearing aids and glasses

Aids such as hearing aids and glasses can improve an individual's quality of life. There can be some embarrassment about needing these, and individuals can resist them as they feel it is a sign of age or having a disability.

It is important to encourage individuals to see this as a benefit and a way to maximise their hearing and sight. Using aids can help them to:

- communicate
- understand the world around them
- keep in touch with family and social networks
- lead a fulfilling and valued life.

AC12.7 The considerations when supporting an individual with loss of taste; smell or touch

Loss of taste (**hypogeusia**), smell (anosmia) or touch (**hypoesthesia**) can have a big impact on individuals' lives. They can affect their ability to enjoy the world around them and can also affect their health, for example, eating a balanced and nutritious diet.

KEY TERMS

Hypogeusia: loss of taste.
Hypoesthesia: reduced sense of touch.

Smell encourages appetite, and a loss of smell makes it harder to smell hazards such as fires or spoiled foods – we all know what sour milk smells like! Our sense of smell also helps to bring back memories which can give us a sense of well-being.

A reduced sense of touch can be the result of illness and diseases that reduce blood flow to nerve endings and increases the risk of falls and burns. Individuals with hypoesthesia need help to maintain good foot care, and they need to take care near hot objects. These individuals may not feel injuries.

When supporting an individual with loss of taste, smell or touch, it is important to be aware of these considerations and adapt your support as necessary. You may need to rely on verbal communication more:

- Explain to the individual what the food is.
- Help them to choose healthy options – even though they may not be able to taste it, they may remember what it tasted like.

You may also need to:

- Put warning signs up to stop individuals touching hot surfaces.
- Make sure fire alarms and CO_2 alarms are tested regularly, as the individual may not smell smoke or gas.

AC12.8 Support available for individuals with sensory loss

Individuals will be able to access initial support through their GP, optician or audiologist and may have access to an occupational therapist who will assist them in accessing and using aids. There are many organisations that also offer advice and support.

RESEARCH IT

There are several services to help those with a sensory loss. Spend some time researching these websites, and note what services and support they offer:

Centre of Excellence for Sensory Impairment (COESI):
www.coesi.org.uk/Home.aspx

Sense:
www.sense.org.uk/

The Royal National Institute for Deaf People:
https://rnid.org.uk/

Wales Council for Deaf People:
www.wcdeaf.org.uk/

RNIB Cymru:
www.rnib.org.uk/wales-cymru-1

Guide Dogs Cymru:
www.guidedogs.org.uk/guide-dogs-cymru/

Sight Cymru:
http://sightcymru.org.uk/

Wales Council for the Blind:
www.wcb-ccd.org.uk/perspectif/index.php

Deafblind Cymru:
https://deafblind.org.uk/about-us/deafblind-cymru/

Check your understanding

1 Where is care for terminally ill people provided?

2 As well as community nurses, which other nurses can provide end of life care in the home?

3 What does the term 'assistive technology' mean?

4 What does the term 'active participation' mean?

5 What is the medical term for loss of smell?

6 What does 'congenital sensory loss' mean?

Question practice

1 A plan detailing how an individual wishes to be cared for during the end of their life is called a:

a living will

b personal plan

c advanced care plan

d medication assessment

2 Which of the following is an example of assistive technology?

a befriending service   c meals on wheels

b hearing aid   d day centre

3 Which two of the following are potential indicators of hearing loss?

a talking louder than normal

b ignoring the telephone

c squinting at the newspaper

d white areas on the pupils

LO13 KNOW HOW LIVING WITH DEMENTIA CAN IMPACT ON THE HEALTH AND WELL-BEING OF INDIVIDUALS

GETTING STARTED

Individuals with dementia will often grow more anxious over time, and become forgetful and withdrawn. It is important that individuals are supported to stay as independent as possible.

What are some ways as a health and social care worker you could support independence with individuals living with dementia?

AC13.1 The term 'dementia'

Dementia is associated with the ongoing decline of the brain's function. It affects 1 in 14 people over the age of 65, and 1 in 6 people over the age of 80. It can be a very difficult condition to live with, and often gets worse over time. However, with early diagnoses, individuals can be supported to live fulfilled and active lives, and to access treatment that can slow the rate of decline. There are many forms of dementia, the most common are:

- Alzheimer's disease
- Lewy body dementia
- vascular dementia.

KEY TERM

Dementia: a group of symptoms that affect how you think, remember, solve problems, use language and communicate. These occur when brain cells stop working properly and the brain is damaged by disease.

AC13.2 Indicators and signs of dementia

Some signs and indicators that an individual may have dementia could be:

- memory loss/problems
- misplacing things
- difficulties with time
- problems processing new information
- problems with decision making
- visual hallucinations
- changes to behaviour
- restless
- mood swings, anxiety, depression
- communication difficulties
- lack of hand–eye co-ordination
- withdrawn or becoming isolated.

AC13.3 Ways in which dementia can affect individuals and how they experience the world

There can be huge emotional, social and psychological impacts for an individual living with dementia. The individual will suffer a series of losses as the dementia progresses.

They can become very confused and angry, leaving them feeling isolated, alone and frightened of the world and people around them. Dementia can affect their independence; as their memory declines they may not be able to remember to carry out simple everyday activities, social networks may suffer as memory and behaviour could impact on their ability to attend their social groups or see friends, and self-esteem can be affected as individuals begin to see themselves decline. Often individuals with dementia will have regressions to childlike behaviours or periods in their past. This means that the world can become a very scary place.

CASE STUDY

Lowri is 70 years old and has just been diagnosed with dementia. Lowri has always been very independent and has an active social life. Her husband passed away some years ago but her two children live nearby, and Lowri enjoys spending time with her grandchildren.

This diagnosis comes as a shock to Lowri and, though very upset, she does not tell anyone as she worries about how they will take it and how they will treat her.

Discussion point: What potential impact could this have on Lowri's health and well-being?

AC13.4 The expression 'living well with dementia'

'Living well with dementia' is a government policy that supports independence and quality of life for individuals living with dementia. It gives guidance on:

- staying socially activity
- informing others about dementia
- looking after their health
- tips to cope with living with dementia
- where support can be found.

It is important that individuals living with dementia know that they are still the same person, despite facing challenges with their memory and concentration. They should know that everyone experiences dementia differently, and their journey will be unique to them.

Ultimately, 'living well with dementia' is about encouraging individuals to focus on the things they enjoy and the things they can do – not the things they cannot do.

Dementia Roadmap Wales is an online platform that provides information about the dementia journey and gives local service information, support groups and information about living well with dementia.

RESEARCH IT

More information on the NHS guidance on living well with dementia can be found here:

www.nhs.uk/conditions/dementia/living-well-with-dementia/

AC13.5. How person-centred approaches can be used to support individuals living with dementia

We have already looked at how person-centred approaches can support individuals who are looked after, and the same applies to individuals with dementia. Person-centred care means putting the person at the centre of planning and decision making. Being person-centred when working with individuals with dementia means they can take part in the things they enjoy.

Alzheimer's Society states the following key points to being person-centred:

- Treat the person with dignity and respect.
- Understand their history, lifestyle, culture and preferences, including their likes, dislikes, hobbies and interests.
- Look at situations from the point of view of the person with dementia.
- Provide opportunities for the person to have conversations and relationships with other people.
- Ensure the person has the chance to try new things or take part in activities they enjoy.

(www.alzheimers.org.uk/about-dementia/treatments/person-centred-care)

CASE STUDY

Enid is 81 and is about to move into a residential care home because of the onset of dementia. She currently lives at home with her husband John, and they have been married for 55 years. They have two children who both live locally.

Dementia is affecting Enid's memory and she is often very confused. She keeps forgetting that she is moving, and shows extreme distress about leaving John.

Mair has been allocated as Enid's key worker to help with her move to the home, and to contribute to the development of her care plan.

Discussion points:

- What should Mair consider when supporting Enid's move into the home?
- How can Mair support the move to limit distress to Enid?
- What could be included in Enid's care and support plan to help support the transition?
- What could be the impact of this move on Enid's well-being?

AC13.6 Considerations needed when communicating with an individual living with dementia

Communication for an individual with dementia can be affected in a number of ways, and can change over time. It is important to understand the individual's communication needs and adapt to these. You should consider the following factors when communicating with an individual with dementia.

- Identify yourself – they may have trouble with their memory, so do not assume they will remember you just because you see them every day. Equally, do not assume that they will forget you; each day may be different.
- Approach them from the front, so they can see you and not be frightened by your sudden appearance.
- Speak slowly and clearly.
- Think about background noise, such as television.
- Make eye contact.
- Keep the conversation simple and focus on one topic.
- Involve them in decisions but keep choices simple.
- Use aids if needed, such as photographs of family, items or places.
- Consider any sensory impairment.
- Use positive body language and note their body language – are they showing signs of being confused or agitated, or are they listening to you and showing understanding?
- Be patient.

AC13.7 The impact that supporting and caring for an individual living with dementia can have on family/carers

It can be very difficult for family members of individuals with dementia. The illness can have a significant impact on their lives, such as having to:

- give up a job to care for a relative which may impact on their income
- move house or adapt their home to support the family member.

It can also be extremely upsetting when a family member, often a parent, forgets who you are. Family who are caring for an individual with dementia can become very stressed, develop anxiety or depression. It can be very difficult seeing their loved one decline in this way and suffer memory problems.

Caring for a family member with dementia can have a physical impact, as this may not be the carer's only work or caring responsibility. Family members caring for someone with dementia can suffer fatigue and other physical strains from manual lifting. There could also be a financial impact if someone must give up work to become the carer. If additional support is needed, there could also be a feeling of guilt.

However, there are positives to caring for a family member. Having that additional time with a loved one in the later years of their life can create lasting memories. People also gain additional skills and challenge themselves in new ways. Being a carer can be incredibly rewarding.

AC13.8 Ways in which carers can be supported to continue their role

There is support for families to continue caring for a family member with dementia.

- They can ask for a free carer's assessment to identify the support needed.
- There are often local and online support groups such as Memory cafés.
- They may be able to access respite care from their local authority or set up flexible working hours from their employers to fit around their caring responsibilities.
- There is financial support through the Carer's Allowance.
- Support can also be accessed through voluntary organisations such as Alzheimer's Society and Dementia UK.
- Dementia nurses can advise and support.
- Social care support may be available to help with personal care.
- Befrienders organisations can also be available to sit with the individual which can mean the family member is able to have some time for themselves.

AC13.9 What is meant by a 'dementia friendly community' and how this can contribute to the well-being of individuals living with dementia

A **dementia friendly community** helps to prevent individuals with dementia becoming lonely and isolated. It creates an awareness and understanding of dementia, so that individuals are not treated differently.

Dementia friendly communities support the well-being of individuals, helping them to stay in their own home for longer. They offer support for carers and understand the needs of individuals with dementia.

Many communities are now working towards being dementia friendly. Local leisure centres may run dementia friendly sessions, and local cinemas will run dementia friendly screenings. It can be helpful to support individuals to access a local dementia friendly group such as a memory café, where people with short-term memory problems can go to speak to a mental health professional or a volunteer. This can be a valuable support network where individuals with dementia can share their experiences and receive support and advice.

KEY TERM

Dementia friendly community: the local community sharing the responsibility for ensuring that people with dementia feel understood, valued and able to contribute.

RESEARCH IT

Check this web page for more information on dementia friendly communities:

www.alzheimers.org.uk/get-involved/dementia-friendly-communities

AC13.10 Support available for individuals living with dementia

An individual with dementia will need a care needs assessment by the local authority. This helps to determine the care needs of the individual and whether the local authority needs to support them.

Based on this assessment, a personal plan will be created. This should be person-centred and include the personal wishes, aspirations and care needs for the individual.

An individual with dementia can also access support from a number of sources including their GP, social services, family members, community and practice nurses as well as charities such as Dementia UK, Alzheimer's Society and the National Dementia Helpline.

Some examples of the support available might be:
- support with personal care
- support to live in your own home
- who will be caring for you and how
- what you might need support with each day.

An individual with dementia can also access support from a number of sources including:
- their GP – initial support and guidance
- social services – responsible for supporting/planning care
- family members – support with day-to-day activities and care, as well as helping with memory and supporting individuals to access support
- community and practice nurses, dementia nurses, community psychiatric nurses – providing specialist nursing care
- charities such as Dementia UK, Alzheimer's Society and the National Dementia Helpline – information about support available for individuals and families.

LO14 KNOW HOW MENTAL ILL-HEALTH CAN IMPACT UPON THE HEALTH AND WELL-BEING OF INDIVIDUALS

GETTING STARTED

Mental health has a huge impact on individuals' health and well-being. Good mental health promotes emotional health and well-being. Individuals with good mental health have the resilience to cope with difficulties and will make positive choices about their well-being.

According to the WHO, people who suffer with severe mental health conditions die prematurely due to preventable physical conditions. For example, depression has been found to have an impact on coronary disease.

Think of some of the ways you support your own mental health. This could be activities you enjoy, food you eat, support networks you access. Why is it so important to access the things that support your mental health?

AC14.1 The term 'mental ill-health'

Many individuals suffer from mental health problems from time to time. These can range from daily worries and anxieties to severe depression and suicidal thoughts.

'Mental ill-health' is when mental health problems become a more serious disorder which causes considerable stress and affects day-to-day functioning. Periods of mental ill-health can be temporary or can cause persistent and long-term difficulties.

Table 2.14 shows some examples of conditions caused by mental ill-health.

Condition	Explanation of the condition
Anxiety disorders	Anxiety is a normal emotion that we all experience, but it can become a disorder when it is felt all or most of the time and coping mechanisms do not work. Anxiety disorders can cause panic attacks.
Schizophrenia	This is a mental disorder that affect the way a person thinks.
Depression	This can range in intensity from mild to severe. Depression is a continued low mood that affects an individual's ability to enjoy their lives. People who are depressed can also have suicidal feelings.
Bipolar disorder (also known as manic depression)	This is a mood disorder that can cause periods of extreme lows (depressions) and extreme high (euphoric) moods.
Eating disorders	This causes unhealthy thoughts, feelings and behaviour about food and body shape.
Personality disorder	This can affect how a person copes with day-to-day life and relationships. It will also affect how they feel and behave.
Psychosis	This refers to a condition that makes a person perceive and see the world in a different way from those around them. They may feel that people who are trying to help them, such as professional health workers, are trying to harm them.
Self-harm	A condition that causes a person to deliberately hurt themselves. It is often linked to intense emotional distress.

▲ Table 2.14 Conditions caused by mental ill-health

RESEARCH IT

Research some of the conditions in Table 2.14 to understand their impact on an individual's well-being. You may find the following websites helpful:

www.mind.org.uk/information-support/types-of-mental-health-problems/

www.rethink.org/advice-and-information/about-mental-illness/learn-more-about-conditions/

AC14.2 Factors that can contribute or lead to mental ill-health

Everyone will go through challenging times throughout their lives, but how we react to them can be very different. There are however some common factors that will affect our mental health and influence how we respond to challenges and opportunities. A person's upbringing and environment as well as their life experiences can impact on how they cope with emotions. Genes also have an impact on mental health, and poor mental health can run in families.

Other factors that can contribute to mental ill-health conditions are:

- personal life and relationships
- traumatic life events
- substance misuse
- health issues
- money, work, housing
- significant life changes
- brain injury/head injury/**epilepsy**
- poor social skills
- discrimination
- unemployment
- domestic violence
- bullying
- low self-esteem
- lack of confidence.

We may not know exactly what causes an individual's mental ill-health, but this does not make it any less important or less serious than any other illness. It is important to recognise all mental illnesses and treat them with the individual at the centre. As mental ill-health will affect everyone differently, their treatment should be personalised to them.

KEY TERM

Epilepsy: a central nervous system disorder which causes seizures, unusual behaviour or sensations.

AC14.3 Potential indicators and signs of mental illness

Signs and indicators of mental illness can vary depending on the disorder and the circumstances around the illness and the individual. Some examples are:

- feeling sad, low mood
- lack of concentration
- confusion
- excessive fears or worries
- extreme feelings of guilt
- mood swings
- withdrawal and isolating from loved ones
- tiredness or problems with sleep
- low energy, lack of motivation
- paranoia, hallucinations or delusion
- inability to cope with daily problems
- inability to cope with stress
- suicidal thoughts
- excessive anger
- hostility or violence
- substance misuse
- change in sex drive
- self-harming behaviours
- emotional outbursts.

CASE STUDY

Bethan is 20 years old. She has learning difficulties and lives in supported housing as she needs help with daily living tasks. Bethan gets on well with the support workers who come in two to three times a day to help her. She also attends a few local classes, including a drama club which she looks forward to all week and where she has made many friends.

Recently the class has had to close temporarily, which made Bethan very upset. She has not been able to meet her friends there and really misses the club. The support workers have told her not to worry – the closure is only temporary and will open again 'in no time'. However, they give Bethan no more information, and she struggles to grasp how long she must wait.

Bethan begins to withdraw from the support staff and says she doesn't want to attend any of her other clubs. Support staff notice that she is not eating as much when they are there, and is not needing to shop for food as regularly. When they ask Bethan what is wrong, she tells them 'My friends don't like me anymore'.

Discussion points:

- What are the indicators that Bethan may be developing mental ill-health?
- How well have the staff supported Bethan in her disappointment?
- What could be done to support Bethan further?

AC14.4 The potential impact of mental ill-health on health and well-being

Left untreated, mental illness can cause severe emotional, behavioural and physical health problems. Mental illness can be life-threatening. Some of the potential impacts could include:

- unhappiness and lack of enjoyment in life
- family conflicts and relationship difficulties
- social isolation – refusing to access support or medical help
- substance misuse – individuals may turn to drugs or alcohol to cope with their illness
- impact on school or work – lack of motivation, feelings of failure or inadequacy
- financial problems or poverty
- weakened immune system from depression, affecting sleep, diet and social isolation
- heart disease and other medical conditions – stress, anxiety and depression can cause high blood pressure, reduced blood flow to the heart and higher levels of cortisol.

REFLECT ON IT

Watch the following video 'I had a black dog' taken from Matthew Johnston's book, and reflect on how:
- mental ill-health impacts on an individual's life
- you can support an individual living with mental ill-health.

https://youtu.be/XiCrniLQGYc

AC14.5 Ways in which individuals can be supported to live well with mental ill-health

There is help available for people living with mental ill-health. There are many services and support networks available. You may have to support individuals to access them and to encourage healthy lifestyles.

The support that individuals need will differ from person to person. Talk to the individual to try to find out what will help them. Some examples could be:

- talking to family and friends
- seeking professional advice
- regular health checks
- recognising the signs and symptoms
- looking after well-being
- regular sleep patterns
- exercise
- mindfulness
- local support groups
- understanding the triggers and how to cope with them
- healthy diet
- drug and alcohol support
- counselling services
- therapies such as CBT or art therapy
- helplines.

AC14.6 Positive outcomes associated with improved mental health and well-being

With improved mental health and well-being come many positive outcomes:

- There will be improved resilience and the ability to cope with difficulties. This in turn will improve mental well-being and help to give the individual a sense of confidence and good self-esteem.
- Physical health will improve – the individual will have more energy to complete physical activities, leading to improved physical health and mental well-being. Sleep may also improve.
- There will be more positivity in work – the individual may be more productive and need less time off sick.
- With a positive sense of well-being comes the ability to think clearly, make decisions and take on new challenges in a positive light.

CASE STUDY

Aled has been experiencing mental health issues and has been seeking help from a counselling service through his GP.

Discussion point: Look at the list below and note down whether you think each point is a sign of improvement or not.

- handing in a sick note
- being very indecisive
- improved sleep
- taking more regular exercise
- drinking more alcohol
- stomach upsets
- relating better to others
- spending time with friends.

AC14.7 Support available to help individuals with mental ill-health

The organisations and charities in Table 2.15 can offer help, advice and support to individuals suffering from mental ill-health and the families that care for them.

Organisation or charity	What they do
MIND Cymru www.mind.org.uk/about-us/mind-cymru/	A charity committed to improving mental health in Wales. They have many Wales-wide initiatives to support people in their community including **social prescribing** and **active monitoring**. 'Side by Side Cymru' is a joint project between Mind Cymru and local Minds in Wales. Its aim is to enable people to feel confident in delivering high quality peer support.
Mental Health Foundation www.mentalhealth.org.uk/wales	This initiative works closely with the Welsh Government to inform policy and improve services for those with mental health problems. They also act as consultant for the Welsh Government to improve individuals' and carers' involvement across Wales.
Hafal www.hafal.org/	A charity covering all areas of Wales, supporting people with mental health problems. They have a special focus on those with a serious mental illness. Their services are underpinned by their unique recovery programme of self-management and empowerment, and looking at all aspects of life.
Mental Health Wales www.mentalhealthwales.net/	An initiative set up by Hafal. This is a website offering useful links and information for mental health professionals, clinicians and individuals living with mental illness, as well as their families and carers.
Time to Change Wales www.timetochangewales.org.uk/en/need-help/	This is an initiative focused on challenging discrimination in society. It aims to remove the stigma surrounding mental health and to create a more open society where mental health problems are not hidden.

▲ Table 2.15 Charities and organisations that support mental ill-health

KEY TERMS

Social prescribing: connecting people to community services to support their health and well-being.

Active monitoring: monitoring the condition but not treating unless proven that condition is worsening.

RESEARCH IT

Choose one or two of the organisations in Table 2.15. Research how they support individuals with mental ill-health.

LO15 KNOW HOW SUBSTANCE MISUSE CAN IMPACT UPON HEALTH AND WELL-BEING OF INDIVIDUALS

GETTING STARTED

Think about harmful substances you come across on a day-to-day basis.

Many of these substances are legal and not harmful when used in the right way and in moderation. However, they can be highly addictive, and can have a very detrimental impact on an individual's health and well-being when misused.

AC15.1 The term 'substance misuse'

'Substance misuse' refers to the harmful and potentially hazardous use of substances such as alcohol, illicit and prescription drugs, glue, aerosols, cigarettes and caffeine.

When a dependency on a substance has developed, it can bring about a strong desire (addiction) to take the substance:

- An individual can find it difficult to control their use of the substance, despite harmful consequences.
- Long-term use of these substances can bring about an increased tolerance, which then means the individual needs to take more and more to get the same effect.
- If an individual does choose to stop taking the substance, they can sometimes have extreme withdrawal symptoms.

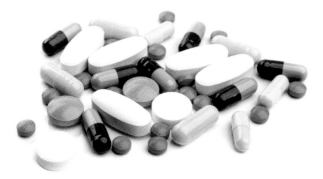

▲ Figure 2.8 Individuals can become addicted to prescription drugs

Due to its controlling nature, substance misuse may have effects on physical and mental health and well-being.

- Long-term effects can include heart disease, cancer, AIDS/HIV and hepatitis.
- Substance misuse and drug addiction can lead to mental illness, affecting the individual's memory and their ability to make decisions and control their stress levels.
- It can affect relationships and employment, and have a devastating effect on an individual's well-being.

AC15.2 Potential indicators and signs of substance misuse

Substance misuse can affect anyone, but there are some individuals who are more susceptible to addictive behaviours which will contribute to substance misuse. This could include individuals who have a family history of addictive behaviours, or who may have suffered abuse, neglect or other traumatic events in their lives. They may suffer from depression or anxiety. Many individuals start misusing substances at an early age and this continues into adulthood.

There are different methods of taking substances. and the method can contribute to addiction. Substances that are smoked or injected carry a higher addiction risk.

Some of the signs that substance misuse may be present for an individual are:

- change in their usual behaviour
- neglecting work
- sudden change in friendship groups
- neglecting family
- withdrawing from activities they previously enjoyed
- risk taking behaviour that was not usual for them
- criminal behaviour
- relationship problems
- aggression

- shaking and other withdrawal symptoms
- dilated pupils
- bloodshot eyes
- sleep problems
- anxiety and depression.

RESEARCH IT

Research drug and alcohol misuse symptoms, including withdrawal symptoms, and what to look out for.

AC15.3 The potential impact of substance misuse on the health and well-being of individuals

As we have discussed above, substance misuse can have a huge impact on all aspects of an individual's physical and mental health and well-being. There is a high risk that their relationships will break down and they might become unemployed and homeless.

Substance misuse can be life-threatening for physical health:

- It can affect a person's weight and make them more susceptible to infections and chronic diseases.
- They may have heart and circulation problems and even organ failure.
- Other physical effects include bad breath and tooth decay, bloodshot eyes, nausea and vomiting, skin problems and rashes.

Substance misuse can also cause mental ill-health.

- It can cause depression and anxiety, psychosis and paranoia.
- Individuals with substance misuse problems can be more aggressive, lose self-control, and suffer cognitive impairment and memory loss.

Substance misuse can take over an individual's life, destroy all or parts of their personal and professional life, and even end their life.

AC15.4 Support available to individuals who misuse substances

There are many local and national initiatives that offer support for those trying to beat drug or alcohol addiction.

- **CAIS Drug and Alcohol Counselling** – for people who are concerned about their own or someone else's drinking or drug taking.
- **Dan 24/7** – a free helpline to talk in confidence about struggles.
- **New Link Wales** – this organisation has developed a programme called First Steps Recovery, aimed at creating individualised services to help recovery.
- **Recovery Cymru** – a self-help and support community.
- **EDAS** – a single point of entry into treatment and support. They also support family and carers looking for guidance and support.
- **Narcotics Anonymous, Alcoholics Anonymous and Cocaine Anonymous** – self-help groups attended by those in recovery from addiction.

RESEARCH IT

Research some of these support initiatives and learn more about the work they do.

Check your understanding

1 What is a 'dementia friendly community'?

2 What is a definition of 'dementia'?

3 When do mental health problems become a mental illness or disorder?

4 Left untreated, how can mental ill-health affect physical health?

5 What does the term 'substance misuse' mean?

6 How can substance misuse affect mental health?

7 Do all substance users become addicted?

Question practice

1 After a care needs assessment is carried out, what document will then be created?

   a a risk assessment

   b a health assessment

   c a personal plan

   d a behavioural plan

2 Which two illnesses shown here are examples of mental health disorder?

   a bipolar

   b epilepsy

   c Parkinson's disease

   d anxiety

3 What can mental ill-health have an impact on?

   a relationships

   b finances

   c immune system

   d all of the above

4 Which type of mental health condition is anorexia?

   a bipolar

   b personality disorders

   c eating disorders

   d depression

5 Substance misuse can cause psychosis. Which of the following categories does it fall into?

   a physical

   b mental

   c financial

   d social

6 Substance misuse can cause job losses. Which of the following categories does it fall into?

   a physical

   b mental

   c financial

   d social

7 Which two of the following early childhood experiences can be a contributing factor to substance misuse?

   a moving schools

   b suffering abuse

   c loss of a parent

   d poor grades

FURTHER READING AND RESEARCH

Weblinks

A document to support the positive impact of physical activity:
www.mentalhealth.org.uk/sites/default/files/lets-get-physical-report.pdf

Mind is a charity that has a lot of help, advice and guidance on supporting physical and mental health and combating mental ill-health:
www.mind.org.uk

To read more about attachment theory, you may find the following websites useful:
www.simplypsychology.org/attachment.html

www.verywellmind.com/what-is-attachment-theory-2795337

To find out more about the Social Services and Well-Being (Wales) Act, you will find lots of useful information on the Social Care Wales website:
https://socialcare.wales/hub/sswbact

The Code of Professional Practice for Social Care can be found on the Social Care Wales website:
https://socialcare.wales/dealing-with-concerns/codes-of-practice-and-guidance#section-29491-anchor

HEALTH AND WELL-BEING (CHILDREN AND YOUNG PEOPLE)

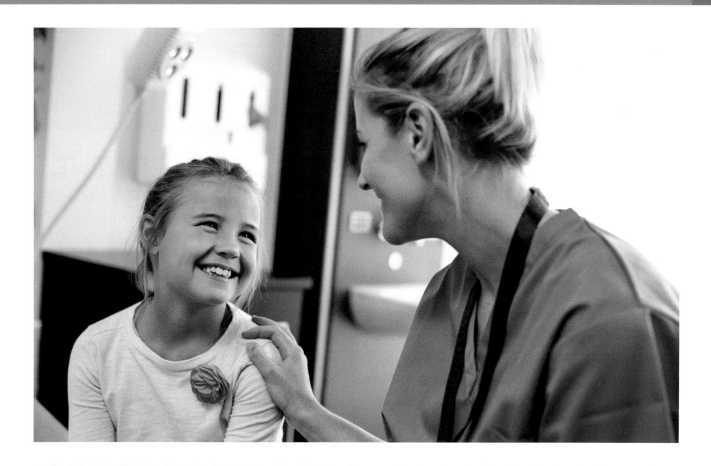

ABOUT THIS UNIT

Guided learning hours: 80 hours

In this unit you will learn about what well-being is and the factors that impact on the health and well-being of children and young people during different stages of development. You will gain an understanding of attachment, resilience and positive relationships as well as how children and young people can stay healthy. During this unit you will:

- look at how environments can support health, well-being and development, gain an understanding of holistic development and how the environment can support this.
- analyse the importance and value of play and how this supports children, through looking at different types of play and the use of environment, equipment and materials.
- develop an understanding of speech, language and communication and the importance of early intervention and different avenues of support available.
- look at how to provide advice guidance and support for making positive choices, and the roles and responsibilities related to administering medication, including legislation and guidance.
- learn about the importance of personal care, nutrition and hydration to health and well-being.

Learning outcomes
LO1: Know what well-being means in the context of health and social care
LO2: Know the factors that impact on the health and well-being of children and young people
LO3: Know the environments that support health, well-being and development of children and young people
LO4: Understand the role of play in supporting the health, well-being and development of children
LO5: Understand speech, language and communication development
LO6: Know how to support the health, well-being and development of children with additional support needs
LO7: Know how to provide advice, guidance and support to children and young people and their families that helps to make positive choices about their health and well-being
LO8: Understand the roles and responsibilities related to the administration of medication in social care settings
LO9: Know how to support children and young people with their personal care
LO10: Understand the importance of nutrition and hydration for the health and well-being of children and young people

LO1 KNOW WHAT WELL-BEING MEANS IN THE CONTEXT OF HEALTH AND SOCIAL CARE

GETTING STARTED

Look back at Unit 003, LO1, section AC1.1 for definitions of well-being and to refresh your learning on this topic.

AC1.1. The term 'well-being' and its importance

When we think about well-being for children and young people, it is important to recognise the role it plays in supporting them to overcome difficulties, grow in confidence, and develop life skills and social skills which will support them into adulthood.

RESEARCH IT

There is legislation and guidance that supports the well-being of children and young people. You may wish to research and read up on the following:

- Well-Being of Future Generations (Wales) Act 2015
- Seven core aims for children and young people in Wales
- Welsh Government Foundation Phase.

AC1.2 Factors that affect the well-being of children and young people

See Unit 003, LO1, section AC1.2 for a list of factors that affect well-being and Table 2.1 for factors that negatively impact on well-being. Other factors that may be relevant for children and young people include:

- Play – children and young people should have access to varied play opportunities. Through play children develop social skills as well as physical and cognitive skills. Play can also be a useful tool for children to express their feelings, concerns and worries
- Home background – if a child or young person is living in a stable, supportive and caring home environment, they are more likely to have their health and well-being needs met. A positive home environment can also be the source of positive role models, which play a huge part in child development. Having access to positive role models can support children and young people to make positive choices about their well-being
- Attachment – attachment, which plays an important role in everyone's well-being, is particularly important for children and young people as it is during their early years that it is formed. A secure attachment will help children and young people to develop and grow resilience which they will take with them into adulthood.

REFLECT ON IT

Watch the following video on ACEs by Public Health Network Cymru:

https://youtu.be/YiMjTzCnbNQ

- What factors impacted on your well-being?
- Were these positive or negative experiences?

AC1.3 The importance of families and 'significant others' in the well-being of children and young people

Families and '**significant others**' are important for the support of well-being for children and young people. As humans, we desire a sense of belonging, and this can be nurtured by our families and significant others.

- A secure attachment to a parent or care giver allows the child or young person to feel safe and protected. They will have a secure base to explore the world from.
- A positive relationship with a teacher can help a child to grow and develop academically, helping them to determine their future path. It will give the child or young person the confidence to try new experiences and believe in their own abilities.

Early childhood experiences will have an impact on later adult experiences. If these are negative early experiences, the child or young person might not develop the resilience and life skills they need for adulthood.

Families and significant others also help to monitor health and well-being and may see signs that something is wrong. They can intervene to get the child or young person the care and support they need. Having someone they trust means that children and young people may open up more about their concerns and fears, or may highlight something is going well for them.

AC1.4 Ways of working that support well-being

When supporting the well-being of children and young people, you can do a number of things:

- Understand the child's likes and interests –do this by talking to the child or young person, and really listening to what they have to say.
- Support their positive relationships and friendships, and encourage them to spend time with these people.
- Encourage respect and diversity, show respect for the young person and encourage them to be inclusive to others.
- Arrange a variety of activities for children and young people to explore.
- Encourage positive risk taking.
- Encourage decision making, and allow children and young people to make their own choices and solve their own problems.
- Support positive routines in order to give consistency and help set boundaries. This helps the child or young person to feel safe and in control.
- Focus on the positives and reinforce this behaviour.
- Give praise and encouragement.
- Encourage a healthy diet, good sleep patterns and exercise to promote good physical and mental health.
- Encourage independence and give appropriate levels of responsibility.
- Set age-appropriate goals and challenges.
- Encourage children and young people to resolve their own conflicts, to negotiate and to solve problems. Support them to be focused on solutions.
- Educate children and young people about the importance of staying safe, including **e-safety**.
- If there is any concern about a child or young person's well-being, refer them to services that can help, such as Children and Adolescent Mental Health Services (CAMHS), health visitor, school nurse, GP.

KEY TERMS

e-safety: being safe on the internet.
Significant others: important people, other than family, in a child or young person's life.

L02 KNOW THE FACTORS THAT IMPACT ON THE HEALTH AND WELL-BEING OF CHILDREN AND YOUNG PEOPLE

GETTING STARTED

It is important to understand the stages of development for children and young people. By understanding these milestones, you are able to see if a child may need additional support. If the stages are not met, you can ask why and analyse what factors may be impacting on the child's development. Through early intervention, you can determine what care and support that child may need.

Think about a child who may not be meeting the physical milestone of walking. Why might early intervention help?

AC2.1 Stages of child development and factors that can affect it

We can look at the stages of **child development** under the following four areas of development:

1 Physical development: physical growth and the ability to use the body.
2 Intellectual development: the growth of the child's ability to think and reason.
3 Emotional development: the growth of a child's feelings and understanding of emotion.
4 Social development: the growth of a child's abilities to understand the world around them and develop relationships with others.

During different stages in a child's life, there are certain milestones they will be expected to hit. These will vary dependent on each child and it is important to remember that just because a child may be later hitting some milestones than others, it doesn't necessarily mean there is a problem. We will look at the above stages of development in the following age groups:

- 0–2 years (infancy)
- 3–12 years (childhood)
- 13–19 years (adolescence).

KEY TERM

Child development: the sequence of language, physical, emotional and thought changes that occur from childhood to adulthood.

Stages of development 0–2 years

Physical development	
Between 0–3 months, a baby can: • slightly lift their head when lying on their stomach • hold their head up for a few seconds with support • open and shut their hands • pull at their own hands • use **rooting** and sucking reflexes	**Between 3–6 months,** a baby can: • bring an object they are holding to their mouths • roll over • grab and play with toys • reach for objects • sit up (with pillows to prop them up) • support their weight on their legs when held up • begin to eat solid food
Between 6–9 months, a baby can: • crawl • grasp and pull objects towards their own body • transfer toys and objects from one hand to the other • keep hands open and relaxed most of the time	**Between 9–12 months,** a baby can: • move easily from crawling position to sitting • sit for long periods • crawl up stairs • walk while holding onto furniture

▲ Table 3.1 Physical development 0–2 years

Physical development	
Between 6–9 months, a baby can: • pick up small finger food • sit up without being supported • reach for objects that are out of the way	**Between 9–12 months,** a baby can: • take first steps alone • stand alone • point with index finger • turn the pages of a book (several at a time) • pick up and throw objects • roll a ball
Between 1 and 2 years, a baby can: • pick things up while standing up • walk backwards • walk up and down stairs without assistance • move and sway to music • colour or paint by moving the entire arm • scribble with markers or crayons	• turn knobs and handles • jump • pull toys behind them while walking • begin to run • kick a ball • build a tower of 5 blocks

▲ Table 3.1 Physical development 0–2 years *(continued)*

KEY TERM

Rooting: a baby's natural reflex to root for their mother's milk.

Intellectual development	
Between 0–3 months, a baby can: • see objects within a distance of 13 inches • focus on faces of caregivers • recognise familiar voices • respond to their environment with facial expressions	**Between 3–6 months,** a baby can: • recognise familiar faces • recognise and react to familiar sounds • begin to imitate facial expressions • coo, squeal, and gurgle • cry according to need • communicate through body movements – waving arms and legs, opening up hands • show boredom by crying or fussing • practise turn-taking when 'talking' with caregivers • start testing cause and effect, such as seeing what happens when shaking a toy
Between 6–9 months, a baby can: • use babbling talk to get attention • use different sounds for different needs • mimic sounds, inflections, gestures • anticipate food on sight • begin to show interest in colours • make 'raspberry' sounds • smile at a reflection of themselves in the mirror • mimic facial movements • follow moving objects with their eyes	**Between 9–12 months,** a baby can: • put vowels and consonants together • use their tongue to change sound • say 'dada' and 'mama' • look for a toy that has been dropped • find partially hidden objects • explore visually and by putting objects in their mouth • understand simple requests • respond to 'no' by shaking their head
Between 1 and 2 years, a baby can: • recognise the names of familiar people, objects and body parts • use 2 words together • follow simple instructions (1 or 2 steps) • begin to sort objects by shapes and colour • tell the difference between 'me' and 'you' • imitate the actions and language of adults	

▲ Table 3.2 Intellectual development 0–2 years

Emotional development	
Between 0–3 months, a baby will: • communicate emotions through crying • feel comforted by someone familiar • have positive responses to touch • become quiet when picked up • show happiness and sadness	**Between 3–6 months,** a baby will: • seek comfort and cry when uncomfortable • express excitement by waving their arms and legs • start laughing aloud
Between 6–9 months, a baby will: • express a number of emotions including happiness, sadness, fear, and anger • show frustration when a toy is taken away • will begin to understand others' emotions (an angry voice, for example, can make a baby frown) • start sucking their thumb or holding a toy or a blanket for comfort	**Between 9–12 months,** a baby: • may begin having separation anxiety • will start to develop self-esteem • will respond to positive feedback by clapping • may cling to one parent or both
Between 1 and 2 years, a baby: • will begin to feel jealousy when not the centre of attention • will show frustration easily • will react to changes in daily routines • may have tantrums and show aggression by biting	

▲ Table 3.3 Emotional development 0–2 years

Social development	
Between 0–3 months, a baby will: • enjoy social stimulation and smiling at people • respond to touch • respond to love and affection • imitate facial expressions	**Between 3–6 months,** a baby: • begins to play with people • may cry when playing stops • will respond to their own name • will raise their arms to signal 'pick me up' • will turn their head towards someone speaking
Between 6–9 months, a baby will: • want to take part in activities with people • point to things for a reason • seek attention	**Between 9–12 months,** a baby will: • hold out their arms and legs while being dressed • mimic simple actions • imitate other children • repeat sounds or movements that make people laugh • always need to be within sight and hearing of their caregiver • display affection in hugs, kisses, pats, and smiles
Between 1 and 2 years, a baby: • enjoys playing alone for short periods • likes to do things without help • has trouble sharing and may hit, push, and grab to keep toys • demonstrates concern for others • is wary of adults they don't know	

▲ Table 3.4 Social development 0–2 years

The stages of development: 3–12 years

Physical developments	
Between 3–5, a child can: • walk backwards and forwards, and turn and stop well • jump off low steps or objects but finds it hard to jump over objects • begin to ride tricycles • skip unevenly • run well • stand on one foot for five seconds or more • use alternative feet when walking down stairs • jump on a small trampoline • hold a pencil in a pincer grip • make shapes out of playdough • use round tipped scissors • start to colour neatly	**Between 6–9,** a child can: • walk backwards quickly • skip and run with speed • jump over objects and from a height • co-ordinate movements for swimming or bike riding • have increased co-ordination for catching and throwing • participate in active games with rules • have improved reaction time in responding to thrown balls • dress themselves and tie shoelaces • be independent in all aspects of self-care • learn to write within the lines
Between 10–12, a child: • will enjoy team sports • will be able to swim • can use adult type tools such as a hammer or saw • will have improved handwriting • will start puberty between the ages of 10 and 14 if a girl	

▲ Table 3.5 Physical development 3–12 years

Intellectual development	
Between 3–5, a child can: • understand two or three simple things to do at once • sort objects by size and type • start to use pitch and tone • start to use the past tense • extend their vocabulary towards 1000–1500 words	**Between 6–9,** a child: • can understand similarities and differences • is beginning to understand more complex grammar • is a fluent speaker, able to make up stories • can handle books well and read for pleasure by 9 • understands that text carries meaning • will take a lively interest in certain subjects • will read aloud • will be able to spell certain words
Between 10–12, a child: • can use and understand very complex language • will become interested in social issues • will ask lots of questions and argue if they disagree with a point of view • will realise that thoughts are private and that people see others differently from how they see themselves • can start to predict the consequences of an action • will begin to use social media, friends and the news to get information and form opinions • will develop a better sense of responsibility • will start to understand how things are connected	

▲ Table 3.6 Intellectual development 3–12 years

Emotional development	
Between 3–5, a child will: • become less egocentric • be more even-tempered and co-operative with parents • express more awareness of other people's feelings • show an understanding of right and wrong	**Between 6–9,** a child: • may begin to develop fears • will be conscious of self-image and may not want parents to kiss them in public • may develop an interest in collecting things • will have a conscious understanding of right and wrong
Between 10–12, a child: • will be uncertain about puberty and changes to their bodies • will be insecure or have mood swings and struggle with self-esteem (especially in girls) • may develop body image and eating problems • will be more aware of their own body and will want privacy	

▲ Table 3.7 Emotional development 3–12 years

Social development	
Between 3–5, a child will: • enjoy dramatic, imaginative play with other children • enjoy competitive games but will want to win • get better at sharing and taking turns with other children • begin to feel more secure and able to cope with unfamiliar surroundings and adults for periods of time • become more co-operative with adults and like to help	**Between 6–9,** a child: • is becoming less dependent on close adults for support • enjoys being in groups of other children of similar age • is becoming more aware of their own gender • develops understanding that certain kinds of behaviour are not acceptable • will have a strong sense of fairness and justice • starts to form closer friendships at about 8 • likes to play with same-sex friends • still needs an adult to help to sort out arguments and disagreements in play • can be arrogant and bossy, or shy and uncertain
Between 10–12, a child: • will be strongly influenced by peer group • will want to fit in with peer group rules • is becoming increasingly independent from family • has a deeper understanding of how relationships with others can include more than just common interests • might have a first crush or pretend to have crushes to fit in with peers	

▲ Table 3.8 Social development 3–12 years

The stages of development: 13–19 years

Physical development	
Between 13–15: • girls' body fat increases • boys' muscle mass increases • girls' breasts enlarge • boys' genitals enlarge • both boys' and girls' voices lower, with boys' voices lowering much more • girls experience their first menstrual cycle • body hair grows • young people may sweat more as their sweat glands become more active • young people may develop acne due to hormonal changes • boys may experience a growth spurt	**Between 16–19:** • boys will grow facial hair • girls are usually at full development • young people will see an increase in strength and co-ordination • young people will have full adult motor skills by 19

▲ Table 3.9 Physical development 13–19 years

Intellectual development	
Between 13–15, young people will:	**Between 16–19,** young people:
<ul><li>start to question school and family rules</li><li>have very distinct views – something is right or wrong, good or bad</li><li>be unable to plan or think into the future</li><li>become confident in their own knowledge</li><li>develop intellectual curiosity</li><li>start to experiment</li><li>have idealistic views</li></ul>	<ul><li>are better at solving problems than younger teens, but are inconsistent</li><li>tend to make rash decisions, even though they weigh the consequences first</li><li>have improved organisational skills and are better at balancing school, activities, social life and work</li><li>will explore job and college options, religion, social and political issues</li><li>will frequently question and challenge rules</li></ul>

▲ Table 3.10 Intellectual development 13–19 years

Emotional development	
Between 13–15, young people are:	**Between 16–19,** young people:
<ul><li>egocentric – 'it's all about me!'</li><li>moody</li><li>full of self-doubt</li><li>becoming aware of their sexual orientation</li></ul>	<ul><li>are more self-assured</li><li>are excited but overwhelmed by thoughts of the future</li><li>can experience depression</li><li>now have a fully developed moral conscience</li></ul>

▲ Table 3.11 Emotional development 13–19 years

Social development	
Between 13–15, a young person will:	**Between 16–19,** a young person:
<ul><li>think that friends are more important than family</li><li>complain about lack of privacy</li><li>fluctuate between clinging to adults and rebelling against them</li><li>start to form an identity, through hobbies, friends, clothes, hairstyles, music</li><li>often push the limits of adults to assert their independence</li><li>spend a lot of time on their phone or social media chatting to friends</li></ul>	<ul><li>is more self-assured</li><li>is excited but overwhelmed by thoughts of the future</li><li>can experience depression</li><li>now has a fully developed moral conscience</li><li>may feel like they are in love</li><li>will begin to have strong sexual urges and may become sexually active</li></ul>

▲ Table 3.12 Social development 13–19 years

Factors that can affect development

There may be a number of contributing factors that affect the stages of development, which has an impact on how and when these milestones are met. Factors include but are not limited to:

- The birth – was there trauma to baby or mother? Was the baby premature? Was their birth weight low?

- Other biological factors – was the mother healthy during pregnancy? Are there any physical health conditions present? Is there good access to health services?
- Environmental factors – such as housing and education.
- Social factors – attachment, parenting styles (see below for more on attachment).

We will look at the following four factors that affect development in more detail in the next section, AC2.2: physical, social and emotional, economic and environment.

It is important to understand that the rate of development and the sequence of development are different.

- The sequence of development tends to focus on the pattern or order of development. For example, it is expected that a child will crawl or walk before they can run.
- The rate of development is the speed in which this order is achieved.

The sequence is a common order in most children, but the rate will vary and is not usually an indicator that there is a problem.

AC2.2 Factors that may affect the health, well-being and personal, physical, social and emotional development of children and young people and the impact that this might have on them

Physical factors that can affect development

Genetic inheritance

Children can be born with a genetic disorder. All children inherit genes from their parents, and a genetic disorder means that there is an abnormal gene in their genetic make-up. However, not all conditions are inherited, for example, Down's syndrome. Some defective genes can cause conditions that cause ill-health, shown in Table 3.13.

Genetic condition	The effect of the genetic condition
Fragile X syndrome	A genetic disorder causing mild-to-moderate intellectual disability as well as behavioural and learning challenges. • Physical features can include a long, narrow face, large ears, flexible fingers. • Males are more frequently affected than females and generally will be more severely affected. • Behavioural characteristics can include ADHD, autism spectrum disorder, hand biting, hand flapping, poor eye contact, social anxieties, aggression, sensory disorders.
Muscular dystrophy	There are two main types of muscular dystrophy: • Becker muscular dystrophy – a genetic disorder causing muscle-wasting conditions. This disorder usually only affects males. Over time, muscles weaken which can lead to severe and increasing disabilities. In some cases, muscular dystrophy can lead to life-threatening health problems due to the heart and breathing muscles weakening. • Duchenne muscular dystrophy – this can be less severe than the Becker. It also affects mainly males: around 100 boys with Duchenne muscular dystrophy are born in the UK each year.
Sickle cell anaemia	A red blood cell disorder which hinders the production of healthy red blood cells which carry oxygen throughout your body. Normally red blood cells are round and move easily; with sickle cell anaemia, they are shaped like sickles or crescent moons, which means that they cannot move as easily around the body.

▲ Table 3.13 Genetic conditions and their effects →

Genetic condition	The effect of the genetic condition
Cystic fibrosis	A hereditary disease affecting the lungs and digestive system. It causes sticky mucus to build up and causes infections in the lungs and difficulties in digesting food. • This disorder is usually diagnosed through the **heel prick test**, and if positive the child will start to develop symptoms in early childhood. • Over time the condition becomes worse, and the lungs and digestive system will become increasingly damaged. • Life expectancy is shortened, despite a number of treatments available to reduce problems and promote quality of life.
Haemophilia	A very rare condition which affects the blood's ability to clot. It is more common in males and is hereditary. • Haemophilia can be mild to severe, depending on the level of clotting factors the individuals have. • Individuals will find they have nosebleeds for longer, bleeding wounds take a long time to stop, their gums are more prone to bleeding and they bruise easily. • They will also have internal bleeding that will cause pain and stiffness.
Hunter syndrome	A very rare, inherited genetic disorder. • It is caused when the body does not have enough of an enzyme called iduronate 2-sulfatase, an enzyme that breaks down complex molecules. • Without enough of the enzyme, the molecules build up in harmful quantities. • This causes permanent damage which affects appearance, mental development, physical abilities and organ function. • It affects more boys than girls, and symptoms normally begin around 2–4 years of age.
Thalassaemia	An inherited blood disorder. • This causes the body to make an abnormal or inadequate amount of **haemoglobin**, which is used by red blood cells to carry oxygen around the body. • This disorder can result in individuals becoming highly **anaemic**. Symptoms include tiredness, shortness of breath and pale skin.
Huntington's disease	An inherited disease that, over time, stops parts of the brain working properly. • This condition becomes worse over time and is usually fatal. • Symptoms usually start at 30–50 years of age and include depression, memory problems, difficulty concentrating, clumsiness, jerking movements of the limbs, difficulties swallowing, speaking and breathing, decreased mobility.

▲ Table 3.13 Genetic conditions and their effects *(continued)*

So how can these physical conditions affect development?

- As well as the physical effects, children may need to miss school due to their condition, which will impact on their intellectual development.
- They may also find there is an impact on their social and emotional development. They may miss opportunities to develop or maintain friendships – friendship groups can move on quickly in childhood, and being away from school and friends may mean that the child is left out.

KEY TERMS

Heel prick test: a small sample of the newborn baby's blood is taken from the heel to carry out testing for rare but serious health conditions.

Haemoglobin: protein found in red blood cells that carries oxygen round the body.

Anaemic: a decrease of haemoglobin in the blood.

RESEARCH IT

Look again at Table 3.13, and research each condition. Can you find a description for each one?

Disabilities

There are several disabilities that can impact on the development of children. These can be disabilities the child is born with, or ones that they acquire at any stage of life due to accident, disease or degeneration. Disabilities can be categorised:

- Sensory disabilities – autism, blindness or poor vision, deafness or hearing loss, anosmia, somatosensory impairment (the inability to feel heat, pain or light touch).
- Physical disabilities – cerebral palsy, spina bifida, dwarfism, muscular dystrophy, multiple sclerosis.
- Learning disabilities – Down's syndrome, Williams syndrome. It is important to note that while autism is **not** a learning disability, some individuals with autism will have some level of learning disabilities.
- Acquired disability – head trauma, spinal injury, post-traumatic stress, loss of limbs, arthritis, multiple sclerosis, mental illness.

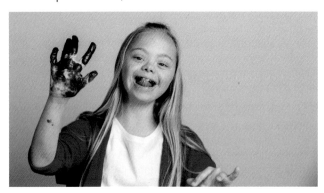

▲ Figure 3.1 A child with Down's syndrome

See Unit 003, AC2.2 for definitions of some of these disorders.

RESEARCH IT

Take the list above and research each area of disability, looking at some of the conditions in more detail.

You may want to refer to these videos about disability awareness:

Sensory disability:

https://youtu.be/LU0dQXJ-YQM

Physical disability:

https://youtu.be/CL8GMxRW_5Y

Learning disability:

https://youtu.be/tfkVA2BKIyY

Diet and nutrition

The benefits of a good, healthy diet cannot be underestimated.

- Through diet we can have increased energy, improved mood, healthy weight, clearer skin, good quality sleep.
- Diet can help to lower the risk of chronic health conditions such as heart disease, cancer and stroke.

Keeping hydrated has positive effects on the body including good oral health, good cardiovascular health, regulating body temperature, helping muscles work efficiently and keeping the kidneys working well.

Table 3.14 shows the effect of breastfeeding and weaning on the physical development of babies.

Stages in a baby's diet	Effect on development
Breastfeeding	It is important that children are given access to healthy diet and nutrition. Health professionals promote breastfeeding for at least the first six months of life: studies have shown that this gives the baby the best start in life and improves the health and development of infants by lowering the risk of: • sudden infant death syndrome (SIDS) • infection • childhood leukaemia • obesity • diarrhoea and vomiting • cardiovascular disease in later life. The benefits of breastfeeding are not just to the baby though. There are benefits to the mother as well, such as a reduction in the risk of: • breast cancer • ovarian cancer • obesity • cardiovascular disease • osteoporosis (weak bones).
Weaning	For the first six months of life, babies should only be given breastmilk or formula. After six months, foods should be introduced gradually. There are some foods that should be introduced one at a time, such as cow's milk, eggs, food containing gluten, soya, nuts and seeds, fish and shellfish. This is because if a baby did have an allergic reaction, it would be easier to determine which food caused it.

▲ Table 3.14 How a baby's diet affects their physical development

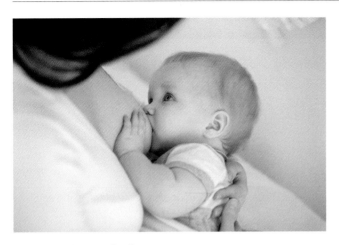

▲ Figure 3.2 Breastfeeding

Physical activity

Physical activity for children is not simply about keeping physically healthy – there are a number of benefits to their development and well-being.

Small children should be encouraged to move as much as possible through active play. This will:

- have positive effects on their co-ordination and muscle development
- support a healthy weight
- improve cardiovascular health
- support learning and social skills.

According to the NHS, as children grow older and move into adolescence, they will need to ensure they do two types of activities a week to stay healthy. For example:

- aerobic exercise – swimming, running, or games such as tag
- exercise for strengthening bones and muscles – gymnastics, dance, bike riding, climbing trees.

(www.nhs.uk/live-well/exercise/physical-activity-guidelines-children-and-young-people/)

CASE STUDY

Ava is seven months old, and her mother started weaning her a month ago. However she is constantly being sick and has diarrhoea. The health visitor asks what food Ava is being given. Her mother blends everything the rest of the family eats with water or milk, and feeds it to Ava.

Discussion point: What advice should the health visitor give to Ava's mother?

Play

Play is essential to the development of babies, children and young people. It is not simply something that gives them enjoyment but also contributes to their physical, social, cognitive and emotional well-being and development.

Play promotes brain development and learning in babies and younger children. It also decreases the risk of health problems such as diabetes, obesity and cardiovascular disease, as play helps to improve physical health through keeping children active.

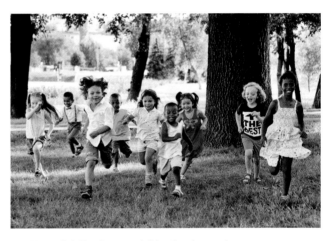

▲ Figure 3.3 Play is essential for development

We will look at play in more detail in LO4 later in this unit, but Table 3.15 shows some of the benefits to health and well-being of playing.

Type of play	How this benefits child development
Outdoor play	This type of play promotes movement. Children have space to run, jump, throw, catch, hide, climb. They can learn about the environment around them, which can spark their interest in nature. Outdoor play supports their physical development, including: • maintaining a healthy weight • developing gross motor skills • improving cardiovascular health • developing co-ordination • improving self- confidence.
Imaginative or creative play	Children can express themselves through arts and crafts, develop an understanding of the world and form friendships through role play. Their cognitive development can improve through playing with puzzles, building blocks and construction toys such as Lego. Some of the developmental benefits include: • improves fine motor skills • builds resilience • promotes cognitive skills • develops social skills and knowledge of the world • promotes mental well-being.

▲ Table 3.15 The benefits of play

Experience of illness and disease

Illnesses can impact on a child's growth and development.

- Minor illnesses such as coughs and colds, tonsillitis and tummy bugs can cause absences from school. These could have a minor impact on the child's intellectual and social development, especially if they happen frequently.
- More serious illnesses such as meningitis and measles can leave the child with a long-term disability, such as sight or hearing loss.

There are other conditions that can affect development opportunities, such as being unable to participate in physical activities or being out of school for multiple hospital visits. Children may feel they are treated differently because of their illness, and this in turn can impact on their mental health.

Some illnesses that can affect growth and development include:

- Crohn's disease
- coeliac disease
- asthma
- congenital heart defects
- cystic fibrosis
- long-term kidney disease.

Social and emotional factors that can affect development

Gender

Issues such as gender stereotypes, gender inequality and transgender issues can all impact on the development of children and young people. Children and their parents are still exposed to gender-based stereotypes, such as pink and blue clothes, boys' and girls' toys. Children might be teased if they choose to play with toys that break the stereotype. It is important to challenge these gender stereotypes and ensure that children are encouraged to have free play and choose whatever toys they wish to play with.

Children who are transgender might experience discrimination, social exclusion and harassment, which can have a long and devastating impact on their mental well-being. However, being able to express their gender identity and being supported to do so can improve their health and well-being.

Types of family

Type of family	How the type of family affects children's development
Single parent	• The parent and child can form a very strong bond, but there can also be feelings of grief, isolation and envy. • Money problems can cause stress and anxiety if there is only one wage-earner in the family. • Single parents often need to seek out others as additional role models in their wider family and networks.
Nuclear	As long as the relationship between the parents is loving and respectful, and they support their children, the children will form strong attachments and grow up with security, resilience and a strong sense of self-worth.
Same-sex	There are very few differences between same-sex and nuclear families.
Foster	Children who move into foster families have often suffered abuse or neglect before they reach their foster family. This can impact on their development and can also mean they have trust issues. However, with the right love and support, children can go on to form positive attachment to their foster families and overcome their problems.
Stepfamilies	Though becoming more common, there are positive and negative aspects to this type of family. • Some children thrive in the larger family, having more children to play with and seeing their parents in happy relationships. • However, there can be resentment and unresolved issues of guilt. • Step-parents can find it difficult to parent the children of their partner.
Childless	• Couples may make the decision to remain childless, for many reasons. This can bring a sense of well-being and strength to their relationship as they made this choice together. • However, if this decision is forced by being unable to have children, it can put a strain on the individuals and their relationship.

▲ Table 3.16 Types of family and their effect on child development

> **REFLECT ON IT**
>
> • What type of family did you grow up in?
> • What were the positive and negative aspects to this for your own development?

Parenting styles

Parenting styles can have a big impact on children's health, well-being and development. This is why the role of the parent is so important for children, and can have a long-term impact right through to adulthood.

There has always been a general consensus that there are four parenting styles (developed by psychologist Diana Baumrind):

• authoritative
• authoritarian (or dictatorial)
• indulgent (or permissive)
• neglectful.

However, more recently newer styles of parenting have emerged, including attachment parenting and free-range parenting.

Parenting style	Effect of this style on child development
Indulgent/permissive	While very loving, there is little discipline with this style of parenting. Children brought up by indulgent parents will have high self-esteem and feel very secure, but can tend to have a strong sense of entitlement and lack problem solving skills. They may struggle to make decisions.
Neglectful	These parents will be emotionally absent and not meet their children's most basic needs. This can affect children's ability to form positive relationships – it can cause mental ill-health through stress and anxiety, and the risk of behavioural problems throughout life is higher.
Authoritative	These parents will set high expectations for their children, but they do so in a loving and caring way. • The home environment is one of support, and children are brought up with clearly defined boundaries and a degree of independence appropriate to their age. • These children will form strong, healthy, successful relationships and are also less likely to give in to peer pressure.

▲ Table 3.17 Types of parenting style

Parenting style	Effect of this style on child development
Authoritarian/ disciplinarian	These parents will also set high expectations but without their loving and nurturing environment. • Children are told what to do and given little decision making options for themselves. • Making mistakes is not tolerated and punishment is often harsh. This type of parenting can make children grow up thinking that obedience gains them love and acceptance. They can develop behaviour problems such as aggression, have low self-esteem and can be anxious around others.
Attachment	Attachment parenting has become popular in recent years and focuses on forming a strong bond between parent and children, with parents being highly receptive and attuned to their child's needs. • Attachment theory was pioneered by psychologist John Bowlby and this parenting style uses that theory, claiming that babies of attachment parents cry less and have fewer behaviour problems. • However, many argue that following the eight principles of attachment parenting is not the only way to form a secure bond with your child. For more on attachment theory, see AC2.5 below.
Free-range	Free-range parenting aims to foster independence in children by giving them greater autonomy and less adult supervision. However, it is not a total disregard for any rules in the way of the indulgent/permissive parent. This style of parenting is believed to encourage problem solving skills and creativity, and helps strengthen personality formation. It can also help children to be more resourceful.

▲ Table 3.17 Types of parenting style (continued)

REFLECT ON IT

- Thinking about the parenting styles in Table 3.17, what do you think the positive and negative impacts could be on the child or young person?
- Do you think there is a perfect parenting style? Why?
- Or do you think a combination of parenting styles might work best? Why?

RESEARCH IT

Read and consider the impact of ACEs on children's well-being, health and development.

Think about the impact this may have on the child in the long term and into adulthood. You may like to look at the following websites:

ACEs and their association with chronic disease

https://bit.ly/ACEs-chronic-disease-report-pdf

The Early Action Together ACEs learning network

www.rsph.org.uk/our-work/resources/early-action-together-learning-network.html

ACEs and their impact on health-harming behaviours

https://bit.ly/ACEs-health-harming-behaviours-pdf

ACE Aware Wales

www.aceawarewales.com/welcome

Relationships

See Unit 003, AC2.2 for information and explanation of an individual's relationships, and the impact of ACEs on children and young people.

REFLECT ON IT

Think about the relationships in your life.

- How have these changed in importance to you over time?
- Why do you think that is?

Education experiences

Education plays a vital role in child development, bringing the opportunity for individuals to lead healthier and longer lives. A positive educational environment helps children to:

- foster a sense of purpose
- explore their interests
- develop the skills they need for future employment and further education.

It is also important that education settings support children and young people to understand the importance of healthy lives and physical and mental well-being. Through education, children and young people can learn to make safe choices.

If a child or young person has negative experiences through education settings such as bullying, difficulties in learning, or not making friends, this can have a damaging effect on their well-being. Exams can also be a source of stress and anxiety.

Culture and racial diversity

Cultural beliefs, customs and behaviours can impact on health and well-being. See Unit 003, AC2.2 for more information on this topic.

Economic factors that can affect development

See Unit 003, AC2.2 for more information on this topic, including the effects of wages, benefits, bills, debts and poverty on development.

Environmental factors that can affect development

See Unit 003, AC2.2 for more information on this topic, including the effects of housing conditions, availability of and barriers to services, and air pollution on development.

CASE STUDY

Nathan, who is 15 years old, lived at home with his parents. His father regularly beat his mother and despite Social Services being involved and offering his mother a shelter, she refused to move. Becoming increasingly terrified of being at home with his father, Nathan ran away from home. After weeks of couch surfing with his friends, Nathan suddenly finds himself with no place to stay and spends a night on the streets.

Discussion point: What could the impact of Nathan becoming homeless have on his development?

AC2.3 The importance of early interventions and partnerships working for the health, well-being and development of children and young people

The earlier we can intervene to help children, the better the chance of a positive outcome. Early intervention means identifying and providing effective support at an early stage before the difficulties become too great.

It is important to understand that a child's brain development can be seriously impaired by the experiences they have in the early years, and these can have a long-term impact if intervention does not occur.

Early intervention means:

1 Identifying risk factors such as poor home environment, developmental delays, problems in school, a disability or a learning need, poverty, substance misuse or domestic violence.
2 Putting in interventions such as home visits, 1:1 support at home or school, mentoring schemes, parent support and GP support. These can all help to bring about positive outcomes.

However, early intervention is a shared responsibility and can involve multi-agencies:

- Health visitors, social services, speech and language teams will all work together to ensure the right support is available.
- It is also vital that intervention programmes work with children and young people and their parents and carers, to ensure they feel involved in the process and that the process is not something that is simply happening to them.
- Partnership working also ensures a consistent approach to the care and support the child is receiving, which results in them feeling safe and secure.

CASE STUDY

Ffion is a teenage mother with little family support. Her baby is 1 month old and suffers with colic. The health visitor is paying a routine visit and notices that the baby is in a soiled nappy and that Ffion is looking unkempt and has been crying. She asks Ffion how things are and Ffion breaks down, explaining she is getting no sleep and her family will not help her.

Discussion points:
- What are the potential risks to Ffion and her baby?
- What additional support could be provided?

AC2.4 The importance of promoting parents' self-confidence in the parenting role and developing their ability to relate positively and engage in play activities with their child

We have already looked at the importance of parenting styles and the importance of involving parents and carers in partnership working. It is vital that parents feel confident in their parenting role and can relate positively to their child and engage with them in play. This helps to form a strong bond between parent and child and helps the parent to be more sensitive to their child's needs.

Parents that can learn to play with their children and that this will help support their child in all aspects of their development. This can also reduce anxiety and stress for both parents and child.

Parents in Wales who are under-confident are offered support through the Flying Start Scheme. This scheme offers:

- **perinatal** and early years support
- early intervention approaches
- support for vulnerable parents and families
- programmes that support positive parenting.

KEY TERM

Perinatal: the short period of time immediately before and after birth, usually a few weeks.

RESEARCH IT

You may wish to look into Albert Bandura's social learning theory. He emphasised the importance of observing, modelling and imitating behaviours. Children learn from their parents, so this theory emphasises the importance of having a confident and capable parent who presents as a positive role model.

What are the benefits to children of having a positive role model?

AC2.5 The term 'attachment' and why this is an important element of development and the ability of children to form relationships

We have already discussed the theory of attachment. Attachment is usually formed in the early years and has a long-term impact on an individual's development, growth, self-identity and future relationships.

Attachment theory is the theory that focuses on this relationship bond and particularly focuses on those bonds between parent and child. John Bowlby first coined the theory, describing attachment as the psychological connectedness between humans.

- He wanted to understand the anxiety and distress of the child caused by separation from their primary caregiver.
- He observed that separation anxiety was not caused by the child's basic needs (such as feeding) not being met but that other motivators were important: for example, when a child is frightened, they will seek out the primary caregiver for comfort and care.
- Bowlby was able to demonstrate that nurture and responsiveness by the primary caregiver are the most important factors for secure attachment.

Attachment is a crucial part of development. It supports the mental foundation the child will use in all interactions with others, and also affects the way they feel about themselves.

- A securely attached child is more likely to have a positive sense of self.
- Attachment can help children and young people increase their independence, safe in the knowledge they are protected.
- Having that early experience means that children and young people will have an inbuilt ability to form positive relationships later in life.

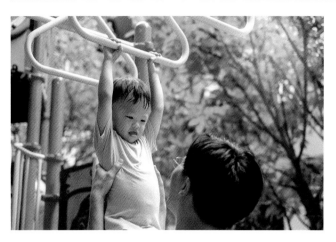

▲ Figure 3.4 Bonding is essential to a child's development

RESEARCH IT

It is important to understand how early childhood experiences can impact on an individual in later life. You may wish to explore attachment theory in more detail. Some useful websites are:

www.simplypsychology.org/attachment.html

www.verywellmind.com/what-is-attachment-theory-2795337

You may also wish to research Mary Ainsworth's 'strange situation', which revealed profound effects of attachment on behaviour.

AC2.6 The term 'resilience' and its importance for the health and well-being of children and young people

Being resilient can help children and young people to overcome adversity, trauma, stress, tragedy and threats. However, children are not born resilient. **Resilience** is learnt over time and through their life experiences.

Parents, carers and other significant adults all share a role in supporting children and young people to develop resilience. This in turn will support their health and well-being as they go through life and deal with difficult situations.

The resilient child will:

- take risks but understand their own boundaries
- explore and be curious
- solve problems and resolve arguments

- know their own limits but push to exceed these
- will build on failure and not give up
- be optimistic and positive.

The child who is not resilient may often:

- have difficulty expressing their emotions
- not engage in activities
- give up when they fail or because they think they will fail
- not take risks, explore or want to try new things
- find it difficult to cope with challenges or changes.

KEY TERM

Resilience: the ability to cope with problems.

AC2.7 The importance of self-identity, self-esteem, sense of belonging for the health and well-being of children and young people

See Unit 003, AC2.10 for more information on self-identity, self-image and self-worth.

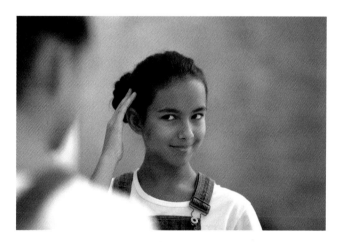

▲ Figure 3.5 Our self-image affects our self-identity

AC2.8 Differences between the medical and social models of disability

See Unit 003, AC2.3 for more information on the medical and social models of disability.

AC2.9 What children need to stay healthy – physically, mentally and emotionally

Physical, mental and emotional health are all essential to ensure overall health and well-being for children and young people.

Physical health

For good physical health, children and young people need:

- A healthy balanced diet – ensuring they have a balanced diet covering all the food groups helps to support physical health and growth. A poor diet can contribute to health problems, poor moods and behavioural problems.
- Good hydration – staying well hydrated helps children with their muscles and joints. It also promotes good cardiovascular health and good energy levels. Poor hydration often leads to tiredness, muscle cramps and dizziness.
- Sleep – a regular, healthy sleep pattern helps energy levels and enhances mood. Poor sleep can cause stress, anxiety, irritability and constant feelings of tiredness and low energy.
- Rest – it is important that activities are balanced with periods of rest so the body can recuperate, and the mind can switch off and relax.
- Activities – it is important to have physical activities and movement to support healthy weight, good muscle tone and development. It supports co-ordination in children and supports motor skill development. Sports and exercise can also improve confidence, and it is proven to help improve low moods through the release of serotonin and endorphins.

Mental and emotional health

For good mental and emotional health, children and young people need:

- Family, friends and a support network – healthy relationships support emotional well-being through giving children a sense of security and belonging. Children have a secure space from which to go out to explore the world around them, safe in the knowledge they have a safe place with involved caregivers to come back to.

- Routine – routines help children and young people to feel in control and give them structure. There is safety in routines, and the child or young person feels secure. Living with little structure and routine can be a scary place for a child who may not be able to provide routines and structure for themselves. This can result in feelings of chaos or being out of control, and can affect behaviour.
- Self-esteem – good self-esteem promotes mental health and well-being. Having poor or low self-esteem can impact all areas of the child or young person's life, and can be very damaging.

CASE STUDY

You are working in a residential setting when a new young person is placed in the home. They have been severely neglected, are undernourished and suffered physical abuse over a long period of time. You are working with a colleague to develop a personal plan with the young person.

Discussion point: What could the setting do to support the young person's health and well-being in the following areas:

- physical
- mental
- emotional?

AC2.10 Agencies and workers that may be involved in supporting the health and well-being of children and young people

Some agencies and workers that may be involved in supporting health and well-being in children and young people might be from the voluntary sector and statutory sectors as well as schools and education provision. They include:

- GP: the first place to contact for diagnosing and referring for support.
- Health visitors: they monitor mothers' and babies' well-being during the first year.
- Family support workers: they can offer support to families who are struggling or who are deemed at risk by social services.
- Social workers: these will be allocated if a referral to social services has been made and a risk identified.

- Education staff – teachers and teaching assistants: they support children in school, and will work with other agencies when needed.
- Educational psychologist: this professional supports schools when children may be struggling with their learning.
- Behavioural specialist: this professional supports children who are experiencing difficulties with their behaviour.
- Dietician: this professional provides advice and information on food and nutrition.
- School nurse: this professional monitors the health needs of school-aged children.
- Dental health services: supports dental health needs.
- NSPCC: National Society for the Prevention of Cruelty to Children. A charity that supports children who have suffered abuse and works to prevent abuse happening.
- Relate: counselling services to support relationships.
- Bereavement services: providing support following bereavements.
- Children's centres: these can be a place for children and families to access support.
- CAMHS: supports children and adolescent mental health.
- Student Assistance Programme: programmes of support for students.
- Changing Minds: psychological services to support positive futures.

RESEARCH IT

Can you find out about any local and national initiatives in Wales?

AC2.11 Links between intellectual, physical and emotional growth and how to support the development from these

Holistic development recognises that intellectual, physical and emotional growth are all linked, especially during the early years from birth to three years. The skills developed during this period set the foundations for further development into childhood and beyond.

It is important to understand that if there is a delay in one area, this could impact another area of development and will be reflected in others.

- **Intellectual development** – this areas covers language and cognitive development, and the growth of the child's ability to think and reason. It helps children to develop the ability to solve problems, organise their thoughts and ideas, and make sense of the world around them.
- **Physical development** – physical growth, development of motor skills, development of muscles and learning to use the body parts for particular skills.
- **Emotional development** – developing feelings about themselves and those around them as well as objects, situations and experiences. This includes the development of the concept of 'self', learning to process feelings and understand emotions. Children cannot always easily manage emotions or find the words to express themselves. It is important that emotions are not ignored or stifled and children learn to accept 'big' feelings when they have them.

CASE STUDY

Maya works in a nursery in the pre-school room. She is planning an activity using a kitchen in the role play area.

Discussion point: Thinking about the three areas of development – physical, intellectual, emotional – can you identify where the children may develop during Maya's activity?

AC2.12 The importance of engagement in meaningful and enjoyable activities on the health, well-being and development of intellectual, physical and emotional growth

If children enjoy something and are engaged in it, then they will learn. It is important to understand a child's interests so that you can develop a programme of support to engage them, keep them interested and therefore motivated to continue. If the child or young person is engaged, then learning will be a natural occurrence and there will be a positive learning atmosphere.

Activities are not just for intellectual development though – they also support physical and emotional development. Activities promote good physical and mental health. They can help children and young people to form strong bonds and friendships.

Engagement in activities can be used to help plan for the next step for children and young people in terms of their development in all areas. You can use their interests to help develop interesting activities, including children and young people as part of this planning process so that they have a sense of ownership.

AC2.13 The importance of creative development and the 'arts' for the health, well-being of children and young people

Creativity can promote confidence, self-esteem and support emotional development. The arts give an individual the freedom to express themselves, and can therefore play a vital role in supporting the health and well-being of children and young people.

Children and young people can often struggle to verbalise emotions, and therefore having a creative outlet can be extremely beneficial. It can help carers to understand what the child or young person is going through.

Health professionals are starting to use creative arts in their overall support for health. Working alongside medication and physical care, the creative arts can also help to support health and well-being. GPs may recommend the arts as a way of supporting their patient's well-being.

CASE STUDY

You have been assigned as key worker to a young girl, Freya, who has recently joined the setting. You notice that she speaks very little and does not join in with activities. Freya has a history of being sexually abused and has missed large periods of schooling, which means she has not developed intellectually at the same rate as her peers.

You notice that while Freya refused to join in with activities, she does like the art room and you will often find her there, alone, sketching and doodling.

Discussion point: How could you use this interest to help Freya in her care and support?

AC2.14 How to use everyday routines and activities to support the health and well-being of children and young people

We have touched on the importance of routine for supporting children and young people's sense of security and having control over their lives. Routines are also important for supporting behaviour: children and young people know what is expected and therefore there is a sense of normalcy to their day. A lack of routine and structure can bring uncertainty and a feeling of chaos and fear.

Consistent routines are important to help children develop healthy habits around eating, sleeping, activity and health.

- Routines, like play activities, also provide learning opportunities: for example, we wash our hands and face and brush our teeth every morning which helps to keep us healthy.
- When children participate in routines, they are learning life skills. There can be an enormous sense of achievement, which promotes good well-being.
- To reinforce routines and behaviour, positive praise and encouragement are essential.

AC2.15 The term 'experiential learning'

KEY TERM

Experiential learning: the process of learning through experience.

AC2.16 How development is supported by experiential learning

Experiential learning relates to the experience of learning through experience. However, just because a child has an experience does not always mean they will learn from it. The learning comes from the ability to reflect, and this is the idea behind experiential learning.

- For children and young people, it is important that they are able to experience failure in order to work through the problem and learn from it.
- Self-esteem and confidence are supported through experiential learning: children and young people are given the freedom to follow their own ideas and overcome challenges as they arise.
- Experiential learning through play often allows children and young people to explore their boundaries and tackle problems in a safe space. Role play and the creative arts help them to learn to express their feelings.
- It can help them to develop social skills and resolve conflict. If you support children to develop solutions and strategies, you will not need to intervene often when they face conflict.
- Experiential play should be unstructured and have no set time or rules. It can occur in a variety of indoor, outdoor and creative activities.

RESEARCH IT

In Wales, the Foundation Phase is the statutory curriculum for all three to seven-year-olds. It is designed to provide a experiential, play-based and developmental approach to teaching and learning. The following websites can provide more information:

https://hwb.gov.wales/curriculum-for-wales-2008/foundation-phase/foundation-phase-framework

www.earlyyears.wales/en/foundation-phase

AC2.17 The role of relationships and support networks in supporting the health and well-being of children and young people

Positive, supportive relationships are critical to the well-being of children and young people. Most crucial to development are the years between birth and two years, when the brain develops and adapts more than at any other stages in a child's development. The interactions a child has in these formative years will have a lasting effect on them throughout life.

We have already discussed the importance of attachment for a child's development. But positive relationships and attachment can also help a child to manage their behaviour and feelings, as they will have positive role models and someone to turn to when they need advice and guidance.

It is important to understand that not all children will find forming relationships easy.

- Children with autism, for example, can find it very difficult to form relationships due to language barriers, anxiety about social situations and rigidity of thinking.
- Poor relationships have also been linked with self-harming behaviour.
- ACEs can affect relationships. During critical early years, children may not have developed the attachment to a caregiver that gives them the basis to form long-lasting relationships.

Children and young people accessing care and support services have often experienced negative relationships, and this means they may struggle forming relationships with foster parents and carers. Serious case reviews have highlighted the importance of professionals forming trusting and positive relationships with the children they support.

Relationships and support networks can have a huge positive or negative impact on the mental health and well-being of children and young people. One significant adult that provides a consistent, positive relationship can have just as much impact as lots of relationships.

AC2.18 Ways of working that develop positive relationships with children and young people based on trust, respect and compassion

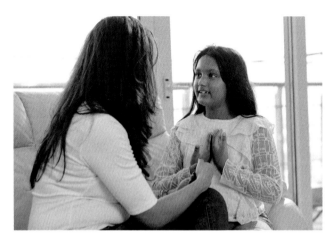

▲ Figure 3.6 Building a positive relationship with children in your care

Bearing in mind what you have just learnt about the importance of positive relationships for children and young people's well-being, you can now look at ways to develop these relationships.

First and foremost, they must be based on trust and respect, and you must have compassion for that child or young person. Developing trust is not always easy when children and young people have been let down countless times during their lives. So how can you develop positive relationships with the children and young people in your care?

- Listen to them – they need to feel valued.
- Think about the language you use – is it age-appropriate? What is the child's first language?
- Patience – relationships take time.
- Eye contact and body language – be open and receptive to the child or young person.
- Respect differences – race, religion, beliefs. However, any form of discrimination should be challenged.

- Use verbal and non-verbal communication.
- Show empathy.
- Do not talk down or patronise.
- Show respect, patience and understanding.
- Give the child or young person age-appropriate responsibility.
- Praise and encourage.
- Reinforce positive behaviour.
- Be a positive role model.
- Give children and young people the opportunity to express themselves – find activities they enjoy.
- Explain to children and young people if information needs to be passed on.
- Always give them a reason for actions, for example, naturally occurring consequences: 'You didn't finish tidying your room, so now we don't have time to go to the park.'
- Keep to consistent routines.
- Give choices and encourage them to make decisions and negotiate.

AC2.19 Type of changes in a child or young person that would give cause for concern

You have already learnt that children develop at different rates and the sequence of development can sometime vary for some children. You have also looked at the importance of early intervention in ensuring that health and well-being needs are met as soon as possible, and care and support is put in place to help prevent long-term negative impact.

Here are some changes that might raise a cause for concern:

- development is not consistent with development milestones
- delays in one area of development which is not consistent with other areas
- regression; for example, child reverts to wetting themselves having previously been dry
- changes in behaviour, such as withdrawal, mood changes, signs of mental ill-health, aggression

- development of fears or phobias
- lacking in energy, more lethargic than usual
- behaviour not appropriate to their age
- changes in sleep, toileting or eating habits
- significant weight changes
- sexualised behaviour is inconsistent with age
- sensory difficulties
- develops a speech disorder
- being dirty, unwashed or hungry
- irregular attendance at schools
- injuries inconsistent with their age or day-to-day activities
- unexplained or repeated bruising.

CASE STUDY

Vivek works in a school for children with behavioural problems. He notices that Josh has started to come to school looking unkept and complaining of being hungry. His colleagues joke that Josh is going through adolescence and not to worry too much. Over the next few days, however, Josh turns up late and does not engage in class.

Discussion points:

- What changes in Josh's behaviour have been noted?
- What should Vivek do next?

AC2.20 The importance of observing, monitoring and recording the development of children and young people

It is important to observe and monitor individuals with a health condition. This can help you to:

- determine the level of care they need
- note any changes in behaviour
- see whether changes indicate any development in their health condition, such as developing mental health issues
- check whether the medication they are taking is working or needs to be reviewed.

Behaviour and mood can often be an indication that something isn't right, and therefore it is important to observe all changes to an individual's behaviour and to record it appropriately.

Clear recording is vital to ensure consistent and safe care. Record keeping also enables you to see any trends or patterns and helps to work towards a decision. It also supports health professionals to obtain a clear picture of the problem.

LO3 KNOW THE ENVIRONMENTS THAT SUPPORT HEALTH, WELL-BEING AND DEVELOPMENT OF CHILDREN AND YOUNG PEOPLE

GETTING STARTED

Think about your different environments – home, education, work.

● What do you like about these environments?
● Why do you think that is?

AC3.1 Features of a positive environment

When we think about environments, it is important to consider both the physical and the emotional environment. The environment has an important role to play for the development and well-being of children and young people. Some features of an effective environment include:

● being stimulating and interesting
● being welcoming and nurturing
● clean, free of clutter and well maintained
● good natural lighting
● temperature and ventilation as appropriate
● good indoor and outdoor spaces for a variety of activities
● comfortable and safe
● interactive and encouraging
● inclusive and accessible (adapted for children with additional needs)
● opportunities to take positive risks and challenges
● opportunities for quiet time and reflection
● personal space, for example, their own bedroom
● welcoming communal spaces.

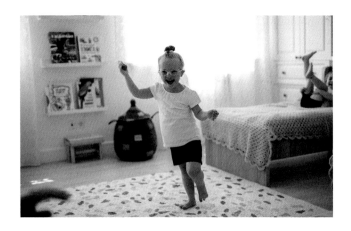

▲ Figure 3.7 What makes a positive environment?

AC3.2 How the environment can support the holistic development of children and young people

Holistic development ensures that all areas of development – physical, emotional and intellectual – are working together. The areas are interconnected and interdependent, and an environment should provide opportunity to support all areas of development.

● There should be a variety of activities to support holistic development.
● The environment should be inclusive, to allow children to engage in a variety of activities, such as creative, physical and imaginative play.
● There should be a mixture of adult-led and self-directed play.
● The environment should be constantly reviewed and assessed to ensure it is fit for purpose.

REFLECT ON IT

Imagine you are working in a day setting for children with sensory needs. Design the environment to promote holistic development.

AC3.3 How the environment can support the inclusion of all children and young people

If the environment meets the features of a positive environment, this creates the foundation for providing an inclusive and welcoming space. An inclusive space should remove barriers that prevent children and young people accessing its services. All children's and young people's needs should be met in the environment.

There are many ways that the environment can support the inclusion of all children and young people:

- An equal opportunities policy should be in place and followed.
- Additional support is provided where needed.
- Adaptations are carried out where needed.
- Staff have a positive and enabling attitude.
- Age, abilities and individual needs are taken into account.
- Specialist equipment is available if needed.
- Alternative methods of communication or assistive technology are available.
- All spaces are user-friendly.
- Staff are trained.

REFLECT ON IT

Look around your learning or work environment.
- What characteristics of a positive environment does it have?
- What could be better?

AC3.4 The importance of ensuring that the environment is welcoming, nurturing, safe, clean and stimulating and takes account of children and young people's needs, interests and preferences

If an environment is welcoming, nurturing, safe, clean and stimulating and takes account of children and young people's needs, interests and preferences, then the children and young people will find being there a positive experience.

This type of environment will help with their development in all areas, and be somewhere that children and young people want to spend time. They will feel safe and secure, and that their voices are being heard.

AC3.5 The importance of balancing periods of physical activity with rest and quiet time for the health, well-being and development of children and young people

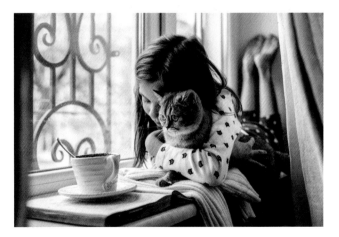

▲ Figure 3.8 A child at rest

We have discussed the importance of having a variety of activities to support development, health and well-being for children and young people. The benefits to physical activity are vast for all areas of development, but it is also important for development that children and young people find time to rest.

- This helps the body to recharge, muscles to grow, the brain to rest.
- Periods of rest help children to develop relaxation skills and mindfulness.
- Rest can improve memory, mood and behaviour.

REFLECT ON IT

Think about your typical week.

- What activities do you do?
- Write a list of your activities, and then analyse if you have enough restful and active periods. What could you change?

AC3.6 The importance of consistent routines for children and young people's health, well-being and development

We have discussed the importance of routines to help children feel safe and secure and to have control over their lives. Consistent routines also help children to develop new skills and support their health and well-being. Children know what to expect and therefore they can focus on the activity without fear of the unknown.

Routines help children to develop their own self-care routines, and promote good mental and physical health and well-being.

Check your understanding

1 What does ACEs stand for?

2 What are some examples of ACEs?

3 Name a legislation that supports well-being in Wales.

4 What is the aim of the Well-Being and Future Generations Act?

5 At what age should you introduce solid foods to infants?

6 What age does the Foundation Phase curriculum cover?

7 What are the three main areas of development?

8 What does holistic development mean?

9 Why are routines important?

Question practice

1 When will a child typically be able to read aloud?

  a 6–12 months

  b 1–3 years

  c 6–9 years

2 When will a child typically start crawling?

  a 0–3 months

  b 3–6 months

  c 6–9 months

3 When will a boy typically grow facial hair?

  a 6–9 years

  b 10–12 years

  c 13–15 years

4 There are many factors that can impact on well-being for children and young people. Which of the following is an example of an environmental factor?

  a having no garden to play in

  b not getting enough sleep

  c parent losing their job

  d fighting at school

5 Which of the following is an example of a physical factor affecting development?

  a play

  b gender

  c parenting styles

  d educational experiences

6 Which of the following is an example of an environmental factor affecting development?

a genetic inheritance

b same-sex parents

c housing conditions

d physical activities

7 What type of disability could Down's syndrome cause?

a physical disability

b sensory disability

c learning disability

d intellectual disability

8 Which of the following is a benefit to the child of being breastfed?

a reduces risk of ovarian cancer

b reduces the risk of SIDS

c increases fine motor skills

d reduces osteoporosis

9 Which of the following is an example of an environmental factor impacting on development?

a asthma

b gender

c air pollution

d family type

10 Which of the following is a benefit to children and young people from having periods of rest and quiet time?

a making new friends

b the body can recharge

c maintaining a healthy weight

d learning how to entertain themselves

LO4 UNDERSTAND THE ROLE OF PLAY IN SUPPORTING THE HEALTH, WELL-BEING AND DEVELOPMENT OF CHILDREN

GETTING STARTED

Think back to your childhood and school.

- Who did you play with? Where did you play?
- Do you remember any of the games you played? How did they make you feel?
- What did you learn from them? What did you find out about the people you played with?

AC4.1 The importance of play for children and young people's health, well-being and learning and development

Play is a very important part of children and young people's development. It supports holistic development in many developmental areas: social and emotional, physical, cognitive, language, problem solving, creative development.

Play also helps children to develop an understanding of the world around them. It supports and encourages the development of self-esteem, self-image and confidence, as well as encouraging self-expression.

- Children will develop motor skills through play, as well as staying fit and physically active.
- Play supports children to build and develop resilience through play, as they have to learn to accept failure and look for solutions.

173

- They may also take risks and overcome challenges through dealing with new situations.
- Children learn how to interact with others through play – they will learn social skills through turn-taking and role play, and develop respect for diversity.

Learning through play is beneficial, as it is less formal than academic work, and children will often relax during their play and learn at their own pace.

Article 31 of the United Nations Rights of the Child refers to the right of children to play. The Welsh Government has a Play Policy, and play is one of their seven core aims for children in Wales.

Children who are not given the opportunities to play will suffer from play deprivation. This means they are deprived of experiences that are essential to their development. They may become both biologically and socially disabled.

RESEARCH IT

Play Wales has some useful information on play deprivation. You may wish to read more about this here, where you will find useful downloads:
www.playwales.org.uk/eng/playdeprivation
You can also read more about Wales Play Policy and The Seven Aims for Children in Wales:
www.playwales.org.uk

AC4.2 Different types of play and their benefits

Play has many forms and can create a variety of activities to support all areas of development. We have discussed how play can support development holistically, and one activity may support more than one area of development.

It is important that children and young people have a balance between activities and periods of rest, as discussed earlier in this unit.

Play can be structured or unstructured, physical or creative. Details of some of the different types of play and their benefits can be found in Table 3.18.

Type of play	Benefit
Physical play	• Supports the development of muscle development, co-ordination, motor skills and social skills. • Helps build confidence and resilience. • Rough and tumble play would also come under this category, and helps children to learn about boundaries and relative strength.
Creative play	• Supports the development of problem solving, imagination, intellectual and social skills. • Helps build an understanding of different concepts and the world around them • Supports self-expression.
Imaginative play	• Supports emotional development. • Helps children and young people to understand and express feelings. • Supports the development of ideas, social skills and negotiation skills. • Helps children and young people to relate to the adult world and a wider environment.
Structured/Adult-led play	• This is play with a purpose and supports the achievement of learning objectives and/or specific skills. • Can focus on the child's or young person's current stage of development to support this stage and provide new learning opportunities. • Can support self-esteem and confidence.
Unstructured/Self-directed play	• Supports learning at the child's or young person's own pace. • The child or young person will make their own choices, solve problems as they arise and experiment. • This builds confidence and self-esteem and helps them to understand their own personal boundaries. • Helps children to develop social skills as they will need to work together.

▲ Table 3.18 Different types of play

AC4.3 How the environment and choice of equipment and materials are used to support different types of play

Let us look at the five types of play from Table 3.19 and look at how the environment and materials can support these.

Types of play	Environment and materials
Physical play	• outdoor areas • space to run, jump, climb • outdoor toys such as ride-on toys, swings, slides, climbing frames
Creative play	• art and craft materials • textures and colours • construction toys • dressing up
Imaginative play	• role play and dressing up • props • outdoor toys such as Wendy houses, tree houses, dens, tents • natural materials
Structured play	• puzzles • games with rules • organised sports • cooking/baking • following instructions to build, for example, with Lego
Self-directed play	Anything to support children to explore in their own time with minimal adult intervention.

▲ Table 3.19 How the environment and resources support play

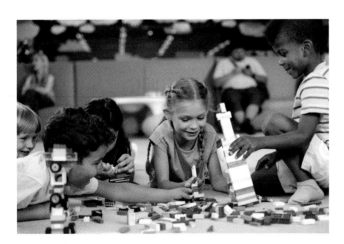

▲ Figure 3.9 Play can be enhanced with materials and equipment

AC4.4 How to support holistic development through play

To support holistic development, you must ensure that children and young people have a variety of play opportunities. It is important to understand the child's or young person's likes and interests, and build these into play opportunities.

CASE STUDY

Teddy is a 13-year-old boy who is new to the setting. Cerys is the staff member allocated as his key worker. Teddy has delayed development due to severe neglect in his early years. Teddy does not like school but will be attending the onsite school once he has settled in.

During a walk around the local area, Cerys and Teddy pass a farm where the farmer is ploughing one of the fields. Teddy is thrilled and wants to stop and watch. Cerys notes this is the most animated Teddy has been since he arrived.

Discussion point: How can Cerys use this to develop play opportunities that support Teddy's development?

REFLECT ON IT

Using the five types of play listed in Table 3.19, think of examples of play that would support development in the following areas:

- physical development
- social and emotional development
- intellectual development.

AC4.5 How play assists children and young people to learn about themselves, those around them and their wider environment

Play encourages social skills and making friends. Children will learn what they like and don't like, as well as what is socially acceptable with their friends. Through role play, children and young people can explore the wider environment and learn more about the adult world.

Children and young people can explore their own strength and their personal boundaries. For example, one child might reach the top of the tree, while another child will feel safer closer to the ground.

AC4.6 How children and young people may use play to express emotions, fears or anxieties or copy behaviour they have observed

Children and young people will often feel more able to express themselves through play. A play situation may therefore help them to explore feelings and emotions in a safe space as they are in control of the play activity.

Play helps children and young people not only to express and explore their feelings, emotions, and fears, but also to develop an understanding of them and ways to control them. It is essential that you pay attention to what children and young people may be telling you through their play.

For young children whose vocabulary is more limited, they may find it easier to express feelings and emotions with toys. They may choose to act out situations that are causing them concern, or use role play to understand it and find solutions.

Children sometimes act out something that they have observed as a way of understanding it, but also to cope with the situation. Sometimes this can give the caregiver cause for concern, and specialist help should be sought.

However, children will also act out situations before they happen, almost as if to 'trial it out' and build their confidence before the event. For example, a child pretends to go to school before they start school; they wave to their parents and take their 'school bag' to another room where they play at school and then come back 'home'. They are experimenting with how it might feel to leave the parent, but learning to understand that they will always come back.

Drawing and painting is another way that children will express their feelings. They can draw things/people/places that have made them happy and sad. Drawing and painting is often used by play therapists to explore what might be causing distress to children and young people.

> **REFLECT ON IT**
> Write a list of what emotions children may be able to express through play.

AC4.7 The importance of risk in play, and how to encourage and support acceptable levels of risk

Risky play promotes physical health, self-confidence, social development and resilience, and plays an important role in supporting health, well-being and development. Through risk taking, children will learn to find their own limits and boundaries and learn to keep themselves safe. These are valuable life skills which they can take into adulthood.

Children and young people who have not learnt to manage risk through play may be more vulnerable in the long term, or have high anxieties about new situations.

It is important that carers and support workers support risk taking, although this must be balanced and child-centred. The caregiver must risk assess the situation, and if the risk outweighs the benefits and there is a high risk of physical or emotional harm, then the activity must not be carried out.

CASE STUDY

Ifan is 16 years old and lives in a foster home. He loves motor sports and enjoys watching these with his foster dad. Ifan has occasionally been quad biking with his foster dad, but has never been on a two-wheel vehicle. After reaching his 16th birthday he is desperate to get a moped licence.

Discussion points:
- Think about Ifan's situation, and discuss the risks and the benefits to the young person.
- What other options might the caregivers think about?

LO5 UNDERSTAND SPEECH, LANGUAGE AND COMMUNICATION DEVELOPMENT

KEY TERMS

Speech: the expression of words, thoughts and feelings by articulate sounds.

Language: talking and understanding – it is not only verbal.

Communication: how we interact with others.

AC5.1 The importance of speech, language and communication for children and young people and how this impacts on health, well-being and development

Speech, **language** and **communication** are important for children's and young people's development, as they need to be able to understand and be understood.

Communication gives children the foundations of friendships and also enables them to learn, play and socially interact. Through speech, language and communication, children learn to build positive relationships, form and maintain friendships, and learn through listening, talking and questioning. These can all have a positive impact on confidence and self-esteem.

However, children and young people who have difficulties with speech, language and communication may find it more difficult to develop reading and writing skills.

- It can also affect their behaviour or cause significant behaviour difficulties, and make it harder for them to make friends and form social connections.
- When children and young people cannot express themselves or are not understood, they can become frustrated, and feel isolated and lonely.

AC5.2 The importance of early intervention for speech, language and communication development delays and disorders

With all areas of development, children are expected to meet certain milestones during different stages of their development. These are usually linked to age, and can give us an indication if there is a problem in an area of a child's development. These milestones are important for supporting early intervention.

Delays and disorders in speech, language and communication can have a significant impact on the child's overall development and well-being. They can also impact on other areas of a child's development and cause problems with behaviour, self-esteem and education.

Early intervention means there is a higher chance of the support having a positive impact and resolving the issue. The longer the problem goes untreated, the harder it may be to resolve. The earlier the intervention, the better the outcome is likely to be.

RESEARCH IT

You may wish to read more about the Welsh Government Talk with Me initiative here:

https://gov.wales/sites/default/files/ publications/2020-11/easy-read-version.pdf

AC5.3 How multi-agency teams work together to support speech, language and communication development

Multi-agency means that people from different sectors with different expertise come together to support children, young people and families, and to achieve the best outcomes for them. There are a number of professionals and individuals who may work together if a child has speech, language and communication difficulties: see Table 3.20.

Professional	Role
Doctors	A GP can identify if there is a medical problem affecting speech and language, such as **tongue-tie** or hearing problems.
Health visitor	Health visitors carry out routine assessments. They can identify problems with speech, language and communication at an early stage.
Speech and language therapist	The speech and language therapist will suggest strategies and interventions to support a child or young person with their difficulty. They will also carry out assessments.
Teachers	Teachers work with other professionals and implement the strategies suggested. They will also help to monitor and review the progress made by the child or young person.
Education psychologist	Sometimes a child with a speech or language difficulty will also have other learning difficulties, so an education psychologist may become involved to assess what might be causing the difficulties and assist in creating a plan of support.

▲ Table 3.20 Professionals who might support children and young people with speech, language or communication difficulties

KEY TERM

Tongue-tie: a condition where the bottom of the tongue is tethered to the floor of the mouth by a short, tight or thick band of tissue.

AC5.4 How play and activities are used to support the development of speech, language and communication

We have previously looked at the importance of play for the support of holistic development of children and young people. Part of a child's development is the development of speech, language and communication. Play can help in a variety of ways: through play, children develop social and language skills by talking, listening, watching, observing and asking questions.

Parents and caregivers are encouraged to verbalise during play activities to help develop language skills. For example, if the child is playing with a toy car, the caregiver may commentate on this play, for example, 'You are playing with the car', 'You are playing with the green car', 'You are making the green car drive on the mat … I wonder where the car will go next?'

Other activities that promote the use of speech, language and communication could be:

- Role play – children use language skills to act out scenarios, talk to each other and express emotions.
- Songs – these encourage learning language patterns.
- Puppets – these can be used to talk about feelings and emotions.
- Story time and books – these encourage listening skills.
- Circle time/registration – the teacher can support children to listen and take turns in talking.
- Show and tell – this time encourages the child to develop language skills and presentation skills.

All types of play – creative, imaginative, physical, unstructured, structured – can allow for conversations about the task, and therefore encourage language and speech development.

REFLECT ON IT

Think about the following play activities and discuss how they could promote speech, language and communication:

- cooking
- sand play
- gymnastics
- Lego
- construction
- arts and crafts.

Check your understanding

1 Name one Welsh Government initiative that recognises the importance of play.

2 What are the five different types of play discussed in this section?

3 What does the term 'early intervention' mean?

4 How does role play help children's speech, language and communication development?

Question practice

1 Which of the following is an example of creative play?

a football

b drawing

c puzzles

d swings

2 Which type of play supports social and emotional development?

a physical play

b creative play

c self-directed play

d all of the above

3 Which of the following is an example of play that allows children to express their emotions, fears and anxieties?

a reading books

b drawing

c playing football

d puzzles

4 Which of these is an example of the speech and language therapist's role?

a diagnose medical problem

b carry out routine assessments

c suggest strategies and interventions

d diagnose a learning difficulty

5 Which of the following is a definition of communication?

a expression of feelings

b how we interact with others

c verbal iterations

d making articulate sounds

L06 KNOW HOW TO SUPPORT THE HEALTH, WELL-BEING AND DEVELOPMENT OF CHILDREN WITH ADDITIONAL SUPPORT NEEDS

GETTING STARTED

If a child needs more, or different, support to what is normally provided by the setting for children or young people of the same age, they are said to have additional support needs.

Can you think of an example when a child or young person might need additional support?

AC6.1 Types of additional support needs that children may have

A child may need additional support at some stage in their lives. This can be long- or short-term support, depending on a number of factors and the reason for the additional support.

- A child may need additional support due to having autism or Down's syndrome, and may need some level of support all their lives.
- Other factors, such as short-term illness and social and emotional factors, for example, bereavement, may need short-term support.

Any child or young person with additional support needs should have an assessment to determine the level of support needed. This can then be reviewed and adapted as needed.

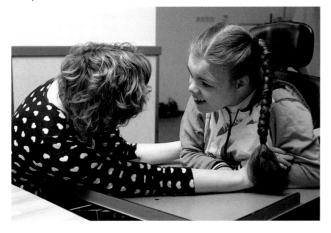

▲ Figure 3.10 A child or young person may need additional support

Table 3.21 shows some of the factors and the support that may be put in place.

Factor causing need for additional support	Additional support
Illness	• extra lessons • tasks sent home so child doesn't fall behind
Speech and language delay or disorder	• speech and language therapy • one-to-one support
Gifted and talented	• individual planning, stretching and challenging
Physical disability or injury	• wheelchair access • one-to-one support • specific aids
Health needs	• one-to-one support • additional time for tasks
Dyslexia	• common word spelling cards • C pen reader (a portable device that reads text out loud)
Hearing impairment	• hearing loop • hearing aid
Behavioural difficulties	• one-to-one support • individual behaviour plan

▲ Table 3.21 Some factors causing the need for additional support, and support that can be provided

AC6.2 Principles of inclusion for children with additional support needs

In any child or young person's setting, inclusion means that all children, regardless of their background, ability or culture, are able to access and participate in services in the same way.

The setting should recognise all children as individuals, including those with additional support needs. There should be a positive attitude to overcoming barriers and ensuring all children are able to access the support they need.

As we have mentioned, the Welsh Government has created seven aims for children in Wales. These are:

1 To ensure a flying start in life and the best possible basis for their future growth and development.
2 Have access to a comprehensive range of education, training and learning opportunities, including acquisition of essential personal and social skills.
3 Enjoy the best possible physical and mental, social and emotional health, including freedom from abuse, victimisation and exploitation.
4 Have access to play, leisure, sporting and cultural activities.
5 Children are listened to, treated with respect, and are able to have their race and cultural identity recognised.
6 Have a safe home and a community that supports physical and emotional well-being.
7 Is not disadvantaged by child poverty.

All children should have the opportunities to achieve their full potential, and settings must work to reduce and remove barriers to inclusion.

RESEARCH IT

Children and young people with a disability are supported in their rights to inclusion under Article 23 of the United Nations Convention on the Rights of the Child. You may wish to read up on this here: **www.unicef.org.uk/what-we-do/un-convention-child-rights/**

AC6.3 How to adapt the environment and activities to enable all children and young people to take part

Sometimes it is necessary to change the environment and activities so that all children and young people can take part.

- The adaptations must meet the needs of the child and should be child-centred.
- Work with the child and their parent/carer to ensure that any adaptation will be suitable.

- Always plan with inclusion in mind.
- Consider how involved the child or young person can be and how much support will they need to participate. Will they be able to participate in some of the activity, even if other parts of the activity will be too challenging?

Adapting the environment

You may need to consider the following:

- Lighting – is it adequate for children with visual impairments?
- Remove barriers to mobility by widening doorways or providing ramps.
- Bring in specialist equipment if necessary.
- Consider noise levels and distraction.
- Adapt height of the equipment that will be used.

Adapting the activity

You should consider how you can make an activity work for children and young people with additional support needs. For example:

- additional sensory materials that stimulate the five senses, such as materials, lights, textures, sounds
- using large letters/pictures
- talking books
- regular breaks
- labelling objects and areas
- transition times
- adapting costumes for role play activities
- respecting diversity – for example, include dolls that have disabilities
- adapting arts and crafts material to make it user-friendly.

CASE STUDY

Joseph has ADHD. You are supporting Joseph in a cookery session.

Discussion points:
- What should you consider when planning for this activity?
- What adaptations can you put in place?

LO7 KNOW HOW TO PROVIDE ADVICE, GUIDANCE AND SUPPORT TO CHILDREN AND YOUNG PEOPLE AND THEIR FAMILIES THAT HELPS TO MAKE POSITIVE CHOICES ABOUT THEIR HEALTH AND WELL-BEING

GETTING STARTED

As a support worker, part of your role is to support children and young people to make positive choices about their health and well-being.

- Reflect on how you could do this.
- What suggestions did you come up with?

Support workers are not experts on all areas of health and well-being. Part of the role is to signpost children and young people to agencies that can provide more specialist support, while supporting them through the process if needed.

AC7.1 Areas relating to health and well-being for children and young people and the agencies that provide information and advice

Areas relating to health and well-being

Children, young people and their families may need support in the following areas:

- substance misuse
- sexual health
- diet and healthy eating
- mental health
- self-harm
- bullying
- online risks
- smoking
- personal, social and health education (PSHE)
- personal and social development
- personal care
- sight and hearing
- gambling.

Agencies that provide information and advice include statutory and voluntary services as well as schools and education provisions, such as:

- GP: can signpost children and young people to relevant services
- Health visitors: can signpost parents and children to services and support
- School nurse: monitors and assesses health needs of school age children and signpost to services and support

- CAMHS: support for child and young person mental health
- Action for Children: a children's charity supporting practical and emotional care and support
- Flying Start: scheme set up by Welsh Government to support early years
- Public Health Wales: can provide information and advice on health needs
- Childline: a dedicated phone line for children to call
- Citizen's Advice: advice on a number of issues such as housing and debt
- NSPCC: works to prevent abuse and support victims of abuse
- Dental health services: support for dental health
- Care Inspectorate Wales (CIW): responsible for inspecting care settings
- Vision UK: support for eye health, vision problems
- Relate: counselling support for relationships
- Social Care Wales: works to lead improvements in social care in Wales, and responsible for the registration of social care workers.

Check your understanding

1 Which Article from the United Nations Convention on the Rights of the Child supports the rights of children with disabilities?

2 What does CAMHS stand for?

Question practice

1 What value is promoted by providing extra support to children with additional needs?

a diversity

b respect

c inclusion

d co-operation

2 Which of the following is an adaptation you can make to the environment for a child with visual impairment?

a adequate lighting

b wheelchair ramps

c labelled objects

d transition times

3 Which of the following is a voluntary service?

a health visitors

b Childline

c Social Care Wales

d CAMHS

LO8 UNDERSTAND THE ROLES AND RESPONSIBILITIES RELATED TO THE ADMINISTRATION OF MEDICATION IN SOCIAL CARE SETTINGS

GETTING STARTED

Look back at Unit 003 to review your learning in this area.

AC8.1 Legislation and national guidance related to the administration of medication

For details of the requirements of this LO, see LO7 in Unit 003.

CASE STUDY

Catrin is 15 years old and has recently moved to a children's residential setting following a child protection case. Catrin has not adapted well, and is having problems with her behaviour as well as flashbacks of the experiences she has gone through.

Catrin is receiving support from CAMHS and has been prescribed an antidepressant which she is refusing to take. Emily is a new support worker and during a team meeting where the issue is being discussed, she suggests crushing the pills and putting them into Catrin's drinks.

Discussion point: What are the potential safeguarding issues here?

L09 KNOW HOW TO SUPPORT CHILDREN AND YOUNG PEOPLE WITH THEIR PERSONAL CARE

GETTING STARTED

The support that children and young people may need with their personal care is likely to be different from the support older individuals may need. It can include personal hygiene, bathing, dental care and menstruation.

You will need to take into account the child or young person's age and abilities when supporting their personal care.

- Think about the difference in needs that a toddler and a teenager might need.
- What factors do you need to consider?

AC9.1 The importance of supporting personal care routines for children and young people

Younger children will need more support with their personal care than older children and young people.

- While children should be encouraged to be independent with their personal care, their age and abilities can mean they are not able to carry out all routines by themselves. They may need help with toileting, toothbrushing, hand washing and dressing.
- It is important to support them to develop more independently in these skills as time goes on.

Supporting young children with care routines also promotes communication, and can help children to develop communication skills and positive relationships.

As time goes on and they need less support, they will also feel a sense of achievement and develop positive self-esteem and confidence. Good personal care can also help promote positive body image.

The routine of personal care for babies and small children also supports a sense of security, as we have seen when looking at the benefits of routines for children.

- Routines also help children to deal better with transitions and new experiences.
- Routines that are similar in the home environment and the care setting help children adapt to new settings.

For older children going through puberty, this is also an opportunity to support good hygiene, health and dignity.

CASE STUDY

Adrian has just moved to a residential children's home following a breakdown of his foster placement. Adrian has had little routine in his life and has moved placement many times. He suffered severe neglect in his early years and it is suspected that some form of abuse took place.

Tim is allocated as Adrian's key worker and he notices that Adrian often looks very unkempt, wearing dirty clothes and forgetting to attend to his personal hygiene.

Discussion points:

- Why might Adrian struggle with his personal care?
- What might Tim do to support a positive personal care routine?

AC9.2 Ways to treat children and young people with dignity and respect when supporting them with their personal care routines, taking into account their background, culture and religion

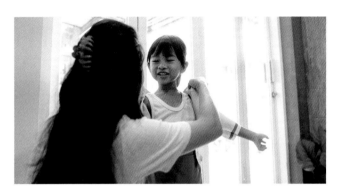

▲ Figure 3.11 Supporting personal care routines

It is important to always treat children with dignity and respect. Some children may need more help than others with personal care, and additional support with eating, drinking, dressing and toileting may be required by children with a disability.

It is also important for a child or young person who needs additional support to feel in control of their personal care routines, so they feel in charge of their bodies and are less vulnerable to abuse.

Religious and cultural beliefs should be taken into account when supporting personal care routines, and it is important to find out the background for each individual child. For example, Hindus like running water for washing in the same room as the toilet, many Buddhists prefer showers to baths, etc.

Examples of how to treat children with dignity and respect:

- Decide with the child on their personal care routine.
- Talk to the child to understand their background.
- Take into consideration, and understand, any religious or cultural preferences.
- Encourage independence whenever possible, and accept that this may take longer.

- Ensure privacy and modesty at all times.
- Request permission and talk to the child or young person throughout the routine.

AC9.3 Ways to support children and young people with their personal care routines in a way that protects both the child or young person and the adult supporting them

It is imperative that both the children or young person and the care and support worker are protected during personal care routines. You must ensure the following:

- Always wash hands before and after contact.
- Wear PPE.
- Support children and young people to wash their hands after using the toilet, before and after eating, before putting in contact lenses if used, and for any other intimate care routine (such as menstruation).
- Support children and young people to change incontinence pads and clothing if they are soiled.
- Changing areas should be kept visible.
- Policies and procedures should be adhered to.
- No phone or recording devices in the changing area.
- Keep all areas clean and ready for use.
- Record and report any concerns, marks or bruises.
- Safely dispose of soiled materials and waste in specific bins for this.

CASE STUDY

Jane is a new worker who has started working at a residential home which offers respite services for children with disabilities. During her first week, she is asked to assist Peter, who has physical disabilities, with his toileting. Jane has been given no training for this, and the colleague who asks her to carry out this task leaves her alone with the boy in his bedroom.

Discussion points:
- What are the risks to the child?
- What are the risks to Jane?

LO10 UNDERSTAND THE IMPORTANCE OF NUTRITION AND HYDRATION FOR THE HEALTH AND WELL-BEING OF CHILDREN AND YOUNG PEOPLE

GETTING STARTED

Think about the children and young people you work with or know in your own life. What sorts of foods and drinks do they consume?

There are currently concerns about the typical diets of many young children in the UK, which are contributing to health problems in childhood and later in life. For children and young people, common concerns are:

- being overweight or obese
- too few vegetables and fruits
- not enough fibre
- too much sugar
- too much salt and processed foods
- iron deficiency.

AC10.1 The terms 'nutrition' and 'hydration'

See AC8.1 in Unit 003 for details of nutrition and hydration.

AC10.2 Principles of a balanced diet and good hydration and government recommendations for a balanced diet and good hydration

It is important to have a balanced diet, as no single food group contains all the essential nutrients the body needs to be healthy and functioning well. A balanced diet, therefore, should include a large variety of foods so that adequate intakes of all the nutrients are achieved.

It is not appropriate to introduce solid foods to infants before six months.

Children have a higher energy and nutrient requirement than adults. They are growing quickly and become much more active, so they should be offered the right foods to meet their needs.

From the age of five, a child's diet should be based on the Eatwell Guide, which sets out guidance on all the food groups and how best to balance these. For more on the Eatwell Guide, see Unit 003 AC8.2.

AC10.3 National and local initiatives that support nutrition and hydration

For details of national and local initiatives, see Unit 003 AC8.3.

AC10.4 The importance of a balanced diet for optimum health, development and growth of children and young people

Children and young people need more energy than adults due to the speed they are growing. It is important that children and young people have the correct foods to support this. They may need to eat more than adults but it is still important that they are eating the right foods. Too little or too much of one element of the five food groups could have a negative impact.

See Unit 003 AC8.4 for further details of balanced diets.

AC10.5 Factors that can affect nutrition and hydration

There are many factors that can affect the nutrition and hydration of individuals. These can include health, environmental, financial, cultural and social factors. See Unit 003, section AC8.5 and Table 2.11 for information on these factors.

For children and young people it is important to note that they may not be able to make choices about their food. Parents and caregivers will be responsible for providing food to their children and young people, and may not always make the best choices for them. Educating children and young people about nutrition and hydration is important to help support them to make healthy choices when they can.

Young people are often influenced by advertising and fads, for example fad diets which are often not based on correct nutritional guidance. They may suggest skipping meals or fasting on certain days. It is important that children and young people are educated about these diet cultures and the dangers they can have on developing bodies.

Other factors to consider are ethics, morals and political beliefs. For example, a child may decide to be vegetarian or vegan and it is therefore essential that they are still maintaining a healthy, balanced diet with foods from all food groups.

Check your understanding

1 What does PPE stand for?
2 Why is it important to understand a child's or young person's religious and cultural beliefs?
3 From what age should children follow the Eatwell Guide?
4 Why do children use up more energy than adults?

Question practice

1 The following statement shows the role of which professional:

'dispense the medication, checking that the medication matches the prescription'

  a doctor

  b pharmacist

  c registered manager

  d care and support worker

2 Which of the following is an example of how to work during a personal care routine that keeps children, young people and carers safe?

  a Report any marks or bruises.

  b Make sure you only use sensitive skin products.

  c Encourage independence whenever possible.

  d Carry out the routine as quickly as possible.

3 Which of the following is an example of a cultural factor impacting on healthy nutrition?

  a neglect

  b halal meat

  c anorexia

  d plate guards

4 Which food group do beans and pulses belong to?

  a carbohydrates

  b proteins

  c fats

  d dairy

FURTHER READING AND RESEARCH

Weblinks

NHS Wales report on ACEs and their association with chronic disease:
https://bit.ly/ACEs-chronic-disease-report-pdf

Royal Society for Public Health's resources on ACEs:
www.rsph.org.uk/our-work/resources/early-action-together-learning-network.html

NHS Wales report on ACEs and their impact on health-harming behaviours:
https://bit.ly/ACEs-health-harming-behaviours-pdf

Well-Being of Future Generations (Wales) Act:
www.futuregenerations.wales/about-us/future-generations-act/

Simply Psychology guide to attachment theory:
www.simplypsychology.org/attachment.html

Further guidance on attachment theory:
www.verywellmind.com/what-is-attachment-theory-2795337

Information from Play Wales on play deprivation:
www.playwales.org.uk/eng/playdeprivation

The Welsh Government Talk with Me initiative:
https://gov.wales/sites/default/files/publications/2020-11/easy-read-version.pdf

PROFESSIONAL PRACTICE AS A HEALTH AND SOCIAL CARE WORKER

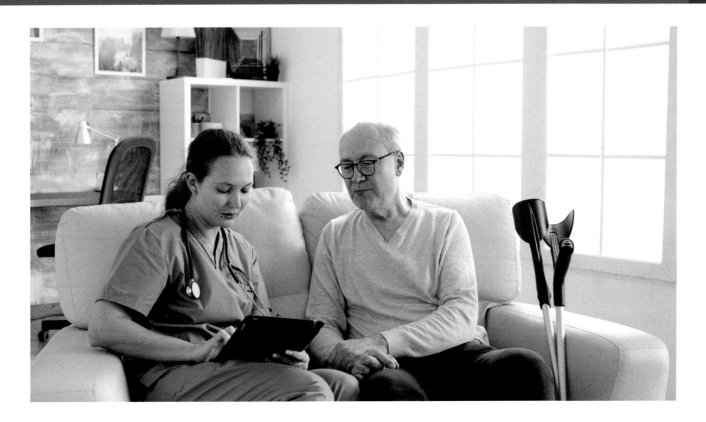

ABOUT THIS UNIT

Guided learning hours: 50

This unit is about your role as a social care worker. It will cover the following topics: your responsibilities and accountabilities, duty of care, standards of professional behaviour required for your job, partnership working, teamwork, handling information and confidentiality, continuing professional development (CPD). You will also understand the importance of reflection to enable you to improve practice.

Learning outcomes

LO1: Understand the role, responsibilities and accountabilities of health and social care workers

LO2: Know how to develop and maintain effective partnership working with others in health and social care

LO3: Know how effective team working supports good practice in health and social care

LO4: Know how to handle information

LO5: Understand the importance of upholding the profession of health and social care workers

LO6: Know how CPD contributes to professional practice

LO1 UNDERSTAND THE ROLE, RESPONSIBILITIES AND ACCOUNTABILITIES OF HEALTH AND SOCIAL CARE WORKERS

GETTING STARTED

In order to carry out your role effectively, you need to know your responsibilities. These are stated in legislation and codes of practice, and you must ensure you meet the requirements of your job as you will be held accountable if you don't. More importantly, not carrying out your job properly could put individuals, children, young people or yourself at risk of danger, harm or abuse.

Why do you think you need to understand your responsibilities and be accountable for your work?

AC1.1 Professional responsibilities and accountabilities within the context of relevant legislative frameworks, standards and codes of conduct and professional practice

A set of standards and guidance is applied to ensure that individuals, children and young people are supported in a way which meets their needs and gives them the best possible service. These standards outline workers' responsibilities and accountability, and should be implemented in everything you do to ensure you are carrying out your job correctly.

You can use these reflections when you come to do the practice qualification, City & Guilds Health and Social Care: Core.

Codes of Professional Practice

The following Codes of Practice describe the standards of professional conduct and practice required of health and social care workers, health workers and health employers in Wales:

- the Code of Professional Practice for Social Care
- the NHS Wales Code of Conduct for Healthcare Support Workers in Wales
- the Code of Practice for NHS Wales Employers.

The codes of conduct outlined above:

- play a key part in raising awareness of the standards required
- promote key values that underpin health and social care
- should be embedded within your working practice.

Individuals, children and young people, carers and family members need to know about the relevant Code. The provision of safe care and support is everyone's responsibility, not just health and social care workers, and it is important that everybody knows what to expect of health and social care workers.

Look back at Units 001/002, AC1.3 and think about how the seven standards of the Code of Practice relate to professional practice.

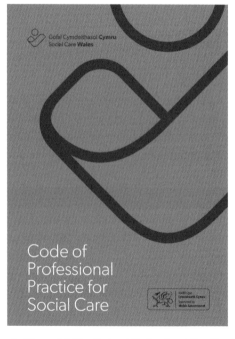

Gofal Cymdeithasol Cymru
Social Care Wales

Code of Professional Practice for Social Care

▲ Figure 4.1 The Code of Professional Practice for Social Care

Practice guidance

In addition to the Code of Practice, there is practice guidance for workers in different settings so that they know what is expected of their role. Practice guidance is available for the following roles:

- social worker
- residential child care worker
- social care manager
- domiciliary care worker
- adult home care worker.

In addition, there is also:

- a domiciliary care worker app which you can download
- guidance on openness and honesty when things go wrong: the professional duty of candour
- guidance on using social media responsibly.

RESEARCH IT

From the list above, decide which guidance is relevant to your role.

Have a look at the link below to the Social Care Wales website, and list the responsibilities you have which are listed within these documents:

https://socialcare.wales/dealing-with-concerns/codes-of-practice-and-guidance

- Is there anything listed here that you didn't know about?
- Is there anything you are not doing at the moment that you need to do?

If so, discuss these with your manager: agree how you are going to do this and whether you need any support.

Legislation

Legislation exists so that people's needs and rights are met, and they are kept safe. Legislation also gives guidance on what you are supposed to do and how to meet people's needs and rights.

Legislation	Your responsibilities	Employers' responsibilities
Health and Safety at Work Act Management of Health and Safety at Work Act	• Ensure safety of yourself and others. • Report accidents and problems. • Attend and implement training. • Use any equipment provided for you. • Follow policies, procedures and risk assessment.	• Ensure policies, procedures and risk assessments are in place. • Protect the health and safety of employees, individuals, children and young people, and anyone else affected by the work of the organisation. • Ensure employees have regular training and supervision. • Ensure appropriate equipment is provided and maintained.
Manual Handling Operations Regulations	• Avoid manual handling where possible. • Follow risk assessments. • Implement training. • Ensure the safety of yourself and others.	• Ensure there are policies and procedures in place. • Ensure employees have appropriate equipment. • Avoid manual handling where possible. • Carry out risk assessment on anything that cannot be avoided. • Carry out individual risk assessments where individuals and employees are at a particular risk of injury.
Control of Substances Hazardous to Health (COSHH)	• Follow policies, procedures and risk assessments. • Ensure the safety of all hazardous substances. • Use, store and dispose of hazardous substances safely in line with risk assessments.	• Ensure there are policies, procedures and risk assessments in place. • Ensure safe use, storage and disposal of any hazardous substance. • Provide information on the hazards and risks associated with any hazardous substances, and what to do if there are problems. • Provide training and supervision.

▲ Table 4.1 Legislation affecting health and social care workers

Legislation	Your responsibilities	Employers' responsibilities
Reporting of Injuries, Diseases and Dangerous Occurrences (RIDDOR)	• Report all accidents in line with policy. • Report near misses and potential accidents.	• Ensure you provide an accident book. • Investigate all accidents to prevent them happening again. • Report RIDDOR reportable accidents to the Health and Safety Executive. • Ensure employees are aware of the accident reporting procedure.
Social Services and Well-Being (Wales) Act	• Follow care and support plans. • Ensure individuals, children and young people are central to their care and support. • Ensure individuals, children and young people have voice, choice and control. • Ensure the well-being of individuals. • Ensure individuals, children and young people are protected from danger, harm and abuse.	• Ensure person-centred support plans are in place, and individuals are involved as equals in the planning of their care and support. • Ensure individuals, children and young people have voice, choice and control. • Ensure the well-being of individuals. • Ensure individuals, children and young people are protected from danger, harm and abuse. • Ensure employees implement care and support plans.
Equality Act	• Ensure you treat everyone equally regardless of their personal characteristics.	• Ensure there are policies, procedures in place. • Ensure all employees and visitors are treated equally regardless of their personal characteristics. • Ensure recruitment procedures do not discriminate. • Ensure all staff have fair access to training and development.
General Data Protection Regulations	• Ensure you keep information confidential and only give access to people if they have a need to know.	• Ensure policies and procedures are in place. • Ensure appropriate storage of data. • Ensure only appropriate people can access the data. • Ensure data is only kept for as long as it is needed. • Ensure people have access to the data kept on them.
The Children Act	• Ensure children are safeguarded from harm and abuse.	• Ensure policies and procedures are in place. • Ensure children and young people are protected from harm and abuse. • Ensure a child/young person's well-being is at the centre of services. • Support partnership working.

▲ Table 4.1 Legislation affecting health and social care workers *(continued)*

You can read more about this and other relevant legislation in Units 001/002 and Units 006 and 007.

REFLECT ON IT

The main pieces of legislation have been detailed above.

• Think of any other relevant pieces of legislation.
• List your responsibilities and those of your employer.

Policies and procedures

Every organisation has a set of policies and procedures or agreed ways of working. These tell you the standards expected while you are at work. They are based on legislation, standards and professional body codes of practice.

You should be given access to these when you begin a new role.

• It is useful to refresh your memory on these regularly to ensure you are still working within the guidelines.
• They also act as a useful guide if you are not sure what to do about something.
• If you think it would be helpful to have a procedure on a particular topic, speak to your manager as this may help other workers too and ensure you are all doing things correctly.

Care and support plans

Individuals, children and young people who receive support in their daily lives will have a care and support plan, which is usually written by a social worker. This gives a summary of their needs and how these will be met.

Care and support plans are usually put together by a team of professionals. The purpose of the plan is to support the individual to achieve what they want in life while ensuring they have the appropriate help to meet their needs.

In addition, organisations will develop support plans or personal plans with individuals, which detail how they will achieve the overall care and support plan.

CASE STUDY

Jayne has a care and support plan which covers the following:

- likes and dislikes
- strengths
- things Jayne needs help with, such as getting up and getting ready for her day, cooking and keeping mobile
- what matters to Jayne – being busy and meeting other people.

The plan will then detail what support Jayne needs help with in order to achieve the things she wants to do. It says that Jayne will have a domiciliary support worker visit twice a day, have physiotherapy once a week and attend a day centre three days per week.

In order to achieve this care and support plan, the social worker, day centre, physiotherapist and domiciliary care organisation need to work together with Jayne.

The domiciliary care service may then have a personal plan for Jayne which tells workers how they support Jayne to get up and get ready for her day, how they support her to cook and keep mobile.

Discussion points:

- How do you think Jayne will benefit from having a care and support plan?
- How will the workers who support Jayne benefit?

Personal plans are a really useful guide to help you do your job. They also ensure consistency among the different workers. If you do something different to what is on the plans, not only are you putting yourself

at risk but you could be putting the people you support at risk.

As you are accountable for your actions, you need to ensure you follow the care and support plans and personal plans all the time.

If you think there is a problem with them or that somebody's needs are not being met, you need to report this to your manager so that it can be put right.

AC1.2 The purpose of job descriptions and person specifications for defining the expectations and limits of roles and responsibilities

Job description

Everybody should have a job description, a contract agreement, a placement agreement or an agreement that sets out how they are expected to undertake their role. If you haven't got one, ask your manager.

Your job description gives you a summary of what is expected of you in your work.

REFLECT ON IT

Get a copy of your job description. Reflect on the following questions about your job.

- Are all the tasks you do summarised within your job description?
- Is there anything you do that is not listed within your job description?
- If you answered yes to the above question, do you think that is because you shouldn't be doing it, or do you think your job description needs to be changed? Discuss this with your manager.
- Likewise, is there anything in your job description you are not doing? Why are you not doing this? Should you be doing it, or do you think your job description needs to be changed? Discuss this with your manager.

Your job description will include:

1 **The responsibilities, tasks or work activities** that you must carry out as part of your job role. These might include:
   - providing support to individuals with daily living activities to meet their needs

- maintaining accurate records of the support provided to individuals
- attending all training provided.

2 **How you must carry out your work activities**. This might include:
- promoting individuals' rights such as privacy, dignity, independence
- maintaining detailed and accurate records while protecting individuals' confidentiality at all times
- putting into practice all training attended by using person-centred ways of working.

3 **Who you report to**, such as your manager or team leader.

4 **Where you must work**, for example, in a variety of settings including in individuals' own homes, in residential care settings or in the community.

REFLECT ON IT

For each responsibility in your job description, think about the things you do in practice that come under each responsibility.

- Discuss your list with a colleague or your manager. How do your responsibilities compare to theirs?
- What do you think might happen if you do anything that is not included in your job description, such as not following policies and procedures?

Person specification

Person specifications detail the knowledge and skills required for your job role. They are usually split into essential and desirable.

REFLECT ON IT

Look at the person specification for your job role.

- Are there any areas you would like to improve your skills or knowledge?
- Discuss these with your manager and agree a development plan.

Job descriptions vary, depending on the job.

They also vary in detail: some may be brief with an outline of the job role and key responsibilities, but good job descriptions will detail the purpose of your role, responsibilities, different tasks you will be required to complete, and also the reasons for doing so. In this way you have a clear understanding of why you are doing

what you are asked, and understand how it affects the individual and setting. For example:

- Instead of saying 'assist at meal times', it would be more helpful to say 'assist at meal times and ensure that the meal meets the dietary requirements and needs of the individual'.
- Instead of saying 'provide good care for individuals', it would be more helpful to say 'provide care that involves treating individuals with compassion, dignity and respect and ensuring that they are involved in their care'.

Adhering to the agreed scope of your job role also involves working within the boundaries or limits of the job role. Basically, if it is not part of your job description, then you should not be expected to carry out the task.

AC1.3 The importance of recognising and adhering to the limits of role and responsibilities

Working in line with your employer's **agreed ways of working** is an essential part of your job role. It ensures that you are carrying out your work responsibilities lawfully, safely and in line with current best practice.

Below are some tips to help you work in line with your employer's agreed ways of working.

1 Find out where your work setting's agreed ways of working are kept, including how to gain access to them. Read them, and if there is something you do not understand, seek advice from your manager.

2 Only carry out work activities that have been included in the scope of your job role.

3 Attend all training and read all information updates provided to you by your employer. If you do not feel confident to carry out a work activity that you have been trained to do, be honest with yourself and talk this through with your manager.

4 If you observe an unsafe working practice, or if an individual, their family or a visitor brings something of this nature to your attention, report it to your manager immediately. You will also need to make a record of these observations. Showing your **courage**

in these situations will ensure that you promote your own and others' health, safety and well-being.

5   Be prepared to explain why you are carrying out your work activities in the way that you do; for example, to the individuals you support with a daily activity or to a colleague when you are working together to assist an individual.

6   Find out who you must report to when carrying out your work activities (this may be your manager or another senior member of the team). Comply with any information or guidance that this person provides.

7   Observe individuals and listen to their feedback (and the feedback of others) on how you carry out the work activities you are responsible for. Reflect on their feedback and use this to continue to improve your work practices.

KEY TERM

Agreed ways of working: the policies and procedures set out by your employer for your work setting.

The 'agreed scope'

Developing effective working relationships with others can only be achieved if you carry out all the tasks that form part of your job role; this is commonly referred to as the 'agreed scope' of the job role.

Working within the agreed scope of your job role is essential for ensuring that you carry out your job responsibilities to the best of your ability. The purpose and importance of working within the agreed scope of your role are set out here.

Work at the correct level

Adhering to the scope of your job ensures that you are working to your ability and doing the tasks that you are qualified to do.

- Doing tasks that you do not have any expertise or qualifications in risks your health and safety and that of those around you.
- You can of course gain knowledge and skills in those areas, but it is best to stick to what you know before you take on responsibilities that are not outlined in your job description and that you have not discussed with your manager first.

You are only responsible and accountable for what you do

All organisations need structures and a clear outline of what everyone does in the setting. In that way:

- You are only accountable for those things that you are responsible for, and not for others.
- It is clear to management who is responsible for which tasks, and so there are no misunderstandings (if you are all doing what you are responsible for).

That is not to say you cannot assist colleagues; it just means you should not take on tasks.

How your employer assesses your competence

During supervision meetings with your manager, and as part of your appraisal at the end of the year, your employer will discuss with you how you have performed in your job role. You will discuss whether you have carried out your work activities to the best of your ability, in line with your job role's requirements and your employer's expectations of you.

By adhering to the agreed scope of your job role, you will be more likely to show that you are doing what is expected of you and doing it competently (to a high standard).

It is part of your duty of care

You have a duty of care to ensure that you provide the best possible care, and that the support you offer is in the best interests of the individual. For example, assisting an individual to move from their bed to their chair on your own when the moving and handling guidelines specify that two staff must be present can have serious consequences, both for you and the individual:

- You may lose your job for carrying out a task on your own that you do not have the agreement from your employer to do.
- You may also injure your back during the move.
- Your actions may cause the individual to fall and fracture a limb.

It ensures everyone's health and safety

You have a responsibility to ensure the safety of everyone you work with. Your responsibilities with regard to health and safety are covered in Unit 007.

Not adhering to responsibilities around health and safety, such as reporting concerns, can have serious consequences. For example, if you do not report concerns about a colleague's unsafe working practices when preparing food:

- It could result in illness such as food poisoning for those in the setting (as well as visitors).
- It could even prove fatal if the individuals already suffer from other illnesses.
- If you do not report your concerns, your colleague will not be able to access the support and training they need.
- Both you and your colleague may also run the risk of losing your jobs.

That is not to say you should spend your days worrying about what *might* happen, but it is a good idea to remember the reasons why you should work within the scope of your job role and responsibilities.

It protects you from untrue allegations

Meeting an individual on a one-to-one basis when it has been agreed that all meetings with this individual will take place in the presence of two members of staff can have serious consequences for everyone:

- You may be accused of something that you did not do, such as shout at the individual.
- Your employer will be required to conduct an investigation into what happened. The incident will also need to be reported to the individual's family and to the CIW.
- This may result in the individual requesting a move to another care setting, you losing your job and could even mean an end to your career in the adult social care sector.

Again, this example is not designed to scare you, but you should remember that your job description has important reasons for everything that it outlines, including the working methods you should follow.

Do
Comply with the agreed lines of reporting. For example:
• If you have a concern about an individual's well-being, should report your concerns to your manager in the first instance rather than going straight to the individual.
• Your job description will outline whom you will report to and you must work within these boundaries and the scope of your job.

Don't
Don't take part in work activities that have not been agreed as part of your job role and that you are not trained to do. For example:
• If your job description does not mention assisting individuals with medication, reviewing care plans or supervision of new members of staff, then you should not be expected to do this.
You may receive training and as a result, your job role and the scope of your role may change, but you should discuss this with your manager before you undertake tasks that are not outlined in your job description.
Don't carry out work activities outside your agreed hours of work. For example:
• Do not assist an individual who wishes to go to the shops after your shift has ended without first seeking permission to do so.
Don't work in ways that are not person-centred. For example:
• Don't impose your views and deny individuals their rights.
• Don't document your opinions when recording the support provided to individuals.
Don't work in locations not agreed with your employer. For example:
• Don't provide support to an individual in your house or in the home of one of the individual's relatives, rather than in the individual's own home.

▲ Table 4.2 Dos and don'ts for adhering to the scope of your job role

AC1.4 How and when to seek additional support in situations beyond role, responsibilities, level of experience and expertise or unsure as to how to proceed in a work matter

There may be times when you do not have experience and the expertise in something and do not know how to respond to a situation. Table 4.3 provides examples of situations when you will need to seek further support, from internal and/or external sources.

When to seek support	The reasons for seeking help
A crime has been committed.	You must seek support from the police if a crime has occurred, such as burglary of an individual's home. You will not have expertise in how to handle this situation and how to preserve evidence.
A situation occurs requiring a medical procedure which you have no knowledge of or skills for.	You may need to contact a medical professional when you do not know how to treat an individual who is suffering from a serious injury, such as a bleed from the head. This will ensure the individual receives appropriate medical care and is not placed in danger.
You are dealing with an individual with an illness you have no medical expertise in.	You may need to contact a medical professional to seek advice about the illness. You could seek a support organisation for information and support, such as Mind.
You witness an individual's family member shouting at their relative during one of their visits.	Seeking support from your manager will ensure the appropriate actions can be taken and the individual can be protected from any further abuse. By doing this: • you are practising your duty of care to safeguard this individual • your safety is also maintained.
You report your concerns of an individual in your care setting being at risk of abuse from a colleague, but your manager is too busy to deal with this.	Seeking support from an external organisation such as the CIW will ensure that the individual is no longer at risk of abuse. By doing this, you will be protecting • this individual's safety • the safety of others who may be at risk in the care setting.
A colleague asks you to use unsafe practices when supporting an individual being hoisted.	Seeking support from your manager will ensure that you will be supported to not carry out these unsafe practices. This will also raise your colleague's awareness of unsafe practices and their consequences. This will ensure the safety and well-being of the individual you are supporting as well as your and your colleague's safety.

▲ Table 4.3 Situations where you may need to seek support

RESEARCH IT

Find out what support is available to help you by:
- speaking to your manager
- researching organisations in your local community that offer relevant support to you or the individuals you support.

If there is ever a situation where you are not sure of what action to take, always speak to your manager. You will then learn the appropriate response so you know what to do in future. It is better to ask than make a mistake which could have serious consequences.

AC1.5 The purposes of policies and procedures for health and social care practice and how to find out about and follow these

As you have learnt, agreed ways of working refer to working practices that have been agreed with your employer and set out how you will carry out your job role and its associated responsibilities.

Social care settings are all different, and therefore agreed ways of working vary between the different settings. However, all social care employers will have the following in place.

Policies

These are the general guidelines for the way you should work. The policies in your setting will comply with legislation and they will reflect the aims of the setting.

For example, in order to comply with the Data Protection Act 1998 and 2018 or the new General Data Protection Regulation (GDPR) 2018, your workplace must have a policy that describes how it will ensure that individuals' personal information will be kept secure at all times when being used, recorded, stored and shared.

Procedures

These set out in detail how you should work, and the ways of working that your employer expects you to follow on a day-to-day basis to ensure the policies are being put into practice.

In your setting, there will be procedures for nearly everything you do, such as:

- moving and handling
- giving medication to individuals
- how to deal with an emergency such as a fire.

Guidelines

These set out *precise* ways of working that your employer will expect you to follow for the care and support of specific individuals and work activities. For example:

- Data protection guidelines may be in place for an individual who has given strict instructions that you are not to tell his family every time he has a fall because he does not want to worry them.
- It is important that you respect his right not to share this personal data about him.

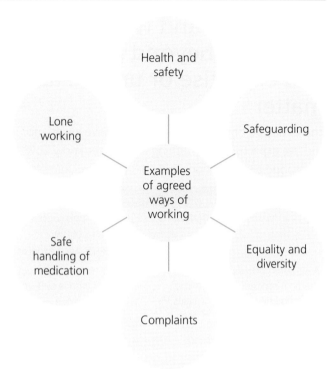

▲ Figure 4.2 Agreed ways of working in health and social care settings

RESEARCH IT

Have a look at your organisation's policies and procedures.

- What implications do they have for your work?
- If you didn't follow them, what could happen?

Most social care organisation's have policies and procedures which cover the following topics:

- health and safety – including first aid, fire, infection control, moving and handling, COSHH, accident reporting, risk assessments
- missing persons
- safeguarding and protection
- equal opportunities
- administration of medication
- concerns and complaints
- whistleblowing
- supporting people's behaviour
- record keeping and confidentiality
- care planning
- dealing with visitors
- staff development and training.

You should have a chance to read policies, procedures and the agreed ways of working in your induction. You will probably need to sign to say you have read and understood these. Updates will be discussed in team meetings or supervision/support meetings.

If there are any aspects of your employer's agreed ways of working that you do not understand or are unsure about, you must seek advice from your manager. Do not sign them indicating that you have understood them if you haven't, as you may not be following them as you are legally required to do. This may mean not only the loss of your job but also that you will be placing everyone's health, safety and well-being at risk.

AC1.6 The importance of reporting practices that are unsafe or conflict with codes of conduct and professional practice, standards or policies and procedures, and how this should be done

It is important to report unsafe and illegal practices to ensure you are following legislation, policies, procedures and codes of practice, as well as ensuring a duty of care and people's safety. Practices that should be reported include:

- bullying or harassment
- not following policies or procedures, legislation or codes of practice
- swearing at individuals, children or young people
- not treating people with dignity and respect
- any form of abuse.

If you feel you are unable to speak to the manager in your care setting, you can report your concerns to someone more senior, or if it is still not resolved, go directly to CIW. All information you share will be treated as confidential – and if you prefer you can do this anonymously (this means that you do not have to leave your name or contact details when you email or telephone).

To whistleblow means to report any unsafe or illegal working practices used in your setting. It may seem scary to report the people you work with, but as long as you have reasonable belief that disclosure is in the interest of the public, then you should.

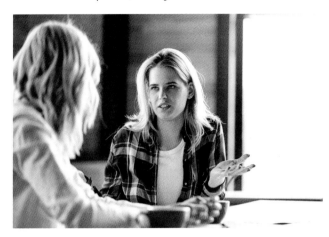

▲ Figure 4.3 It is important to speak out to report any concerns you may have

Whistleblowers receive protection. For example:

- The employment rights or career of a whistleblower will not be affected as a result of them reporting unsafe practice.
- Legislation is also in place to protect a whistleblower.
- Your care setting will have a whistleblowing policy, and procedures in place for advice on what to do.

See the end of this unit for links to useful websites regarding whistleblowing.

- Anything you suspect that is of a criminal nature should still be discussed with your manager first. Your manager will then contact the police, or you may need to do this.
- If you have serious concerns about the setting where you work and not just a colleague, such as the setting's failure to care for individuals, you may need to go directly to the CIW.

Look at your organisation's policies or the internet for some examples of issues that should be reported in a health and social care setting.

AC1.7 The term 'duty of care'

Everyone who works in health and social care settings has a legal duty or responsibility to support individuals, children and young people and also other people they come into contact with (including their employer, colleagues and individuals' families and friends), so that danger, harm or abuse are avoided.

This means placing the best interests of all those people at the heart of everything you do, and making sure that they are kept away from harm.

Fulfilling your duty of care and supporting an individual's rights can be difficult at times, as dilemmas may arise which you will need to be able to handle or know where you can access support and advice.

Think about someone you care about, such as a family member or a good friend.

- How do you show that you care about this person?
- Do you treat them differently from other people you know? If so, how?
- Can you think of an occasion that you were worried about this person? Why were you worried?
- What did you do to show the person you cared about them?
- How did that make the person feel? How did it make you feel?

Promote best interests and safety

A duty of care means you must always:

- act in the best interests of others when carrying out your responsibilities
- make sure that they are kept safe from any harm.

This means considering what will be best for individuals you support – supporting them to make their own decisions but ensuring that they are aware of the risks associated with any decisions before they make them.

Examples of implementing your duty of care vary, such as:

- supporting an individual to decide on the best course of action
- reporting that the carpet in the entrance hall is frayed so that visitors and your colleagues do not accidentally trip over it.

Take action to prevent harm

Duty of care also requires you to take action to prevent harm. For example:

- If you see that the person you support is leading an inactive lifestyle and drinking heavily, it is your responsibility to make them aware of the consequences of this.

Your duty of care to individuals, your colleagues and visitors to the setting means that you must say something if you see unsafe practice. For example:

- If a colleague spills something on the floor and doesn't mop it up, you need to take action immediately so people don't slip. Not reporting unsafe practices can lead to others slipping over or the spread of infection, if the spillage contained, for example, bodily fluids.

This also goes hand in hand with promoting individuals' safety, by ensuring individuals are kept safe not only from harm and injury but also from being abused. Report any changes in an individual's behaviour that concern you. For example:

- You may notice that they become withdrawn or very tearful every time a specific family member visits them. This could possibly be a sign that the visitor is abusing them. This will not always be the case, of course, but not reporting this may result in the individual continuing to be subjected to abuse.

Promoting individuals' well-being

This goes hand in hand with working for the best interests of the individuals you support. Here you can exercise your duty of care by supporting individuals' rights to choice, privacy, dignity and respect, by working in person-centred ways that indicate that you genuinely care about individuals and aim to always provide good quality care.

Sometimes individuals are unable to make decisions for themselves because they do not have the capacity to do so, perhaps due to a learning disability or a mental health condition. In these situations, decisions can be made on their behalf and these are referred to as 'best interest' decisions.

It is still very important to record the reasons why the individual lacks capacity to make a decision and what has been done to maximise their capacity so that you can show the reasons behind your actions. It is your duty of care to work within the Mental Capacity Act. Remember that a duty of care is a legal requirement that you must fulfil when supporting individuals.

See AC5.5 for further information on best interest decisions.

AC1.8 Conflicts and dilemmas that may arise between duty of care and the rights of individuals

Ensuring a duty of care can cause dilemmas and conflict. Examples might include:

- Ensuring confidentiality versus passing information onto those that need to know – for example, when you think there might be a risk of harm or abuse.
- Supporting choice versus thinking about what is in the best interests of the individual – for example, if an individual continues to drink alcohol when this goes against medical advice.
- Supporting positive risk taking – if the person wants to carry out an activity that has significant risks.

It is not always the case that one duty automatically has priority over another. In these situations, you need to think about what is in the best interests of the individual and which option respects their rights. This is explored in Table 4.4.

Example of scenario or situation in the setting	What is your duty of care?	How might you address this situation?
A person you support is obese. She eats a lot of sugary food and consumes sugary drinks. What conflicts are there?	Your duty of care is to ensure that the individual is aware of the dangers that her diet poses to her health. You cannot force her to change her diet. However, you should make her aware of the information that is available about healthy eating and the dangers to their health of eating too much sugar, by speaking to them about this.	Speak to the individual about the dangers and risks that her lifestyle poses. Ensure you give her information on healthy eating and the dangers of eating too much sugar. You should offer and encourage healthier alternatives. If her eating habits are severely affecting her health, then you should also consult your manager, who will advise whether you should speak to the individual's GP for further advice.
You need to assist an individual with mobility problems to have bath. He tells you he doesn't want a bath, but he hasn't had one for two weeks. What conflicts might you face?	Your duty of care is to ensure somebody is clean and support their personal hygiene. If he does have a bath, you need to ensure he is safe whilst getting in and out of the bath, and provide any other support to ensure his safety.	Even though you have a duty of care to support personal hygiene, if the person is deemed as having capacity then he has a right to choose. It may be that he would prefer a shower or a wash or he might prefer to have one at a different time or day or with a different worker supporting him. Discuss the options and what support is available, and give information about the consequences of not having a bath if he still insists he isn't going to look after his personal hygiene.
Your colleague asks you to assist them with moving an individual from their bed to their chair but you have no skills and previous experience in this. What conflict might you face?	As you have no experience with the moving procedure, the best course of action is to speak up and say so. If you decided to go ahead, just because you have been put on the spot, you risk the safety of the individual being compromised. By speaking up, you have fulfilled your duty of care to the individual by ensuring they are not at risk and shown that you have their best interests at heart. You have also fulfilled your duty of care to the setting where you work as you could have potentially breached your job role, responsibilities and the agreed ways of working.	Speak up and say you cannot carry out the moving and handling procedure. Inform another colleague and ask someone who has the skills to complete the task. Inform your manager of what has happened and explain your reasons for not wanting to complete the task. Ask for training in moving and handling so that you are able to gain the knowledge and skills in order to complete these tasks.

▲ Table 4.4 How to exercise your duty of care

CASE STUDY

Duty of care

Sally supports two people in a mental health setting. She has just gone on shift at 1 p.m. and the individual she is supporting is still in bed. She has noticed this has happened a number of times, and each time a support worker Jeff has been on shift. When she asks Jeff how the morning has gone, he says that the person wanted to stay in bed.

Discussion points:

- What should Sally do in this situation?

Sometimes there is a conflict between supporting choice and implementing duty of care. In this situation, you would need to ask the following questions:

- Does the person have capacity – are they making an informed choice?
- Does it happen with other workers, or is it just with Jeff, as Sally seems to think?
- How often does it happen?
- Could there be an underlying health problem, such as depression?
- Has the person got enough going on in their lives to motivate them to get up?

It might be that the person does have capacity and it has only happened twice. (It just so happens that Jeff was on shift both times.) Both occasions were at the weekend when the person didn't have to get up for a particular reason. If this is the case then you wouldn't need to take any action.

However, if it was a regular occurrence, it wouldn't be in the individual's best interests to stay in bed on a regular basis unless a health condition necessitated it. In this instance you would need to discuss it with the team, so that guidance can be agreed on what to do in the best interest of the individual.

AC1.9 The term 'duty of candour' and state why it is important to be open and honest if things go wrong

The 'duty of candour' is your legal duty to be open and honest with individuals and their families when something goes wrong that appears to cause harm or has the potential to cause harm. We have already introduced this concept in Units 001/002, AC1.4.

This duty applies to all health and social care settings and social care workers. It is important to be honest if mistakes have been made so they can be prevented from happening again and trust can be maintained.

Duty of candour was introduced and recommended as a result of the Francis Inquiry report published in February 2013 into Mid-Staffordshire NHS Foundation Trust. The inquiry examined the causes of serious failings in care over a period of 50 months, between 2005 and 2009, at a Staffordshire hospital where a disputed estimate of 400–1200 patients died because of poor care.

The report made 290 recommendations, including the statutory or legal duty of candour for all health and social care workers and services. As a result of the report and its findings, health and social care workers have a legal responsibility to ensure the following:

- Openness – you must enable individuals and others to raise concerns and complaints freely without fear.
- Transparency – you must only share information about the care of individuals with, for example, team members and regulators such as the CIW.
- Candour – you need to ensure that any individual who is harmed by care or support services is informed of this, as they may not realise it. For example:
  - An individual may have been assisted with their personal hygiene by a worker who has since found out they had an infection; the risk of potential infection must be explained to the individual.
  - An appropriate solution must be offered, regardless of whether the individual or someone else acting on their behalf has made a complaint or has raised any queries.

Implementing the duty of candour

1 **Tell individuals or their representatives when their care or support has gone wrong, has caused significant harm or has the potential to cause significant harm in the future.** In this way you will be promoting individuals' rights to be safe and free from harm and acting in their best interests.

2 **Inform individuals and their representatives what happened as fully as possible.** This must also be put in writing, and include an apology and the actions that will be taken next. For example:

- the safety measures that will be put in place
- sources of support available for those affected.

In this way you will be promoting individuals' and others' well-being by upholding their rights to being informed, communicated with and treated with respect, like an equal partner in the working relationship.

3 Be open and honest about all incidents that appear to have caused or have the potential to cause significant harm to individuals and others. In this way, you will not be failing to act when care or support goes wrong by working in line with the agreed scope of your job role. By being honest about any mistakes you have made, you can then ensure you learn from these and make sure they don't happen again.

As we saw in AC1.6 of this unit, if it is not just you who has made a mistake, and you have concerns that the care setting is not complying with the duty of candour, you must in the first instance follow your agreed ways of working for making a complaint. If you are dissatisfied with the response you receive from your complaint, you can raise your concerns directly with the CIW.

If organisations and care settings fail to comply with the duty of candour, they can face serious consequences such as being closed down, heavy fines and even criminal prosecution.

AC1.10 Accountability for quality of own practice

As a social care worker, you will have to register with Social Care Wales. In order to be a registered practitioner, you will need to adhere to the standards required of you, including the Code of Practice. Failure to adhere to these could result in your registration being taken away from you – this would mean that you wouldn't be able to work in the health and social care sector again. You are also legally accountable to individuals you support for any errors you make or procedures you omit to follow which result in harm.

In order to be accountable for your practice, you will need to work in ways which maintain best practice. You can achieve this by doing the following:

- Read, understand and follow your employer's agreed ways of working. If you are unsure about any aspects of your work activities, raise this in the first instance with your manager.

CASE STUDY

Duty of care and duty of candour

Jennie has been a care and support worker for many years, and now works weekends in a residential service. Jennie is very hard working and takes her responsibilities as a care and support worker very seriously.

Today, Thursday, Jennie has come into work because it is the monthly staff meeting and all staff must attend. As Jennie has arrived a little early, she has time to have a coffee break in the office where she meets with some of the other members in her team. As discussions among the staff ensue, some of the team members comment that as Jennie is only a weekend worker, she doesn't really have a duty of care towards the individuals she supports (or the others she works with), because duty of care only applies to those team members who work full-time (as they are the ones who see the individuals who live in the home regularly and know them best).

Jennie joins in the discussion and begins by saying that she thinks that everyone who works in the home has a duty of care towards the individuals as well as others they work with. Jennie adds that having a duty of care has nothing to do with how often you work with an individual or how many hours you do.

Having a duty of care, Jennie states, is about working in a way that does not put individuals' or others' health and safety at risk. It also means being responsible and supporting individuals to take the lead and be in control of their lives. Sometimes, Jennie explains, this may also mean recognising when the care provided is not effective and being honest about this with individuals and others involved in their lives.

Discussion points:

- How would you have felt if you were Jennie in this situation? Why would you feel this way?
- Would you have acted in a different way? Why?
- Is there anything else that Jennie could have included about the meaning of duty of care?
- Does Jennie say anything about the duty of candour?

- Familiarise yourself with the standards expected of you, and take these into account when you practise.
- Seek information, guidance and support from your manager and colleagues in relation to how you can improve and develop your work practices.
- Always follow the guidance given to you in training.
- Implement person-centred practice at all times.
- Implement principles of care into everything you do.

AC1.11 The importance of reflection and how to use this to improve practice

What is reflection?

To reflect means to think. Being able to reflect is an important skill to have at work. It involves thinking honestly about your practice, both the positive and negative aspects, and not being afraid to question your practice. When you reflect, you:

- take a 'step back' from your day-to-day activities and spend time thinking about a work activity you have carried out or a situation you have experienced
- examine in detail the reasons why and how you carry out your work practices
- assess the knowledge and skills you have and the behaviours you show, including their impact on you, the individuals you provide care to and others
- identify your strengths and weaknesses
- identify areas of your work practice that can be improved
- develop different ways of working that can improve your working practice
- develop new areas of learning such as different or new approaches to situations that may arise.

Reflection can be thought of as a continuous cycle. Gibbs' reflective cycle (1988) is often used by social care workers for reflecting on their work activities. It shows the different stages in the reflection process and the questions you should be asking yourself: see Figure 4.4.

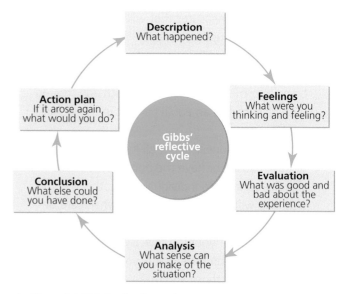

▲ Figure 4.4 Gibbs' reflective cycle

Reflection is an important part of your practice qualification. You will be required to keep a reflective log throughout the qualification. The next activity will help you prepare for this.

REFLECT ON IT

Skills for reflecting

Think about the different skills that are involved in reflection.

- Are you a good reflector?
- What skills do you think you need to develop to become a better reflector?
- Do you currently reflect on your practice?
- How can you build reflection on practice into your working practice?

Handovers, team meetings, supervisions and support meetings are all times when you can reflect on your practice.

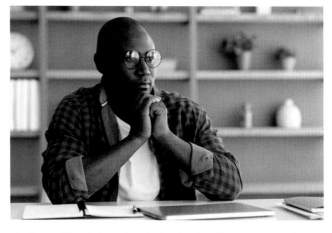

▲ Figure 4.5 It is important to be able to reflect on your work

Why is reflection important?

Reflecting on your work activities does not just happen once a week or at the end of the month. It is a continuous process that you will use throughout your career and in the different roles you undertake. Reflecting on your work activities is an important way to:

- **Get to know yourself** – the personal qualities you have, the areas of knowledge, understanding, skills and behaviours you have and those you need to develop.

  Gaining a greater understanding of who you are will help you to recognise how your practices influence others.

  This will also lead you to know more about the individuals you provide care and support to, so that you can adapt your working practice to meet their unique needs and preferences.
- **Develop yourself** – by identifying opportunities to address gaps in your knowledge, skills and behaviours.

  For example, you may do this by accessing additional training from the care setting where you work or working closely with a more experienced colleague. Doing so will improve your competence and your work practice.
- **Develop best practice** – by finding out about the practices and approaches that are not working, you and your colleagues will be able to develop new ways of working and approaches that will have a positive influence on the care and support that you provide to individuals.

Essentially, it is only by reflecting that you can look at a situation and decide if you need to change your approach or actions, either during the situation or the next time you are faced with a similar one.

Tips for reflection

- Think about your successes and the things that you have done well so that others can learn from them.
- Thinking positively can also improve your performance and positively affect your behaviour when you are with individuals.
- Take some time to step back and decide how you will approach the situation you are faced with, to ensure you have thought this through and it is a sensible approach.

- At the end of the day, reflect on what has happened during that day (what has gone well and what you could improve). Making this a part of your daily routine for improving your role can improve the experiences of people you support.
- Remember that everyone makes mistakes, and there are always areas where we can improve. It's important to admit this.
- Don't focus too much on the weaknesses and things that have not gone well, as this will leave you feeling demotivated. Balance the positives and the areas for development.
- Don't think that you are too busy or too tired to reflect at the end of the day. Reflection will enhance and improve things for you and the people you support by improving your work practices.

RESEARCH IT

There are a number of reflective practice models. The Gibbs Model is mentioned above but you may find another model suits your learning style better.

Look on the internet for other reflective practice models, and reflect on an activity you have carried out recently. This will help you if you progress to the City & Guilds Health and Social Care: Core.

AC1.12 The term 'confidentiality' and how this can be maintained by health and social care workers

KEY TERM

Confidentiality: to keep something private or secret.

Confidentiality is an important principle for those working in health and social care settings with children, young people and adults, as you will come across personal, private and sensitive information in your role. It underpins every aspect of your job role, duties and responsibilities. As a health and social care professional, this will mean that you will need to:

- respect the personal information of individuals and their families

- respect individuals' and their families' rights to privacy
- share information only with those who need to know
- gain permission from individuals' before you share information
- instil trust between you and individuals and/or their families
- share personal information only with others when there is a reason to do so
- keep all personal information in a secure location
- password-protect computers
- only hold records for as long as they are required in line with your organisational policy.

Demonstrating confidentiality requires social care workers to follow the agreed ways of working as set out in their confidentiality policy and procedures in their work settings. Legislation such as the Data Protection Act, GDPR and the Freedom of Information Act is also relevant, because they set out how to work with personal information about individuals and their families.

Confidentiality in day-to-day communication refers to all personal information that is held about or obtained from individuals and their families such as name, address, date of birth, employment history, current and past health conditions, care and support needs.

It includes all personal information that has been shared verbally, in writing, electronically or in other formats such as photographs, signs and symbols.

Table 4.5 shows the dos and don'ts of confidentiality.

Do	Don't
Make sure you only share individuals' personal information with those who have authorisation or those who are allowed to know it, for example, your manager. If there is a health emergency, a GP or hospital consultant may request personal information about an individual's health. You will need to seek guidance from your manager about this, or the GP may need to speak directly with your manager, who will only disclose the information that is required.	Don't share individuals' personal information with other individuals in the care setting unless you have permission or consent to do so from the individual. If the individual is unable to consent, then you must have permission from their representative. For example, don't disclose personal information about individuals to others accidentally, such as mentioning that an individual is diabetic and therefore cannot have a piece of chocolate cake like everyone else.
Store individuals' records securely in the care setting. They should be stored in a locked cupboard when no longer being used.	Don't discuss individuals when out of the setting and in public places. If you are upset by a situation and need to discuss it, do so in a way that keeps all personal and private information confidential. <ul><li>Never mention names, personal details, appearance, where the individual is from or anything that may reveal the identity of the individual.</li><li>Don't discuss individuals in a negative way.</li></ul>This will not only mean that you are following confidentiality rules and guidelines, but it will also mean that individuals, colleagues and those outside the workplace know that you can be trusted and relied upon.
Complete individuals' written records in a private area – in the office and out of view from others.	Don't discuss individuals with other individuals you care for. Think about how you would feel if people you knew discussed you with others. Creating and maintaining trust between yourself and the individual you care for is key to your relationship and the care that you offer them.
Make sure that individuals' electronic records are only accessed by those who have permission to do so and are password-protected.	Don't leave individuals' records lying around when not in use, as they may be accessed by those who do not have authorisation to do so.
	Don't give confidential details over the phone if possible. If you do need to give details over the phone, check the identity of the person who has called you. You may need to take their number and call them back so that you are able to take some time to check their identity.
	Don't speak about individuals where other members of staff can overhear you.

▲ Table 4.5 Dos and don'ts for maintaining confidentiality

AC1.13 Circumstances when 'confidential' information must be passed on and who this should be passed on to

Individuals have the right to have all personal information held about them kept private. However, sometimes there may be occasions when it is necessary to share their personal information with others **in confidence**. This process of sharing confidential information with others is referred to as doing so on a **'need to know'** basis. This means that only relevant information is shared with those who require it. Below are some examples of when you may need to breach confidentiality:

- if the individual poses a risk of harm to someone else
- the notification of infectious diseases
- the prevention of terrorism
- because of a police investigation
- if the person is at risk of abuse or has been abused.

When passing on confidential information, there are certain things you will need to think about:

- Check the identity of anyone you give confidential information to – it is important to check the identity of anyone who has requested the information, especially people you do not know outside the setting. This is to make sure that confidential information is not then passed on to others to misuse.
- Dealing with family members or relatives – remember that just because someone is related to the individual, it does not mean that they are automatically entitled to see the individual's records. You must ensure you have consent from the individual.
- You may need to pass information to somebody when the individual has requested you not to, such as in a safeguarding situation. You should inform the person that you need to pass the information on to protect them.

KEY TERMS

In confidence: when sharing information, this means to trust that it will be kept confidential.

'Need to know': you should only pass on information when it is absolutely necessary in order to protect an individual's privacy and ensure their safety.

CASE STUDY

An individual you support is found unconscious in their bedroom. You call an ambulance. In order to treat the individual effectively, the paramedic will require personal information about the individual, such as whether they have any current health conditions and whether they are taking any medication.

A young person who visits a mental health drop-in centre and wishes to have lunch will need to inform the staff there about their allergy to nuts, so that their dietary needs can be met and they can be kept safe from becoming unwell.

Tom lives in a residential care setting, and shares information with his key worker that he observed a visitor shouting at another individual who lives in the same setting. Tom will need to be informed that the worker is required to pass this information on 'in confidence' to their manager, who will inform social services in order to protect the individual from any further harm or abuse.

Discussion point: These are examples of situations where confidential information will need to be passed on. Can you think of any others?

REFLECT ON IT

Confidential information
Reflect on the importance of sharing confidential information about individuals when providing care and support.

What are the consequences of not doing so?

AC1.14 Potential conflicts and dilemmas that can occur between retaining confidentiality and safe practice

Conflicts and dilemmas can occur when deciding whether information should be passed on:

- Something may happen that makes you suspect that there might be a problem, but you are not sure, or an individual may tell you something and ask you not to tell anybody.
- You may not report something as you know that this might cause a lot of problems for yourself, a colleague or someone you support.

Anything that gives you a cause for concern should be reported to your manager, who can decide on appropriate action. If you think someone is at risk of harm or abuse, you should report it even if the individual asks you not to. You should tell the individual you will need to pass this information on.

Remember that you have a duty of care to people you support, so by not reporting something you could be held accountable. Even though you might not feel comfortable reporting something, you are protecting the person so it is in their best interests and yours to do so.

We will look at safeguarding in more detail in Unit 006.

CASE STUDY

An individual you support goes home for the weekend. When they return, you notice they have bruises on their arms. When you ask them what happened, they say that they walked into the corner of a cupboard. They say you don't need to make a fuss about it as it is only a bruise. You are concerned but you are not sure whether it should be reported as you know the individual likes going home.

Discussion point: What action should you take?

AC1.15 Why it is important to discuss with individuals and/or carers any 'confidential' information that must be passed on

If you need to pass on information about individuals to others, you must make sure that you discuss this with the individual. In some cases, you will need to obtain their consent. In other cases (see AC1.13) you should pass it on even if they do not consent. It is important to discuss this with them so you can:

- get consent where required
- ensure you have a true picture of what happened
- be open and honest in implementing your duty of candour (if you have to pass this on and they do not consent)
- maintain trusting relationships
- let people know that you are trying to protect them.

When an individual lacks capacity and is unable to give consent, permission must be sought from their representative.

Telling the person you are going to pass on information will mean you are not breaking confidentiality agreements. You should tell the individual or their representative what you will need to pass on, who you are going to pass it on to and how. Also, you should explain the reasons why you need to pass this information on.

LO2 KNOW HOW TO DEVELOP AND MAINTAIN EFFECTIVE PARTNERSHIP WORKING WITH OTHERS IN HEALTH AND SOCIAL CARE

GETTING STARTED

Working in partnership with individuals, children and young people, families, carers and other professionals is an essential part of your work in the health and social care sector. Developing and maintaining effective relationships with others is crucial so that you can all work together to meet individuals' needs.

Think about all the people you might work in partnership with in a health and social care setting.

AC2.1 The principles of working in partnership

Your job role in health and social care will involve working alongside a wide range of different people and organisations that have different roles and responsibilities. This may include:

- the individuals you provide care or support to, their families, friends, advocates or others who are important to them
- your colleagues and other team members such as your manager
- professionals from other organisations such as social workers, mental health nurses, dieticians, dementia care nurses and GPs.

Working in partnership with others is more than just working alongside them. It involves becoming 'a team'. This can only happen when you are all committed to:

- **sharing a common set of values** – to support individuals' independence, to safeguard individuals from harm, to respect individuals' unique differences
- **agreeing goals** – to enable positive outcomes for individuals (which may be agreed over both short and long periods of time)
- **communicating effectively** – communications must be open and honest, timely and regular, and can be verbal or written.

Working in partnership brings many benefits for you, the individuals you support, and others both inside and outside

the organisation. Most importantly in a setting, working effectively as a team and in partnership means that you all have the shared goal of providing the best support possible for individuals. Working in partnership and working effectively together can have the following benefits:

- You all improve and develop your understanding of different ways of working, share knowledge and best practice. For example, a colleague may show you a more effective way of communicating with an individual who has hearing loss.
- A stronger team creates a better working environment where you all feel supported.
- Understanding one another's roles and responsibilities will avoid duplicating your work, so that you make better use of your time. You may also share resources, such as meeting venues, which can reduce costs and encourages everyone to meet together.
- You all work together to provide person-centred care. Individuals receive care that is co-ordinated and meets all of their needs.

AC2.2 The term 'co-production' in relation to partnership working with others

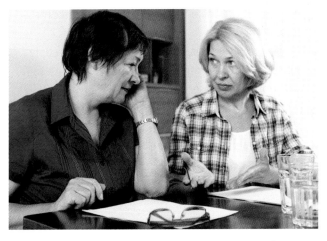

▲ Figure 4.6 How do you work in partnership with others?

Co-production is one of the key principles of the Social Services and Well-Being (Wales) Act 2014. We have already looked at co-production in Units 001/002, AC1.1 and AC3.2.

Co-production means that a group of people work together in an equal partnership to achieve a goal. In health and social care, this means that professionals, individuals, children and young people as well as people important to them all work together to achieve the best outcomes for the person who needs support. This will enable them to live the best life they can in line with their wishes, needs and abilities.

The principle of co-production is based on:

- mutual respect
- equality
- networks of mutual support
- sharing of skills
- building on strengths
- outcomes-focused
- trust and reciprocity
- partnership work
- shared responsibility.

Traditionally, services were designed by managers, social workers and other professionals. Co-production means individuals are in an equal partnership, designing their own service with the appropriate support. In the past, services were based on the idea of doing things 'for' or 'to' individuals. Co-production is about doing 'with' them.

Benefits of co-production

Co-production:

- recognises that people know best what matters to them
- creates opportunities for people to access support when they need it
- creates opportunities for social change
- provides more meaningful, flexible and outcomes-focused services
- recognises individuals, children and young people have a positive contribution to make to the design and operation of services
- supports and empowers people to get involved in the design and delivery of services
- empowers people to take responsibility for their own lives
- ensures that professionals work together
- gives people a stronger voice
- builds individuals' resilience
- makes effective use of resources.

Think about the organisation you work in or imagine a residential service for young people or for people with dementia.

- Can you give examples of co-production in action?
- Think of how this could be developed. Discuss this with your manager.

AC2.3 Roles of other workers and professionals in health and social care

Working together with other people is part of your day-to-day role as a health and social care worker. Every professional relationship you have will be different, so it is really important to know the roles and responsibilities of everyone you will come into contact with.

There are many different professionals involved in health and social care services. Each has their own role and contribution to meeting an individual's needs. Knowing people's roles will help make the best use of resources and the team's strengths. It will enable people to work together in the best interests of the people they support.

- **Care and support worker** – supports individuals with all aspects of day-to-day living.
- **Activities worker** – organises social activities for people who need care and support. This can include trips, days out, craft activities and entertainment. Activities workers will also support people while undertaking these activities.
- **Rehabilitation/reablement worker** – supports people to develop their skills to enable them to live independently often following an illness, such as a stroke.
- **Shared Lives carer** – opens up their home and family life to enable someone who needs care and support to come and live with them. This can be permanently or just for a few hours a week.
- **Advocacy worker** – are either volunteers or paid. Their role is to represent individuals, children and young people so their voices are heard and their best interests are considered when decisions are made which affect their lives.

- **Social care manager** – manages a service such as a domiciliary care service or a residential service. Managers register with Social Care Wales and have certain responsibilities as a 'registered person' in relation to ensuring quality and implementing the code of practice.
- **Social worker** – draws up the initial care and support plan so that a package of services can be accessed to meet the individual's needs.
- **Occupational therapist** – works with people with disabilities to ensure they have the right equipment for daily living. They also help with physical rehabilitation.
- **Physiotherapist** – works with individuals with physical disabilities or injuries, and designs a treatment and exercise plan to help those individuals improve their movement.
- **Safeguarding officer** – works for the social services department, and receives and investigates reports into actual or potential abuse.
- **Foster carer** – provides a home to children and young people when their own parents cannot.
- **Playworker** – develops and creates opportunities for children to play. They could work for a local authority or in health or educational settings.
- **Dietician** – supports people to maintain a healthy diet.
- **Nurse** – there are different types of nurses including community nurses, mental health nurses, stoma nurses, Marie Curie cancer care nurses, who support people with different health needs.
- **Inspector** – works for CIW, and inspects and takes action to improve the quality of care in Wales. They will visit services regularly to ensure they meet standards.

REFLECT ON IT

Find out about the people you may come into contact with in your job.

- What role do they play in the lives of the individuals, children and young people you support?
- Looking at the list above, is there any other job role that you can think of which is not listed? Find out about what they do.

AC2.4 The importance of multi-agency working

Multi-agency working protects individuals and ensures their rights are met. The Social Services and Well-Being (Wales) Act 2014 provides a framework for health and social care services to be integrated.

Safeguarding in particular requires all professionals to work together in the best interests of the individual. Agencies should have shared values so that person-centred services are delivered in a way which keeps people safe.

Benefits of multi-agency working

If all the appropriate agencies are working together to meet the needs of individuals, children and young people, and their carers and families, this will ensure:

- the right people are able to provide the necessary care and support
- workers have the skills and expertise required to meet individuals' needs
- everybody involved in a person's care and support knows what is going on
- an individual can access the services and equipment they need
- effective and responsive communication
- individuals are safeguarded and protected
- there is a joined-up approach.

When working together, the following components ensure effective multi-agency working:

- an environment in which people can work together effectively
- professionals who understand each other's roles and responsibilities
- professionals who support and challenge each other
- continuous learning and development
- effective systems for information sharing
- effective leadership focused on the individual, child or young person across the partnerships
- effective communication built on mutual respect and trust
- no power struggles
- no protecting one's own job role
- commitment to ensuring you complete agreed tasks
- taking responsibility for your part in the team.

AC2.5 The importance of developing good relationships while maintaining clear professional boundaries when working with other workers and professionals, carers and families, as well as individuals

In order for multi-agency working to succeed, positive relationships must be formed as described above. This ensures effective partnership work in order to meet people's needs.

CASE STUDY

Rosie was involved in a serious road traffic accident and suffered severe brain injuries. She was in hospital for six months following the accident. After Rosie left hospital, she needed 24-hour support. She had limited communication, problems with memory and couldn't walk. She lived at home with her husband and two children.

Before her discharge from hospital, the social worker, physiotherapist, occupational therapist, nurses and surgeon were all involved in her care.

The occupational therapist carried out an assessment of her home and ensured she had the right equipment to help her with her mobility and day-to-day living.

The physiotherapist worked intensively with Rosie to try to improve her mobility and co-ordination. She also developed a long-term rehabilitation programme to help Rosie regain as much mobility as possible. She worked with Rosie and her husband to show them the exercises they needed to do daily. The physiotherapist was planning to visit Rosie once a week to continue her physical recovery.

The social worker developed a care and support plan with Rosie and her husband. Rosie's husband, who was self-employed, had been off work for the last six months looking after the children. Rosie and her husband however felt it was important for him that he aimed to go back to work over the next few months, even if it was only part-time.

A domiciliary care agency was contracted to provide support to Rosie from 7 a.m. to 10 a.m. to help her get up and do some housework in the mornings so that Rosie's husband could get the children off to school.

The surgeon was planning to perform a series of operations over the next two years, to try to improve Rosie's mobility and some of the health problems she was facing.

Discussion points:

- What are the benefits of multi-agency working to Rosie?
- What are the benefits of multi-agency working to Rosie's family?
- How should the multi-agency team that are supporting Rosie work together over the next year to ensure Rosie's and her family's needs are met?
- Are there any other agencies that may need to be involved in supporting Rosie and her family?

When working with other agencies, it is important to always remain professional. This can sometimes be difficult for a number of reasons:

- being asked to do things outside your job role
- personality clashes between professionals
- relationships not built on trust and mutual respect
- not feeling confident working with professionals who use complicated terminology
- power struggles.

If you have any difficulties, open and honest communication with the professional or your manager will help to resolve the problem. Your manager can support you in whatever way you need to help resolve any issues. You should always work in the best interests of the people you support. That will help to ensure positive multi-agency work.

Remaining professional with individuals you support

Developing a positive, professional relationship with people you support is key to the success of ensuring their well-being. The Social Services and Well-Being (Wales) Act requires you to have conversations with the people you support in order to discover their wants, needs and desires. In order to do this effectively, you must have effective communication built on a foundation of mutual trust, professionalism and respect.

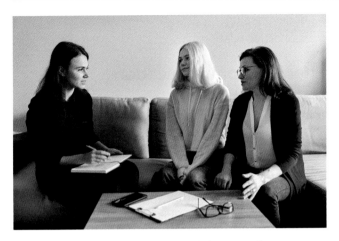

▲ Figure 4.7 Effective communication is important for professional working relationships

When supporting people in health and social care settings, relationship-centred working is crucial, but this can cause uncertainty for some people as it can be difficult to know where the boundaries of these relationships are. Being aware of the professional boundaries of the relationship will help.

Sometimes you might be one of the most important people in an individual's, child's or young person's life. This might mean they see you as a friend. It is important to ensure people know where the boundaries are, and that you are not their friend but are a professional worker who is there to support them.

Setting boundaries at the start of a relationship helps both parties to understand and explore the nature of that relationship. It helps ascertain what is acceptable or unacceptable, and sets people's expectations about the relationship and how they can best work together.

Principles for maintaining professional boundaries

- The relationship you have with people you support can be seen as similar to a friendship. However, it is a professional relationship with the purpose of supporting someone to ensure their needs are met. You can be 'friendly' but you are not their friend.
- Health and social care workers should work in a way that promotes professionalism, clarity, consistency, fairness and transparency.
- The needs of the individual should be paramount. Your own values should not affect the way you support an individual. Your aim is to support the individual to have an active part in their lives as much as possible.
- You should be responsible for maintaining your own professional boundaries. Sometimes this can be difficult, such as during end of life care. You should reflect on and identify when you are having difficulties maintaining these professional boundaries, and seek extra help so you can discuss your own feelings and access specialist advice.
- Professional boundaries include all forms of communication including social media. Don't accept people you support as 'friends' unless it is for a group related to supporting them and is part of the individual's care plan.

You should always remain professional when using social media, even for personal use, and you should not present the organisation you work for or your job in a negative light. Don't share confidential information about people you support or the organisation.

- If an individual misunderstands or becomes confused about a relationship, you should report this immediately and seek advice about how to proceed.
- Supervision is a crucial aspect of supporting professional practice, as it enables you to reflect on your practice, seek feedback from others and develop actions you can take to improve.
- If you already have a relationship of any form with an individual you support or their families or friends, you should report this to your manager immediately so there is no conflict of interest and professional boundaries can be maintained.
- When individuals, children and young people start using a service, they should have information on the aims and objectives, roles and responsibilities of all parties and limits of the service. This will support professional boundaries.
- You should know the limits of your role as detailed in your job description, and know when to signpost people to other services if they are outside the scope of your role, such as a counselling service.
- You should support individuals, children and young people to develop and maintain their own relationships and friendships within their community, so that you are not seen as a replacement for friends.

- Individuals and their families should know how to complain and the appropriate channels of communication.

Unacceptable practice

Some practices are clearly unacceptable and are a breach of legislation and the Code of Professional Practice. These include:

- causing physical harm to individuals
- sexual contact with individuals, children and young people
- being aggressive or showing anger to individuals
- inappropriate touching or hugging
- seeking personal information that is unnecessary
- sharing own personal or intimate information where it is unnecessary
- not reporting accidents or important information to managers and colleagues
- abusing your role in any way
- accepting gifts in return for favours
- misusing an individual's money or belongings
- treating some individuals more favourably than others, having favourites or being over-involved with a particular individual
- providing care and support that you are not qualified to do
- trying to impose your own culture or religious beliefs and values on others
- providing support that will not achieve the personal care plan

Can you think of any other examples to add to this list? There are more examples and further discussion of unacceptable practice in Unit 006 on Safeguarding.

AC2.6 Ways of working that build trust

Effective working relationships must be built on openness, honesty and trust. There will be times when you are able to all work successfully to meet an objective, but there will also be times when you disagree with one another. This is all part of being in a team.

In order to work well with others, remember that good working relationships have key features, including:

- effective communication
- shared values

- understanding
- supportive relationships.

Effective communication

This includes both verbal and non-verbal communication, and means communicating clearly with colleagues, clarifying your understanding of what has been communicated.

When working in a team, you will need to ensure that everybody understands their role in order to offer the best possible care to individuals in the setting. This will include:

- effectively communicating in any discussions
- making sure that you value what everyone else has to say, their views and opinions
- working together to reach a decision which is in the best interest of the individual.

In writing, this involves using respectful language and ensuring what you have written is true.

Shared values

In working relationships, this involves treating others how you would like to be treated. In other words, treating the people you work with respectfully, being honest, polite, responsible and trustworthy. For example:

- You can show respect by being considerate of the opinions of colleagues, valuing their views and advice.
- You can show that you are trustworthy and honest by communicating correctly and accurately something that you have done wrong.

All of this helps to create strong relationships, where people are open and supportive of one another.

Understanding

This involves getting to know one another, knowing each other's strengths and limitations, and being willing to understand and learn more about each other's roles and responsibilities.

Supportive relationships

This means supporting one another to work together as a team. This may involve putting a colleague's needs before your own, or being prepared to give your time to a colleague who is finding it difficult to learn a new skill.

Support involves giving and receiving, sharing knowledge and experiences and also showing or displaying support for one another. You not only work together to resolve issues, but also demonstrate your support for colleagues by speaking up. For example, if you feel a colleague has made a good point, then you can say 'Yes, I agree with X. I think X has made a good point'.

Of course, there will be times when there will be disagreements in the team, but the best way to approach this is to listen carefully to all viewpoints and work together to reach a solution.

A good tip is to think about how you like to be supported at work, by your manager or by other colleagues:

- Do you sometimes want help and support when you are struggling with a task?
- Do you sometimes struggle with your workload and wish a colleague would help you?
- Do you wish someone would say 'well done' when you have done a good job?

Remember that your colleagues feel the same way too. They might sometimes feel that they have too much work to do, and might appreciate some encouragement on days when they are not at their best.

Empathising can help to create strong professional relationships. This will lead to a more productive and happier workplace if people feel supported and motivated to do their job.

AC2.7 The importance of respecting diversity and recognising cultural, religious, ethnic and linguistic differences when working in partnership

Think about a large group that you belong to. It could be the organisation you work for, or your school or college. Think about how diverse the group of people are.

There may be people with different backgrounds, culture, language, sexual orientation, religion and socio-economic status.

There are many benefits from living in a multicultural society where diversity is supported. Look back at Units 001/002, LO4, where we explored what diversity means.

It is important to respect diversity and difference when working in partnership for the following reasons:

- It enriches the partnership through shared experiences with different people.
- It promotes tolerance and understanding between partners from different cultures.
- It supports teamwork and fosters effective communication.
- It demonstrates professionalism, dignity and respect.
- It ensures we work within the requirements of legislation and codes of practice.
- It ensures individuals, children and young people's needs are met as they are the focus of the partnership with a strong team to support them.
- We can learn different perspectives.
- It is enriching to get to know other cultures better.

REFLECT ON IT

- How can we support diversity in social care settings?
- Is there anything more you can do in the setting you work in?

If we did not respect diversity when working in partnership:

- individuals' needs would not be met
- effective communication would not take place as individuals wouldn't feel respected and valued
- ultimately, you would not be doing your job in line with legislation and standards.

Check your understanding

1 Apart from legislation, name two other documents that outline your roles and responsibilities.

2 List two responsibilities you have under the Code of Professional Practice for Social Care.

3 What are the benefits of a job description?

4 How can you use a person specification?

5 What are the consequences of not adhering to your job role?

6 List three ways of getting additional support.

7 Why is it important to be honest when things go wrong?

8 Give three examples of when you might be held accountable for your practice.

9 What are the benefits of reflective practice?

10 When might you need to pass on confidential information?

11 List three people that you will work in partnership with.

12 What are the benefits of partnership working?

13 What are the benefits to individuals from multi-agency working?

14 List five ways you can build trust with your colleagues.

Question practice

1 Which of the following is your responsibility under the Health and Safety at Work Act?

  a Write a risk assessment for everything you do that is dangerous.

  b Ensure the safety of yourself and others.

  c Write policies and procedures to ensure safety.

  d Follow procedures for your safety only.

2 What is the main purpose of a job description?

  a to show the accountability of an employer

  b to list the legal requirements of an employee

  c to outline the overall requirements of a role

  d to manage staff disciplinary actions

3 Why should you seek support if you don't understand something?

  a so you will know what to do

  b so you can tell others how to do something

  c so your manager can help you

  d so you don't look ignorant

4 Policies, procedures and agreed ways of working must be followed. What is the main reason for this?

  a Your manager asks you to.

  b Legislation says you must.

  c It says you must in your induction handbook.

  d You will do what you are told.

5 Which of the following would be raised by a whistleblower?

  a a personal family problem

  b a change to an individual's support plan

  c an incident or unsafe practice

  d a disagreement between colleagues

6 What is a duty of care?

  a being open and honest with people

  b ensuring the safety of people you come into contact with

  c being caring towards individuals

  d making sure you tell people what you are doing

7 What should you do when there is a conflict between duty of care and the rights of individuals?

  a Don't say anything to your manager.

  b Ensure people's rights are always upheld.

  c Do what is in the best interests of the individual.

  d Do what your manager tells us to.

8 Confidentiality means:

  a never passing information on

  b passing information on a need to know basis

  c telling other professionals about people you support

  d ensuring people are confident in the service

9 A definition of co-production is:

a producing documents with others

b working with your manager on a task

c being on the same level as your co-workers

d working with the individual and others as equals

10 Why does a working relationship differ from a personal relationship?

a Your job is a paid position and has boundaries.

b You call individuals by their first name.

c Because you need consent.

d Because individuals see you as their friend.

LO3 KNOW HOW EFFECTIVE TEAM WORKING SUPPORTS GOOD PRACTICE IN HEALTH AND SOCIAL CARE

GETTING STARTED

Teamwork is essential in any workplace. As a health and social care worker, team work will be a big part of your job.

Think of a team that you have belonged to in the past. This could be a sporting team, a team at work, a team in school or college.

- What made it successful?
- What problems did you face?

AC3.1 Types of team working and how teams may differ in structure, purpose and constitution

When people come together to work towards a common goal, a team is formed. All team members have a purpose within the team, and are equals. Teams work together to achieve the aims for the good of individuals and the organisation. You might belong to a number of different types of teams at work, as shown in Table 4.6.

Type of team	Explanation
Permanent	This is a group of people who work with each other for a long time, and the team is not dissolved once a task is completed. A team of social care workers supporting individuals, children and young people in their own homes would be an example of a permanent team. Individual members within the team may change, but the team and its structure remains.
Temporary	This type of team disbands once the task has been completed. For example: • An individual coming out of hospital following a serious accident or illness may have a team of people supporting them, such as a physiotherapist, an occupational therapist, a social worker, a social care team and healthcare professionals. • Once the individual has undergone a period of rehabilitation, the team may disband as the individual's needs have been met.
Task group	This is a team designed for a specific purpose. It is sometimes known as a 'task and finish' group. • An example could be an organisation, which has a number of services across Wales, setting up a task and finish group to look at how the organisation can improve in a particular area of work, such as how they can increase the use of Welsh language in the workplace. • The task and finish group may consist of workers from all levels of job roles across the organisation.
Committees	This type of team can be permanent, temporary or work on a particular task. For example: • In a care home environment, individuals living in the home can form a residents' committee to put their views forward. • They might form a temporary committee to decide on a single task, such as redecoration of the home.

▲ Table 4.6 Different types of team

Type of team	Explanation
Self-managed	This type of team works together on a common purpose without a leader. Everybody in the team is accountable for their own actions. • An example would be a multi-disciplinary team at a care and support meeting. There may be a chair in meetings but there is no manager or leader.
Cross-functional	These types of teams may be formed to work on a particular task. For example: • A manager of a social care setting is moved temporarily to another role to work with others from across the organisation on a particular task, such as implementing and training staff on a new care and support planning and digital recording system.
Virtual	A virtual team is separated by distance but still works on tasks together, meeting online and through the use of digital communications.

▲ Table 4.6 Different types of team *(continued)*

All teams have a structure which identifies who is a member and who they report to. You usually see these in visual form as an organisational chart. Most organisational charts are hierarchical, as seen in Figure 4.8.

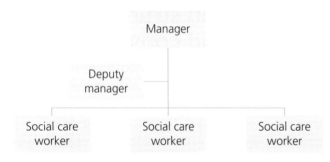

▲ Figure 4.8 Organisational chart

Some structures can be more organic, and have a circular form with links between a number of different people.

REFLECT ON IT

• Find a copy of the organisational chart in the organisation you work for.
• Check you know who everybody is and what their roles are.

There are different roles within teams. Dr Meredith Belbin was a management consultant who identified a number of team roles. He said that people have a natural tendency towards one or more roles. These roles include:

• The **resource investigator** always seems to know who can help. They are good at networking and exploring potential opportunities. They are extrovert, but can lose interest after the initial enthusiasm has worn off.

• The **shaper** is dynamic, determined and courageous. They thrive under pressure and have natural leadership skills. They can however be easily provoked and often don't think about the feelings of others in the team.

• The **co-ordinator** is mature, confident and a natural chairperson. They clarify goals and support decision making, but they can be manipulative and controlling.

• The **plant** is creative, imaginative and takes risks. They can solve difficult problems but they can be too immersed in a task to communicate with other team members effectively.

• The **team worker** is good at co-operating with others and is keen to build effective working relationships. They are sensitive and diplomatic. They usually don't like confrontation and might not be very good at making decisions in a crisis.

• The **monitor evaluator** is strategic and shows good judgement. They look at different options and weigh up difficult decisions. They monitor work processes and strive for quality. They can lack leadership, inspiration and drive.

• The **implementer** is reliable and disciplined. They act on ideas and are efficient. They can however be inflexible and slow to see opportunities.

• The **completer finisher** is keen to get the job done. They have a good eye for detail, and finishes and delivers a job on time. While they are reliable, they can be a worrier and reluctant to delegate.

Every role has positive aspects and areas they find difficult. None are better than others but a team should ideally have at least one of each role within the team. Most people naturally lean towards one or two of these roles.

RESEARCH IT

- Look online for a free Belbin questionnaire, and complete it to identify what role you are.
- Ask the colleagues in your team to also complete one, to see how your team is made up.

REFLECT ON IT

Imagine a team where everybody was a natural chairperson or a natural shaper. Imagine how that team would function.

- How do you think a team might perform if they didn't have one of the roles, such as a completer finisher?
- What do you think a team can do if they have too many people in one role and nobody in another role?
- Think about the team you belong to. Can you identify people who naturally fit these roles? What role do you think you might belong to?

AC3.2 Core principles that underpin effective team working

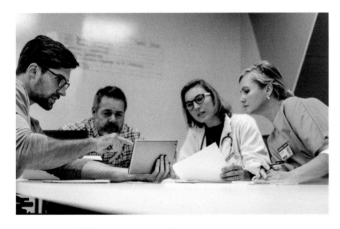

▲ Figure 4.9 Effective team working

Teamwork is one of the most essential qualities for the success of any organisation. If teamwork is not present then the organisation is far less likely to achieve its goals. Maintaining effective teamwork is an ongoing process and one that needs commitment from all members.

There are a number of core principles that ensure effective team work:

- **Clear vision, aims and objectives** – all team members should know the aims and how they are going to achieve them.

- **Commitment** – everybody in the team should be committed to the aim. If there is a lack of commitment, this will cause tension and it may cause the team to fail.
- **Ensure everyone is clear of individual roles** – this ensures tasks get done and people aren't expecting other team members to do what they themselves should be doing.
- **Ensure high levels of participation** – everyone should be involved. If people don't feel their contribution is valued, they won't be as committed
- **Effective communication** – communication will not only ensure things go right, but it will also ensure that problems can be resolved.
- **Establish clear leadership** – an effective leader ensures cohesion and co-ordinates action.
- **Maintain a positive, supportive culture** – the culture within a team is crucial to the success of the team. A positive culture supports effective relationships. Team members should feel able to admit if something has gone wrong and ask for help when they need it.
- **Encourage reflection and growth** – a team that constantly evaluates what it does is a team that improves and develops.
- **Trust** – team members must be able to trust each other, otherwise tasks will not be shared out equally and members will be checking up on what others are doing.
- **Have an action plan** – effective teams not only need goals but also a plan as to how they are going to achieve these goals. Realistic deadlines and everyone's roles should be agreed in order to achieve the goal.
- **Respect** – team members must respect each other. This will ensure a positive culture and effective communication. A lack of respect will create an atmosphere of paranoia, fear and anger.

REFLECT ON IT

Think about the team you belong to and the principles listed above.

- How well do you think you perform as a team?
- Is there anything you think you could do better?
- Think about a problem you may have had in your team. What would you say was the cause of the problem?
- Are there any other principles you think could be added to the list?

AC3.3 Ways effective team working contributes to the well-being of individuals

Team working brings together the skills, experience and knowledge of all members within the team, to meet the needs of individuals accessing services. Effective communication ensures everyone knows what is going on, so that a seamless service can be provided.

CASE STUDY

Maisie has learning and physical disabilities, and lives in a house with 24-hour support from a team of workers. The house always seems a happy place. The workers are all very friendly to Maisie and to each other. There is lots of laughter in the house as Tom, one of the workers, is a real joker.

The staff team provide excellent support to Maisie. They agree goals with her every month and they all support Maisie to achieve these goals. They record her progress on a chart on the back of her wardrobe door, which she likes as she can see how she is doing. Other staff know exactly where Maisie has reached as well.

The team have meetings which Maisie also attends. She can share her thoughts and opinions. If the team need to get authorisation for activities due to finances, they will usually discuss it with Karen the manager the same day and get back to Maisie straight away.

Maisie gets on well with all the workers as they are all so helpful. At the change of a shift, Maisie will often be involved in the handover and tell the workers who is starting their shift and what has been going on that morning. The workers always know what is happening even if they have been on leave, as they keep good records and always have a detailed handover.

Discussion points:

- What examples can you see in the case study above of effective team work?
- How does this support Maisie's well-being?

REFLECT ON IT

Think about the examples below of ineffective team work. How might these examples affect the people who are receiving services, and also other team members?

- One member of staff doesn't often write in the communication book.
- Some team members don't support individuals in the service to do the daily cleaning.
- One member of the team had an argument with another member last month and hasn't spoken to him since.
- One member of the team hates taking the young person swimming, and does their best to get out of it.
- Janet always likes to have weekends off and complains if she has to work over the weekend.

RESEARCH IT

There is lots of interesting information on teamwork. Theories of stages of team development are helpful to identify reasons for potential issues in a team. They can also be helpful in understanding some of the issues the individuals you are supporting may be going through, if for example they live in supported housing and somebody new moves in.

- Research stages of team development on the internet.
- How can you apply this to teams you work in?

LO4 KNOW HOW TO HANDLE INFORMATION

GETTING STARTED

Handling information in social care settings is a big responsibility. There is a lot of information to document about every individual in a care setting, and this is held in different files and reports.

The information about individuals is personal and private to them, so it is very important that these documents are handled with care. These are legal documents and need to be completed, stored and shared by following agreed ways of working and legal requirements.

- Make a list of all the records you keep at work.
- Why do you keep these records?

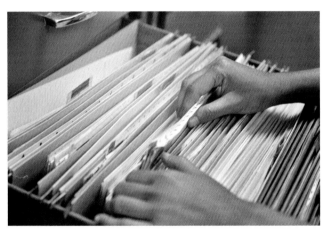

▲ Figure 4.10 Documents must be handled and stored responsibly

AC4.1 The term 'handling information'

Handling information means the storing, recording and passing on of information. In social care settings, you will come into contact with a lot of information on a daily basis. You have some responsibilities in relation to this information.

REFLECT ON IT

Think about all the conversations that you and your friends or family have.

- Do they ever tell you something private or personal about themselves that they do not want others to know?
- Do you make sure that you keep that information safe and not tell others?
- How would they feel if you told someone or passed on that information without asking them?
- Think about how you would feel if you told your friends something private about yourself and did not want them to tell anyone else.

Now think about the information that you tell people about yourself, and more specifically, official, private and **personal information** that you tell your doctor or a nurse.

- How might they record, store and share this information? You may not want them to pass this on to others without your permission.
- Why do you think it is important that they record, share and store this information in a safe way? Is this because the information is personal and private? Is it because you do not want others to have access to this information?
- Have you ever wanted to see the information that they have recorded about you?
- How would you feel if you asked to see the information that the people who care for you had recorded, only to be told you are not allowed to see it?

Thinking about these issues will help you to understand why it is important to handle information securely in care settings.

KEY TERM

Personal information: information that is personal to the individual such as their name, date of birth, weight, care needs.

Reasons for effective handling of information in a social care setting include:

- accountability
- shows how decisions were made
- supports the delivery of services
- helps to respond to complaints
- helps to identify risk
- supports effective clinical decisions
- supports person-centred practice

- ensures effective communication
- provides documentary evidence of outcomes
- promotes effective sharing of information in a multi-disciplinary team.

AC4.2 Legislation and codes of conduct and professional practice that relate to the handling of information including storing, recording, confidentiality and sharing

Legislation in relation to recording, storing and sharing information is very important because it:

- sets out the **rights** and **responsibilities** of all those who live and work in care settings
- requires accurate information to be recorded about individuals
- requires information about individuals to be shared securely.

In your role as a social care worker, you will need to know and understand the different pieces of legislation that exist in relation to the recording, storing and sharing of information so that you are able to carry out your duties to the best of your ability. Showing your **competence** involves putting into practice your knowledge and skills of how to record, store and share information effectively.

KEY TERMS

Rights: legal entitlements to something; for example, to have the information held about you by an organisation kept secure.

Responsibilities: the legal and moral duties and tasks that you are required to do as part of your job role. Examples include writing information in an individual's record book clearly, only noting factual information, completing records fully and accurately so that they can be read and understood.

Competence: to effectively apply the knowledge, skills and behaviours you have learnt.

Legislation	Implications for social care
General Data Protection Regulation (GDPR) 2018	This Act ensures that: • information is gained with the individual's consent • proof is kept that you have gained consent • individuals can remove consent when they wish • information is removed when it is no longer needed • individuals' rights and interests must be safeguarded • information is accurate and kept up to date • information is used and held only for the reasons given • information is adequate, relevant and not excessive • information is kept safe and secure • public authorities must have a data protection officer
Human Rights Act 1998	Under the Act: • Individuals have the right to respect for their private and family life, home and correspondence such as letters, telephone calls and emails. • Personal information about an individual must be kept securely and not shared without their permission, except in certain circumstances, such as in a medical emergency where information about an individual's condition is required.
Freedom of Information Act 2000	This Act promotes the right of people to request information held about them by public bodies. Under this Act, as a care worker you must: • Support individuals' rights to access and view information that has been recorded about them (unless there are reasons to keep it confidential), such as care files, medical reports, documents, letters, test results, minutes of a meeting held about their care needs. • Remember this when you are recording information about individuals, as they may access the files and will be able to read what you have said.
Code of Professional Practice for Social Care	Under the Code, you have a responsibility to respect confidential information and clearly explain policies about confidentiality to individuals and carers.

▲ Table 4.7 Legislation relating to storing, recording and sharing information, and confidentiality

AC4.3 The meaning of 'secure systems for recording and storing information'

Recording and storing information must always be done in ways that ensure the security of the information being held. This is because individuals have a right for their personal information to be kept private and safe, and you have a duty to uphold this.

Secure systems for hard copy or paper files

What is the meaning of 'secure systems'? What do they look like in a care setting? Below are some key features of secure systems for paper and electronic records and information.

The consequences of losing information could be serious. 'Identity theft' is a crime, and has become a substantial problem in recent years. This is when people steal other people's personal details to commit fraud. They may pretend to be that person in order to buy goods or get loans in that person's name.

To make sure that the systems in your setting are secure, you should make sure that private information and files are:

- **kept locked** – make sure that files are kept in a filing cabinet, or a drawer that is locked, and not left where others may be able to see or access them. Keys should be held with a named member of staff to ensure that only those who have permission can access the information.
  It is also important that you do not take personal information about individuals anywhere with you as you could accidentally misplace or lose it, which would potentially give other people access to the information. For example, if you are supporting an individual to learn how to travel independently on public transport, do not complete your daily records while travelling; you can do this safely on your return.
- **safe from damage** – files should be protected from water, fire damage and theft. Keep them in waterproof document folders or in locked filing cabinets.

- **easy to retrieve when required** – you should easily be able to find what you are looking for. You can do this by, for example, by using an index, listing individuals' surnames in alphabetical order, in a named file.
- **understood by those who have access to it and those who will be using it** – files and the information in them must be presented in a format that can be understood clearly. Handwriting, for example, must be neat and legible; it should be dated so that it is clear when the records were written.
  Even if you make quick notes on a notepad, transfer them to a safe place before destroying them so others cannot read them, for example, by shredding them.
- **monitored regularly for their effectiveness** –you and your colleagues should review and feed back on how well the systems in place are working. What is working well when it comes to recording and storing information? What is *not* working well? What else do you need to do to improve?
  Your setting will have its own policies in this area, and you should make sure that you are aware of these.

Secure systems for electronic files

The storing of records electronically and the potential to share private information on the internet means that the protection of all personal data has become a very important issue. Where files are stored electronically, for example, on a computer, tablet, or phone, you should make sure that private information and files are:

- **password-protected** – if files are stored in a computer, the computer and files should be password-protected, and with different passwords for those with different levels of access to ensure that only information that is needed is accessed by those with permission to do so. Passwords should be changed regularly and should not be written down.
- **firewall-protected** – computers that store personal details, data and information should be protected by a 'firewall'. This is a piece of software that protects the computer and its information from people who do not have permission to access the network or the information.

It can also stop people 'hacking' into the computer and possibly stealing information. Hacking occurs when people access a computer without permission, and possibly misuse the information.

- **protected by anti-virus software** – firewalls can also stop other internet viruses from infecting the computer. They can be installed as part of anti-virus software which will stop any harmful virus from entering your computer.

  You may know from experience of having a virus on your laptop or computer that viruses can harm documents or files that you have stored. You may even have had your computer or laptop repaired or fixed and lost files. How serious might this be if a virus infected a computer in your care setting?

  While anti-virus software may not stop all viruses, it is definitely something that should be installed on computers in your setting, as this can stop important information and files from being lost.

- **backed up** – you must make sure your computer is regularly backed up or saved into another location as well. This is usually in a secure location on the internet.

- **easy to retrieve when required** – you should easily be able to find what you are looking for, by setting up files and folders which are appropriately named.

AC4.4 The importance of secure systems for recording and storing information in health and social care

It is important to have secure systems in place for recording and storing information in a social care setting to comply with legislation. Not doing so will mean that you are not carrying out your responsibilities competently.

If you are not recording and storing information properly, the information that others in the setting may need to access about individuals will be of poor quality. If the information is not accurate or correct, this can lead to mistakes happening, and unsafe care and support being provided to individuals.

The individuals that you support also need to be confident that the information that they give to you will be recorded and safely secured. This involves showing **compassion** when handling their personal information – in other words, thinking about how you would feel if it were your personal and private information, and how safely and securely you would want it to be handled. If the people you support do not trust that this will happen, it could stop them from giving you information, or affect the things that they decide to tell you.

It is important that individuals, children and young people understand that you will only share the information they have given you if you have their permission to do so, unless you need to share it to protect them from harm or if they have been harmed.

- Any information that you do share about them with your colleagues, or other professionals, will only be shared in private to ensure its confidentiality and on a 'need to know' basis.

- When making a decision about information to be shared on a 'need to know' basis, the individual's personal situation must always be taken into account, as well as their best interests. You can only do this if you know the individual. Explore the pros and cons of sharing information, for the individual's best interests.

- For example, if an individual tells you that they are going to harm themselves or someone else, you would need to share this information without their permission, probably with your manager, because not doing so may mean that they will put themselves and others in danger.

You will also need to keep in mind any capacity issues – does the individual have capacity to make the decision to share details?

> **KEY TERM**
>
> **Compassion:** this is central to keeping individuals' personal information secure, as doing so shows your kindness towards individuals in upholding their rights to dignity, respect and being taken seriously.

AC4.5 Features of manual and electronic information storage systems that help ensure security of information

All the records that you access and complete in the setting where you work are legal documents. This is because they fully document the care and support provided to individuals, record all decisions taken and how those decisions were made.

Because records may be referred to in the future, it is important that they are **up to date**, **complete**, **accurate** and **legible**. This will also be helpful to the next person who accesses the records:

- Not only will your notes inform the support they give to the individual, if they are up to date, accurate, complete and neatly recorded, it will also save them time from having to find out when the information was recorded or trying to make sense of what you have written.
- The information that these contain is very important for ensuring the provision of high quality, safe and effective care to individuals.

All the information that is maintained and stored must also adhere to legislation because individuals' information contains personal details. For example, the information may be about:

- an older adult who is returning home after being in hospital
- a young adult who has developed mental health needs
- an individual with learning disabilities who would like support to find a job and there are concerns about their safety.

Those issues/details would need to be recorded so that the appropriate actions can be taken to ensure that individuals' safety and well-being can be safeguarded.

KEY TERMS

Up to date: records contain information that reflects the current situation.

Complete: records contain full details and all the information that is necessary.

Accurate: records contain factually correct information.

Legible: records are written in a way that can be easily read and understood.

AC4.6 Information that needs to be recorded, reported and stored

Many different records and reports are kept in care settings. Examples of some of the main ones are:

- care or support plans that detail individuals' needs, choices and support required
- daily reports that provide information on the daily tasks completed with individuals
- health profiles that provide information on individuals' health needs, conditions and allergies
- medication records that provide details on individuals' medication, including the dose, how often they are taken and how to take them
- menus that provide information on individuals' nutritional requirements and preferences
- fluid balance charts that provide information on individuals' fluid intake and output
- moving and handling charts that provide information on the equipment individuals use, and the support required to move from one position to another
- activity records that provide information on the activities completed with individuals
- risk assessments that detail the potential and actual risks to individuals and others, and how to manage them safely
- accident reports that document accidents that have taken place in the work setting
- health and safety checklists that provide information on the health and safety checks completed in the care setting
- a visitors' book that provides information on people that have visited.

AC4.7 Ways to record written information with accuracy, clarity, relevance and an appropriate level of detail in a timely manner

Keeping records up to date

This is important because individuals' needs and preferences can change. If individuals' information becomes out of date, it does not provide a true picture of the support they require, the care needs they have, their preferences for how they want to live their life.

This may mean that the care and support that you provide does not meet an individual's needs and can result in it being unsafe.

If documents are dated, then it will be clear for you or the next colleague who accesses the record to see when the information was recorded. They can update the record by adding a new entry, signing and dating this.

You can keep records up to date by recording all information:

- as soon as possible – making an entry into an activity record or whatever you use in your setting as soon as you have completed an activity, such as cooking a meal with an individual
- regularly – making an entry into the daily report at the end of *every* shift
- consistently – documenting information about individuals in *all* records that you use.

Keeping complete records

This is important because not doing so can mean that important information about an individual may not be recorded. The individual might not be provided with the correct care, and a health condition may worsen as a result. Not writing down records completely can therefore have serious consequences for individuals, but can also mean that you risk putting your own job and career at risk.

You can ensure records are complete by recording all information:

- with all the necessary details – for example, write out a **risk assessment** in full, identifying clearly the **hazards**, potential risks and the ways you have agreed with the individual to manage these before supporting them to go shopping.
- with the date, time and your signature – include these at the end of your daily report entries as it will be clear that this is your record in full and no one else can add to it. It also means the next person to access the record can see who added to it and when.
- as soon as possible – completing records as soon as possible after you have finished a task or after an accident has occurred will ensure that you do not forget to include important information, and will provide a true picture of what happened.

Writing accurate records

You can ensure records are accurate by recording all information:

- with the facts only – information recorded in an accident report must be based on what you have seen and heard (**fact**), not on what you think or feel (**opinion**). Make sure that you can justify what you have written – you should have clear reasons for what you have recorded. Avoid using jargon and abbreviations.
- with the relevant details only – you have a duty of care to communicate fully and effectively with colleagues, ensuring that they have all the information they need to support individuals, children and young people effectively. Relevant information on an individual's support plan will mean that the key areas of support are clear and easily understood by your colleagues, so that they can provide consistent care and support
- relating to the individual only – only write about the individual and not anyone else in their notes, so it is clear that the information relates to that individual only.

KEY TERMS

Fact: a fact is something that is true. It can be proven and measured using evidence or documentation. Fact relies on observation or research.

Opinion: a person's view of something which may or may not be true. Their view may be different from another person's view about the same thing.

Ensuring records are legible

This means that individuals, your colleagues and others accessing your records must be able to read your handwriting and understand what you have written. Not doing so may mean that important information about individuals is not understood, that misunderstandings arise and that the required care and support are not provided when individuals need this. It also means that colleagues may spend more time trying to work out what you have written.

How would you feel if you accessed a record and could not read what was written? Would this make you worried that you may miss important information, simply because the writing was not clear and legible?

You can ensure records are legible by recording all information:

- clearly – information recorded on an individual's care plan must be written using neat handwriting so that it can be read easily.
- correctly – use correct spelling and grammar so that the information can be easily understood by those who access and read them.
- in permanent ink or typed – use permanent ink that cannot be erased or altered. If you make an error on a paper-based record, put a single line through it, so that the error is still legible and what you wrote is clear.
- concisely – try not to write too many paragraphs. Bullet points are often a good way to convey information and will save time for the next person who needs to read the records. You should cover all important and correct information and be clear, but if you can be concise, even better!

AC4.8 Differences between fact, opinion and judgement and why understanding this is important when recording and reporting information about individuals and their families or carers

When writing reports, it is crucial to record fact and not include any opinion or your own **judgements**. Records should be free from any personal bias. This is very important for ensuring that the information provides a true picture of what really happened. Not doing so can mean that important decisions about individuals are made based on inaccurate information.

For example:

- Recording that you feel that an individual was looking 'a bit down' when you supported him to get dressed in the morning is your opinion, and may not lead to any further action being taken.
- Recording that the individual told you he was feeling 'a bit down' when you supported him to get dressed in the morning is fact, and would lead to further actions being taken. This might include asking the individual to find out the reasons why he was feeling 'a bit down', booking an appointment with his GP and closely monitoring how he was feeling by the team.

You should therefore ensure that the records are facts, not your own personal thoughts and opinions. This will help to ensure your records are accurate.

Records may have to stand up in a court of law, for example, in a safeguarding case. Opinions and judgements would be irrelevant here.

KEY TERM

Judgement: a decision which takes everything into account. You look at the facts and people's opinions and then make your own judgement.

AC4.9 The importance of sharing recorded information with individuals and knowing when and why this cannot occur

Sharing information with individuals you support is important for the following reasons:

- The information is more likely to be accurate, as the individual can tell you if something is not true.
- It ensures dignity and respect, and that individuals are seen as equal partners in their care and support.

- It focuses the worker's mind to report respectfully and sensitively.
- It fosters a spirit of co-production.
- Involving individuals, children and young people in record keeping will ensure the records are written in a way they can understand and access.
- It builds a culture of trust and openness.
- Legislation states that individuals can have access to their own records.

There may be times when you shouldn't share records with individuals you support. These times include:

- when there is a safeguarding issue
- if the reports are part of a legal case
- if the reports contain personal information about somebody else.

We will look at this in more detail in Unit 006.

Check your understanding

1 What information do you need to handle in a social care settings?

2 Give one example of how to store information safely.

3 Explain why records should be up to date, complete, accurate and legible.

4 List five reasons why information should be factual, accurate, legible and concise.

Question practice

1 What is most likely to promote effective team working in a care setting?

   a Ensure team members update support plans.

   b Record all medication given.

   c Provide feedback to the individual.

   d Pass information to other team members consistently.

2 Josie's team were put together a month ago to develop a new induction programme for the company. In the team are members of other services across Wales. What type of team is this?

   a a self-managed team

   b a committee

   c a permanent team

   d a task group

3 Which legislation relates to the storing of information?

   a Reporting of Injuries, Diseases and Dangerous Occurrences Regulations

   b General Data Protection Regulations

   c Management of Health and Safety at Work Act

   d Social Services and Well-Being (Wales) Act

4 Which of the following is the most important when recording information?

   a facts

   b opinions

   c judgements

   d ideas

LO5 UNDERSTAND THE IMPORTANCE OF UPHOLDING THE PROFESSION OF HEALTH AND SOCIAL CARE WORKERS

GETTING STARTED

As a health and social care worker, you belong to one of the most important professions in your community. Supporting vulnerable people hasn't always been given the importance it deserves. The coronavirus pandemic showed the importance of the health and social care work profession, and its valuable contribution to society.

There has been a move over more recent years to professionalise the workforce, ensuring workers are registered and qualified. This ensures accountability and improved care and support.

The Code of Practice requires you to uphold the health and social care profession by acting in line with legislation and standards and implementing a person-centred outcome-focused service which supports individuals' needs and well-being.

Why do you think it is important that social care is seen as a profession by society?

AC5.1 The term 'positive role modelling' in health and social care

A positive role model is someone who acts with integrity, optimism and compassion. They always try to do their best for themselves and others. They are often high-achievers, as they are usually successful and inspire others. People admire role models and want to emulate them.

In health and social care, it is important to be a positive role model so you can influence the behaviours of individuals we support and other workers. Acting in a professional manner will gain the respect of people in wider society as you come into contact with them.

How positive role modelling can affect individuals we support

Children and young people, or people who have had troubled backgrounds, often haven't had positive role models in their lives. Aspirations and hope are vital to the achievement of children and young people in care. They can often have low self-esteem, so having positive role models around them who value and respect them and treat them as equals can have a positive effect on the individual.

Positive role models can help people to build resilience so they can achieve their goals and potential. When you support people to have control over their lives, you are showing them that there is a choice, that failure isn't the only option, that they can achieve their hopes and dreams.

How positive role modelling can affect other professionals

Your behaviour can have an effect on the people you work with, particularly people with less experience or who are new to the sector.

When new workers start, they will have a period of shadowing more experienced workers, to see how things are done. The way you communicate and support individuals will have an important impact on fellow workers. If you treat people with dignity and respect, then your less experienced colleagues will learn to do the same. Supporting and helping less experienced colleagues and explaining how you work will ultimately improve the quality of the service individuals receive.

REFLECT ON IT

Think about role models in society today.

- Who are they, and how have they influenced others?
- Are all role models positive, or can you think of negative role models?
- How do they influence others?

Think about people you support or your colleagues.

- Have you influenced them?
- Could you be a better role model?

Social media has played a crucial role in providing role models for society. People now become 'influencers' on social media, have millions of followers, make a career out of it and become famous. This shows the impact role models can have on people. Many young people are far more aware of environmental issues, for example, due to role models in society.

- What are the positive and negative aspects of influencers?

AC5.2 Reasons for not behaving in a way, in work or outside work, which would call into question your suitability to work in the health and social care profession

As discussed above, you have a responsibility to uphold the credibility of your profession so that you are valued and respected by society and build and maintain the trust of the community, your employers, individuals you support and their families and carers.

REFLECT ON IT

Table 4.8 includes real examples of behaviour that brought charges against health and social care workers. For each example, think about how the worker's behaviour could impact on individuals they support.

Behaviour	Impact on the worker
Exchanged inappropriate messages with colleague about having sex with a child	The worker was deemed unsafe to practise. They received a 12 months' reviewable suspension from being a care worker, and had to undergo safeguarding training.
Failure to properly record work undertaken, follow advice given or communicate with manager in a transparent way	The worker showed blatant disregard for the Code of Professional Practice, so was removed from the register and not allowed to work in social care again.
Failed to give appropriate information in a safeguarding investigation	The person was removed from the register and was not allowed to work in social care again.
Behaved in an aggressive way to a young person	
Shared an inappropriate video of a young person with colleagues on a WhatsApp group and inappropriate behaviour towards a colleague	
Dishonesty and delayed reporting that a young person had absconded	
Shouting at a young person and pushing them	
Did not ensure money was properly accounted for	
Failure to carry out checks on a night shift and falsified records to show they were carried out	

▲ Table 4.8 Unprofessional behaviour and its consequences for individual workers

AC5.3 The relationship between the use of social media and personal and professional conduct

Many of us use social media to communicate with others personally and professionally, as there can be lots of benefits to doing so. It can however blur the boundaries between our professional and personal lives.

When using social media, you should follow the same guidelines as you would when communicating in writing or face to face with people. You should follow the good practice guidelines listed below:

- Remember legislation and codes of conduct.
- Ensure privacy and confidentiality – don't mention people you support or work with to people outside work.
- Demonstrate respect and professionalism.
- Work within your organisation policies – if the policy doesn't say you can communicate with colleagues to share information on social media, then you shouldn't do so.
- Don't use social media in a way which could be seen as bullying or intimidating behaviour.

- Think carefully about accepting friends. You should not be friends with people you support or their families, unless it is on a professional account and in line with policies and procedures.
- Check your privacy settings.
- Be careful who you associate with on social media. If you acknowledge a radical post, it could look like you endorse those views.
- Don't mention your workplace or talk about work on social media.

AC5.4 Reasons for not forming inappropriate relationships with individuals, their families, carers, colleagues or others

So far in this LO, you have looked at how to form professional relationships with people you support. There are a number of reasons why you shouldn't form inappropriate relationships with individuals, their families, carers or colleagues:

- to ensure you maintain appropriate personal and professional boundaries
- to protect individuals and others from abuse
- to protect yourself from allegations of abuse
- to ensure you implement codes of practice and legislation
- to uphold the profession of health and social care workers
- to ensure effective communication
- to ensure person-centred support and ensure individuals' needs are met
- to give people the right impression of your relationship with them
- to protect your privacy
- to protect yourself from investigations into inappropriate relationships
- to protect yourself from disciplinary action.

> **REFLECT ON IT**
> - How many examples of inappropriate relationships can you think of?
> - Think of the consequence of each example.

AC5.5 The importance of recognising and sensitively using the power that comes from working with individuals and carers and not act in any way that abuses this power

There are inherent power imbalances in relationships with individuals, their families and carers, who often take a subordinate role or think the carer knows best. This is caused by a number of reasons including:

- People are very grateful for your support, so they see your position as one of power.
- Individuals are used to receiving support, so they accept whatever happens.
- Individuals have potentially been in unequal power relationships in the past, so this is the norm for them.
- Individuals, children and young people, and their families, see you as a trained professional, so you must know best.

It is important that you recognise this imbalance and take action to manage and reduce it.

You can do this by informing people at the start of your relationship how you see your role in their care and support:

- You are equal partners.
- You are there to help them achieve their goals and to meet their needs.
- They are in control of their care.

This way, power imbalances are being managed from the start.

Reflecting on your practice and ensuring you are not putting your own values onto others is another way of ensuring there are no power imbalances.

Implementing person-centred care and support in a spirit of co-production will also ensure equality. There will be times when you do have knowledge and skills that you need to pass on to people you support or their families, which can be seen as putting you in a position of power, but think sensitively about how you do this. Discussing options with individuals and involving them in decision making and gaining consent are all ways of reducing power imbalances and ensuring equal partnerships based on mutual respect.

LO6 KNOW HOW CONTINUED PROFESSIONAL DEVELOPMENT CONTRIBUTES TO PROFESSIONAL PRACTICE

GETTING STARTED

It is important to constantly improve your practice. Without ongoing development, you can lose motivation and get 'stuck in a rut'.

Can you think of some other reasons why your own development is important?

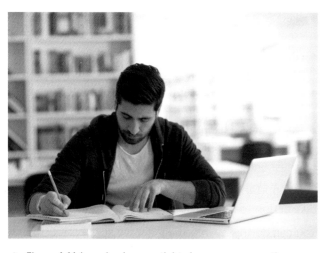

▲ Figure 4.11 Learning is essential to improve your practice

AC6.1 The term 'continuing professional development'

Continuing professional development (CPD) means developing your knowledge, practice and skills in order to improve your practice. You should do this throughout your career, so that you are constantly improving.

CPD is not just about going on training courses. It can include reflection on practice, e-learning, self-study, research, receiving and acting on feedback, and shadowing others.

Lifelong learning has many benefits. Learning is essential to our existence:

- It keeps our brains sharp.
- It develops our skills.
- It improves self-confidence.

CPD is available to all workers in health and social care, and you should utilise it to your best advantage.

AC6.2 Legislative requirements, standards and codes of conduct and professional practice that relate to continuing professional development

The Code of Professional Practice for Social Care sets out requirements for social care workers to

'be accountable for the quality of your work and take responsibility for maintaining and improving knowledge and skills'.

Some pieces of legislation and national minimum standards also require you to have regular training, such as health and safety, or safeguarding.

- To work in health and social care, you need to register as a worker with Social Care Wales.
- To register and remain on the register, you will need to undertake the Level 2 Health and Social Care Core Qualification, followed by the Health and Social Care Practice qualification at either Level 2 or 3, depending on your job role.
- As a registered worker, you must complete 90 hours learning every three years. This must be recorded on your Social Care Wales online account. The resources section includes links to a toolkit to help you do this.

AC6.3 Ways used to evaluate own knowledge, understanding and practice against relevant standards and information

This qualification contains a set of standards which are taken from the national minimum standards in health and social care. Through completing case studies and a multiple choice test, your knowledge will be assessed against the qualification standards.

- When you complete the practice qualification, your assessor will observe you in your workplace to assess whether your practice meets the standards. You will also complete a reflective journal to evaluate knowledge and practice, and look at ways to improve.
- Supervision and appraisal are tools to evaluate knowledge and practice against your job description and organisational policies and procedures.
- Handovers, team meetings and team discussions are useful ways of reflecting on practice to ensure you are meeting individuals' needs as detailed in care and support plans.
- CIW will carry out inspections of the service you work in. They will assess the work of the service in line with national standards. Their report can then be used to assess your practice as a team and identify areas for improvement. You can find the inspection reports at:

https://careinspectorate.wales/how-we-inspect-adult-and-childrens-services

You can refer to any of the standards mentioned above for self-reflection, to see how well you think you are meeting standards.

REFLECT ON IT

Using one of the methods listed above, look at the standards involved and assess your own practice. You could get feedback from somebody else if you wish, as this might give you further information.

- In which areas do you do well?
- Can you make any improvements? If so, discuss these with your manager so you can access any support you need.

AC6.4 Responsibilities of employers and workers for CPD

Under the Code of Practice and legislation, employers have a responsibility to provide suitable instruction, supervision, training and development, as is necessary to create a safe, qualified and skilled workforce. This includes:

- induction training
- training to ensure you are prepared for any changes in job role
- workplace assessment of practice
- providing support to employees when they need it
- providing regular effective supervision to support development through reflective practice
- regular refresher training
- statutory training, for example, health and safety training.

Social care workers have a number of responsibilities under the Code of Practice and legislation in relation to professional development. These include the following:

- You must implement any training into your practice.
- You must meet relevant standards of practice, follow procedures and work in a safe, lawful way.
- You must take responsibility for maintaining and developing your knowledge and skills.

AC6.5 Learning opportunities available to health and social care workers and how these can be used to improve knowledge and practice

Your setting and colleagues are not the only sources to keep yourself up to date with good practice. There are many other learning opportunities to help you improve your practice:

- Pay attention to what is happening around you, and how health and social care issues are being reported in the media.
- Ask if you can observe or shadow an experienced senior colleague who can demonstrate good practice, to see how they perform in their role and learn from their expertise. This will allow you to increase your knowledge in areas in which you may not be confident or have little experience.
- Do not be afraid to ask for advice and feedback on how you are doing. A motivated, enthusiastic and

competent workforce that seeks such opportunities helps to maintain high standards.

- Training is also a good way to ensure that you are up to date with your skills and to gain new ones. You can also share any new knowledge with colleagues, which will again encourage good practice.

- Issues around social care are often a topic of debate in government, and there are often changes to legislation which will be documented in the news. Television programmes sometimes focus on issues in the health and social care sector. The news often tends to cover some of the more negative issues in care homes, but it is important that you use this as motivation to do your best to achieve good practice. You may also read stories in newspapers and magazines.

- Approach external agencies and charities that have a specialist knowledge of a particular condition, such as a charity which supports people with dementia. You can gain a greater understanding of new developments in this area by asking if they can provide further information or direct you to other useful sources.

AC6.6 Ways to access and use information and support on knowledge and best practice relevant to role

RESEARCH IT

Have a look at the Social Care Wales website and their learning hub:

https://socialcare.wales

https://socialcare.wales/hub/home

There is a lot of information here to help you.

Your manager will play a crucial role in supporting your development. They can:

- help you reflect on your practice
- provide development opportunities you need
- support you to implement any new knowledge and skills into your practice.

A personal development plan is a useful way of supporting and recording your development. Your organisation may have their own personal development plan. If not, there are many templates available on the internet or you can devise one yourself. It should include as a minimum:

- personal information – name, date, manager
- what you want to learn or develop
- how you will achieve it
- what support you need
- how you will assess and provide evidence of your achievements
- your target date for achieving this
- a date to review your progress.

Your plan can look at short-term goals over the next month, medium-term goals over the next three to six months, or long-term and career goals.

REFLECT ON IT

Obtain a copy of your organisation's personal development plan or find an online template.

- Record at least three goals for yourself.
- Discuss these with your manager.

AC6.7 Ways to apply learning to practice and transfer knowledge and skills to new situations

In order to gain the maximum benefit from your learning and development, it is essential that you record what you have learnt as you go along, and reflect on how you can use it in your everyday work. The following checklist is useful to ensure you apply your learning to practice:

- What have I learnt?
- How does this apply to my practice?
- How does it affect me and the people I support?
- How can I implement it in my practice?
- What action am I going to take, and when?
- What support do I need?
- Do I have any other development needs as a result of this activity?

Add any action you have planned to your personal development plan.

AC6.8 The importance of seeking and learning from feedback on practice from individuals, families and carers, colleagues and other professionals

You can ask for feedback from colleagues, individuals and families in order to assess how you are doing. This feedback can be:

- formal – through appraisals and meetings with colleagues, or questionnaires for individuals and families, or
- informal – in a conversation.

You may find that you receive both compliments and criticism, but it is important to receive both aspects constructively and learn from the experience.

By seeking feedback from others, you can learn new things about yourself that you didn't previously know, as others may see things differently from you. We can find out new information to help us in our work; for example, an individual you support may tell you something else that they would like to achieve.

You should get regular feedback from individuals, children and young people about the support they receive. This enables you to know that the support is meeting their needs or whether there are any problems. If you don't have feedback, then you only have your own view of the situation.

Receiving feedback may help you to identify further development goals to include in your personal development plan. It will also tell you what you are doing well, and allow you to measure your progress against standards and previous action plans. This will help to build confidence in yourself and your work.

AC6.9 Principles of reflective practice and why they are important

To reflect means to think. Being able to reflect is an important skill for your work. It involves thinking honestly about your practice, both positive and negative aspects, and not being afraid to question your practice. When you reflect, you:

- take a 'step back' from your day-to-day activities and spend time thinking about a work activity you have carried out or a situation you have experienced
- examine in detail the reasons why and how you carry out your work practices
- assess the knowledge and skills you have and the behaviours you show, including their impact on you, the individuals you support and others
- identify your strengths and weaknesses
- identify areas of your work practice that can be improved
- develop different ways of working that can improve your working practice
- develop new areas of learning, such as different or new approaches to situations that may arise.

You will look in more detail at reflective practice when you start your practice qualification. It is useful therefore to start some reflective practice now, to prepare you for this.

RESEARCH IT

There are a number of reflective practice models online.

- We looked at Gibbs' reflective cycle earlier in this unit: look online for more detail on his theory, and also Kolb's work.
- Think about what you have learnt so far undertaking this qualification. Reflect on it, using one of the models above. You can use this for your practice qualification.

AC6.10 The purpose of supervision and appraisal

Your manager will meet you to assess your performance at work. This process is referred to as formal **supervision**, and its purpose is to support you with planning and monitoring your personal development. For example, in the care setting where you work, you may have regular performance reviews, where you discuss and evaluate your performance at work with your manager.

During a supervision with your manager, you will have an opportunity to discuss any issues and receive feedback on what has been going well, and what improvements you need to make. Because these meetings may happen only every few weeks, it is a good idea to note down things that you want to discuss beforehand. This is the time to:

- discuss specific issues and individuals you are working with
- discuss career progression
- identify sources of support and training courses you would like to undertake.

Appraisals are another source of formal support, where your employer (not necessarily your manager) assesses your performance with you over a much longer period, such as one year. It provides you with the opportunity to:

- discuss and reflect on your work performance
- identify your strengths and areas for development
- discuss how you can progress in your role with training and development opportunities.

KEY TERM

Supervision: a worker, usually a manager, working with another worker in order to support them to meet organisational, professional and personal objectives.

AC6.11 The role and responsibilities of employers and workers for undertaking supervision and appraisal

According to the Code of Practice and national minimum standards, health and social care employers have a responsibility to carry out supervision and appraisal.

Supervision meetings should be held every two months as a minimum or once every three months for domiciliary care workers. This is in addition to regular day-to-day supervision. If there is no regular day-to-day supervision, then supervision meetings should be held every fortnight. This can be pro rata for part-time staff.

Appraisal is usually an annual process which reviews the performance of the worker over the year and identifies areas they need to develop over the next year.

All workers, regardless of whether they are full-time or part-time, volunteers or apprentices, need supervisions and appraisal. This should foster a culture of learning within the organisation. It encourages employees to reflect on their practice, and identify their training and development needs in order to improve practice.

During supervision, employers have a responsibility to:

- follow organisational policies and procedures
- ensure that supervision is free from bullying and harassment
- make time for and prioritise supervision
- plan and prepare for supervision
- identify areas of good practice in the worker
- identify areas the worker can develop and improve
- obtain feedback from the individual
- provide support and guidance to the individual
- record minutes of the meeting for future reference
- maintain confidentiality.

Workers have responsibilities during supervision and appraisals, such as to:

- attend planned supervisions and appraisal meetings
- plan and prepare for the meetings
- maintain a positive attitude towards meetings
- implement any agreed actions
- identify areas of practice to develop
- take feedback constructively
- reflect on any learning and development undertaken and look at this being implemented into working practices
- report any problems or concerns.

AC6.12 The use of reflective practice in supervision and appraisal

Supervision and appraisal are great opportunities to reflect on your practice. In LO1 we saw the importance of reflective practice in social care.

Supervision is an opportunity to think about what has worked well since your last supervision meeting. If things didn't go as planned, why was that? Could you have done anything differently? Did you face any problems over the last month? If so, why did they occur, and what could be done to prevent them happening again?

If mistakes are made but you are open and honest about what happened and take action to prevent these happening again through reflective practice, this reinforces a positive culture and ensures quality. It can help you to identify patterns, trends, assumptions and beliefs, and highlight areas where teamwork needs to be improved.

AC6.13 The importance of effective supervision, reflective practice and relevant learning opportunities on the well-being of individuals

In order to provide a quality service which meets individual needs and ensures well-being, social care workers need to be professional, trained and competent. They need to have appropriate skills to deliver a service which meets people's needs. They must be open and honest when things go wrong and look at how these can be put right.

Reflective practice, supervision and relevant training support this, and ensure people's needs are being met and ultimately their well-being. They enable workers to:

- be clear about their roles and responsibilities in meeting individuals' needs
- understand the legislation and organisational policy which affects their role
- know how to implement this.

AC6.14 Areas of work where own literacy, numeracy and digital competency skills are needed to support professional practice and ways to develop them

Literacy, numeracy and digital literacy are essential skills that workers use in everyday situations at work.

> **REFLECT ON IT**
>
> Copy and complete the table below, noting all the times you use **literacy**, **numeracy** and **digital literacy** in your normal day's work.
>
> | Literacy | Numeracy | Digital literacy |
> |---|---|---|
> | | | |

> **KEY TERMS**
>
> **Literacy:** includes reading, writing, summarising information, using grammar and correct spelling and punctuation. It also includes the ability to speak and listen effectively to ensure effective communication.
>
> **Numeracy:** the ability to understand and work with numbers, such as adding, subtracting, working out percentages and multiplying figures.
>
> **Digital literacy:** the ability to read, write, find and evaluate information on any digital platform, such as computers, mobile phones, audio and other technology. It also involves keeping yourself safe online.

It is good to develop essential skills in these areas as this will help you in your work and also in everyday life. For example, going to the shops uses numeracy skills, such as working out percentages if there is a 10 per cent discount on products in a sale.

If you are doing an apprenticeship, you will be required to undertake Essential Skills qualifications which include literacy and numeracy. Many training providers and colleges use e-portfolio systems where learners upload work into their portfolio and their assessor gives feedback and adds review records.

When you start an apprenticeship, you will probably have carried out a literacy and numeracy assessment on Wales Essential Skills Toolkit. This identifies your levels of literacy and numeracy. You can return to this and carry out short activities to help you improve in the areas you didn't do so well on. This will help you prepare for your Essential Skills qualifications and improve your skills, so you can cope better with literacy and numeracy tasks at work and in everyday life.

- If you are not on an apprenticeship, there are lots of other ways of improving your skills. There are some useful websites in the resources section at the end of this unit.
- In the workplace you can develop your skills by taking your time when writing reports and using spellchecks to help you. When using spellcheck, you should still reread your work, as sometimes incorrect words are used.

- You can also ask for feedback from colleagues on your report writing. Sometimes people write as they speak, but this is not appropriate for a report as it should be written in a professional manner. Getting feedback from someone who is used to writing reports is a good way of developing your skills here.
- If you have to use computers at work, a good way of learning is by having a go and trying things out. Having someone more experienced to mentor you when using computers is a good way of developing your skills.

Check your understanding

1 How can you be a positive role model to other workers?

2 Give three reasons why it is important to update your knowledge regularly.

3 How can you benefit from supervision and appraisals?

4 How can you use reflective practice in supervision?

5 Describe three ways in which workers can ensure that individuals, children and young people are treated with dignity and respect.

Question practice

1 Dave has received a social media friend request from a young person he supports. What is the best action Dave could take?

   a Ignore it and suggest colleagues do the same.

   b Accept it but don't post comments about work.

   c Explain to the individual why they cannot accept.

   d Decline it and amend security settings.

2 Why is feedback from your manager important?

   a Managers can then report back to inspectors about your performance.

   b It is your responsibility to know what you are doing wrong.

   c You can identify areas of competence and development areas.

   d They can monitor and observe your practice.

3 Why is reflection on practice in supervision important?

   a It informs workers when they get things wrong.

   b It requires little or no preparation.

   c It supports workers to improve their performance.

   d It gives instructions so workers know what to do.

FURTHER READING AND RESEARCH

Weblinks

A video outlining the Code of Professional Practice for Social Care:

Advice on whistleblowing from the Children's Commissioner for Wales:
www.childcomwales.org.uk/whistleblowing

Guidance on whistleblowing from CIW:
https://careinspectorate.wales/contact-us/whistle-blowing

Safeguarding procedures in Wales:
https://gov.wales/safeguarding-guidance

Belbin's team roles theory:
www.belbin.com

Professional boundaries with children living in residential child care for residential child care workers from Social Care Wales:
https://socialcare.wales/service-improvement/professional-boundaries-with-children-living-in-residential-child-care

This page includes a useful toolkit for social care workers:
https://socialcare.wales/learning-and-development/continuing-professional-development-cpd

How CIW inspects adult and children's services:
https://careinspectorate.wales/how-we-inspect-adult-and-childrens-services

A useful guide to supervising and appraising for employers and employees:
https://socialcare.wales/cms_assets/file-uploads/Supervising-and-appraising-well-social-care.pdf

Free literacy and numeracy resources for adults:
www.bbc.co.uk/teach/skillswise

Free literacy, digital literacy and numeracy resources for adults:
www.skillsworkshop.org/maths

Wales Essential Skills Toolkit:
www.walesessentialskills.com

Free literacy resources from the National Literacy Trust:
https://literacytrust.org.uk/free-resources/

These literacy and numeracy resources are aimed at children but are also helpful for adults:
www.bbc.co.uk/bitesize

A list of available resources for literacy and numeracy:
www.read-write-now.org/resources/literacy-and-numeracy-information/useful-numeracy-links

SAFEGUARDING INDIVIDUALS

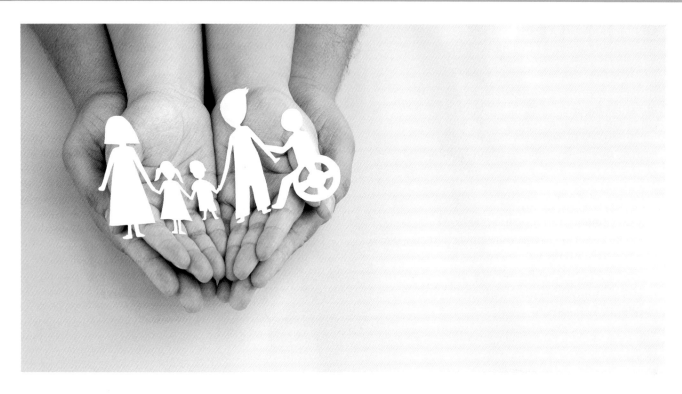

ABOUT THIS UNIT

Guided learning hours: 40

Safeguarding children, young people and adults from harm, abuse and neglect is everyone's responsibility. This unit will provide you with an understanding of the purpose of legislation and national policies and how they underpin workers' practices when safeguarding individuals.

You will learn about the main types of abuse and neglect, their associated signs and symptoms, and ways of working that keep both individuals and workers safe. Understanding the actions, behaviours or situations that could lead to individuals being harmed, abused or neglected will raise your awareness of how you can protect individuals.

Knowing how to respond, record and report safeguarding concerns will further equip you with the knowledge of what to do when individuals are being or are at risk of being harmed, abused or neglected.

Learning outcomes
LO1: Understand the purpose of legislation, national policies and codes of conduct and professional practice in relation to the safeguarding of individuals
LO2: Understand how to work in ways that safeguard individuals from harm, abuse and neglect
LO3: Understand the factors, situations and actions that could lead or contribute to harm, abuse or neglect
LO4: Understand how to respond, record and report concerns, disclosures or allegations related to safeguarding

LO1 UNDERSTAND THE PURPOSE OF LEGISLATION, NATIONAL POLICIES AND CODES OF CONDUCT AND PROFESSIONAL PRACTICE IN RELATION TO THE SAFEGUARDING OF INDIVIDUALS

GETTING STARTED

Think about an occasion when you or someone you know heard about a child, young person or adult being abused or harmed. You may have heard about this by watching a television programme or read about it online.

Where and how was the person abused or harmed?

AC1.1 The term 'safeguarding'

Everyone who works with children, young people and adults has a responsibility to keep them safe from **harm**, **abuse** and **neglect**. Doing so forms an essential aspect of working in the health and social care sector. Safeguarding means:

- promoting individuals' health, development and well-being
- promoting individuals' rights to live safely and free from harm, abuse and neglect
- recognising the signs and dangers that an individual is being harmed, abused and/or neglected
- understanding what to do when an individual is being or is at risk of being harmed, abused and/or neglected.

Protection of children, young people and adults is also part of safeguarding, because it involves identifying and preventing harm, abuse and neglect as well as promoting their welfare. Safeguarding children, young people and adults is essential for:

- providing safe care that prevents harm, abuse and neglect from taking place
- empowering individuals to make their own decisions and be in control of their care
- enabling individuals to access care that gives them the best outcomes in life.

KEY TERMS

Harm: any type of abuse or neglect that can have a negative effect on an individual's well-being.

Abuse: when someone is mistreated in a way that causes them pain and hurt.

Neglect: a failure of others to care for and meet an individual's needs which results in harm being caused to the individual. An individual can also cause harm to themselves if they fail to care for themselves, such as by not taking prescribed medication or not eating and drinking healthily.

AC1.2 The main categories of abuse and neglect

Abuse and neglect can happen anywhere, including in an individual's own home, and even in places such as health and social care settings that are meant to be safe and protect individuals from harm.

To safeguard individuals from harm, abuse and neglect, you need to be aware of the main categories of abuse and neglect so that you can recognise when these happen. The Social Services and Well-being (Wales) Act 2014 sets out the main categories of abuse and neglect as physical abuse, sexual abuse, psychological abuse and neglect. You will learn more about these as well as other types of abuse of adults, children and young people in the next section.

It is also important to understand that:

- abuse and neglect can take many different forms
- individuals may experience one or several types of abuse and neglect at the same time – or at different times.

The Social Services and Well-being (Wales) Act 2014 also supports individuals' well-being and the Welsh

Government has published a well-being statement to explain what well-being means:

- having your rights
- being happy, physically, mentally and emotionally
- protection from abuse, harm and neglect
- having education, training, sports and play
- positive relationships with family and friends
- being part of the community
- having a social life and enough money to live a healthy life
- having a good home.

In relation to a child, well-being also includes physical, intellectual, emotional, social and behavioural development. In relation to an adult, well-being also includes control over day-to-day life and participation in work.

(www.gov.wales, Social Services and Well-being (Wales) Act 2014, The Essentials, 2015)

The main types of abuse and what they mean

Financial abuse

This is the illegal theft or use of an individual's finances, assets or possessions. For example, an individual might be:

- pressurised to give their money to someone else, such as a carer, relative, friend or worker
- threatened to make changes to their will, inheritance and the assets that they own.

Financial abuse can also involve:

- misusing an individual's benefits
- not giving an individual access to their money
- controlling how the individual spends their money without the individual's permission
- taking an individual's money and/or debit card or credit card.

Fraud and scamming are other examples of financial abuse. For example, some fraudsters target vulnerable and elderly people at home, by posing as council officials to gain entry to their homes and as sellers of fake goods.

Financial abuse of children and young people also happens and may include getting the child or young person to spend their pocket money on items to then give to their abuser. If the abuser is another child, then this may involve taking the child's dinner money or getting them to buy sweets and give them to the abuser.

Physical abuse

This is unwanted contact that causes an individual pain, injuries or other physical suffering. For example, it can include hitting, kicking, slapping, shaking or pulling hair. Physical abuse can also involve other unlawful physical acts such as:

- withdrawing an individual's medication
- giving an individual medication that they don't need
- rough handling an individual
- withholding an individual's food
- stopping an individual from walking around by locking them in their bedroom
- restraining an individual by not allowing them to get up from their bed by keeping the bed rails up
- female genital mutilation (FGM).

Sexual abuse

This is unwanted sexual contact and involvement in sexual activities and relationships. For example, it can include rape, sexual assault, inappropriate looking or touching, sexual harassment, making an individual watch pornography or sexual acts and indecent exposure. Sexual abuse can be defined as any sexual activity that the individual

- has not consented to
- was forced to consent to
- is unable to consent to
- is tricked into consenting to.

In August 2020, NSPCC Cymru reported that child sexual offences in Wales have doubled in the past five years. In total, there were 3,715 recorded offences including rape, online grooming and sexual assault against children in Wales between 1 April 2019 and 31 March 2020, representing a 107 per cent rise since 2014–2015.

(NSPCC, News and opinion, *Child sexual offences jump 57% in 5 years*, 10 August 2020)

Emotional or psychological abuse

This can be defined as actions that make an individual feel worthless and humiliated, and cause emotional distress.

This type of abuse underpins the other main types because all types of abuse will cause the individual distress and suffering. For example, it can include:

- verbal abuse such as swearing, shouting or name calling
- bullying (including cyber bullying)
- humiliation
- intimidation
- denying an individual's rights to privacy (for example, by opening their post without their permission)
- denying an individual's rights to dignity (for example, by deliberately removing their walking aid so they can't mobilise)
- denying an individual's rights to choice (for example, by making choices for the individual over what to eat or wear)
- preventing the individual having contact with their family or friends
- denying the individual access to services such as their local GP, dentist, leisure centre.

CASE STUDY

Is it abuse?

Marshall is a night care assistant in a care home providing care to 60 residents. One of the residents, Georgina, asked Marshall at the end of his last night shift whether he minded buying her some more toiletries as she had run out completely. Marshall happily agreed as he is always very keen to help the residents in any way he can.

Upon arrival for his night shift today, Marshall went to see Georgina and showed her what he had bought for her: shampoo, shower gel and toothpaste. Marshall explained to Georgina that when he bought these items from the local supermarket they had a 'buy one get one free' offer and so he decided to keep the free items for himself. When Georgina asked Marshall whether she could have the free items, Marshall replied 'No, because I have bought these in my own time and have used my car to go to the supermarket for you.' Georgina tells Marshall that she's not happy about this. Marshall leaves the items he bought for Georgina in her room and upon leaving, tells her that she's ungrateful and that he will no longer be helping her out anymore.

Discussion points:

- Is there any type of abuse happening here? Why?
- How do you think Georgina is feeling? Why?
- What actions should Marshall have taken in this situation? Why?

Other types of abuse and what they mean

Institutional or organisational abuse

This is when an organisation has inadequate systems, policies and procedures in place that do not meet individuals' needs – they lead to poor care and support and also deny individuals' rights to privacy, dignity and independence. For example:

- In a health and social care setting, this may involve having strict routines in place that specify when individuals can have their meals or go to bed so that staffing resources can be maximised.
- These practices are not in the interests of individuals; they are in place to meet the organisation's needs.

This type of abuse can occur in any setting such as in an individual's home, in a care home, in hospital.

Modern slavery

Modern slavery is the exploitation of a person in order to serve others (domestic servitude) without being paid. This includes slavery – human trafficking where individuals are exploited by others and sold as slaves. Slaves do not have a choice, it is forced and compulsory labour. Slaves, including children, may be forced into work where they are sexually exploited.

Slavery has occurred throughout history but it still occurs today in the UK. The Modern Slavery Act 2015 is in place to prevent the enslavement and trafficking of people.

Discrimination and hate crime

Discrimination is the unfair treatment or denial of a person's rights. For example, this may include:

- withholding care or support to an individual because of their sexual orientation
- not providing care to an individual in line with their religious beliefs.

Discrimination and/or any other type of abuse can become a hate crime if it takes place because of hostility towards a perceived, or an actual protected, personal characteristic as defined in the Equality Act 2010 (see AC1.4 in this unit for more information).

Hate crimes can take place because of hostility towards:

- age
- disability
- gender reassignment
- marriage and civil partnership
- pregnancy and maternity
- race
- religion and belief
- sex or sexual orientation.

Hate crimes can include:

- verbal and physical threats
- assault, harassment
- inciting others to commit hate crimes
- damage to property.

Domestic violence or domestic abuse

This is any incident or repeated incidents of controlling, coercive or threatening behaviour between family members and partners. Domestic violence and abuse could include:

- humiliation
- threats
- intimidation
- isolation (such as from their friends)
- exploitation
- **honour-based violence**
- **female genital mutilation (FGM)**.

Abuse by a stranger

This type of abuse occurs when a person not known to the individual deliberately targets them. For example, this could include:

- a builder putting pressure on the individual to buy something that they don't want
- a solicitor overcharging for services that they provide.

This type of abuse relates to fraud and scamming as part of financial abuse.

KEY TERMS

Honour-based violence: domestic violence committed in the name of perceived immoral behaviour, that is seen as having brought shame to a family or community.

Female genital mutilation (FGM): a practice where the female genitals are deliberately cut, injured or changed, which might be done because of cultural beliefs.

The main types of neglect and what they mean

Neglect by others

This is a form of abuse where the person providing care to an individual does not provide it or fails to provide care that meets the individual's needs. Therefore, neglect by others can be deliberate, or can occur as a result of a person not understanding an individual's needs. It can include:

- not providing an individual with support to eat, drink, take their medication or mobilise
- not ensuring the individual is provided with a warm, clean and comfortable environment
- denying the individual access to their friends, family and or others such as their GP or dentist or optician.

Self-neglect

This refers to when an individual fails to care for themselves emotionally and/or physically. This could be because their mental health has declined, or could even be as a result of other illnesses.

Self-neglect can also include withdrawing from having contact with others, by not accessing family, friends and/or other services.

CASE STUDY

Types of abuse

Identify for each of the following scenarios whether abuse is happening and if so the types of abuse you recognise.

1. Cadwallen throws one of the toy cars at the children's centre worker who was standing nearby. The children's centre worker shouts at Cadwallen that he won't be getting any lunch.
2. Charlie has a heart condition and his sister Amy, who is Charlie's main carer, does not allow Charlie's friends to visit the house because she doesn't like them.
3. Beca has a learning disability and her mum doesn't give her access to her money because she thinks others might take advantage of her.

AC1.3 Common signs and symptoms associated with harm, abuse and neglect.

As you will have learnt, understanding the main types of abuse and neglect is essential for safeguarding individuals from harm, abuse and neglect. In addition, recognising common **signs** and **symptoms** associated with harm, abuse and neglect as shown in Table 5.1 will also help you to identify when abuse and neglect may be happening.

Remember that these are the main signs and symptoms you should look out for, and may not be present in every individual or be evidence of abuse.

The most effective way that you can safeguard individuals from harm, abuse and neglect is by getting to know every individual so that you can notice and act upon any unusual changes that they show.

KEY TERMS

Signs: something that can be seen by others, such as bruises, sores and malnutrition. Signs can also include changes in behaviours and moods.

Symptoms: these are experienced by individuals. They are an indication that something is wrong, for example, feeling upset, angry, scared or alone. Symptoms could be the result of an illness or abuse.

Type of harm, abuse and neglect	Common signs and symptoms
Financial abuse	• Unexplained loss of money and inability to pay for essential food shopping items or household bills. • Unexplained loss of personal belongings such as jewellery. • Sudden changes in how an individual manages their finances, such as regular or large sums of money being withdrawn and given to others or a sudden change made to their will. • Fear and anxiety shown by the individual when discussing their financial affairs, or the individual unusually refusing to talk about their financial affairs. • Fear and anxiety shown by a child or young person around an adult, or appearing to be under the influence or control of an adult. A child or young person may also have an unexplained lack of dinner money or pocket money or be unable or reluctant to spend their dinner money or pocket money.
Physical abuse	• Unexplained or unusual bruises, cuts, scratches, sprains or fractures. • Injuries may include burns and scalds, bite marks and finger marks on different areas of the body. In addition, long sleeves may be worn in hot weather to cover up any visible injuries. • Other signs and symptoms may include loss of weight, being in pain and discomfort, showing fear, anxiety and/or being withdrawn, particularly in the presence of a specific person.
Sexual abuse	• Unexplained or unusual bruises particularly around the upper arms, thighs, buttocks, breasts and genital area. • There may also be unexplained bleeding, repeated urinary or genital infections, stained or torn underwear. • The individual may be distressed, feel guilty or ashamed and/or become withdrawn. • The individual may have difficulties walking or sitting, concentrating and/or sleeping. • Being alone with a specific person or receiving assistance with personal hygiene makes the individual fearful. • Unusual changes in behaviour may occur such as aggression, mood changes or self-harm. • A child or young person using inappropriate language or exhibiting overtly sexual behaviour.
Emotional or psychological abuse	• Unusual changes in behaviour and mood, such as becoming angry towards others, feeling anxious, becoming upset and tearful easily. • Disturbed sleep patterns and an unusual change in eating habits, leading to weight loss or weight gain. • Emotional abuse may also result in low self-esteem, depression or withdrawal.

▲ Table 5.1 Common signs and symptoms associated with harm, abuse and neglect

Type of harm, abuse and neglect	Common signs and symptoms
Institutional or organisational abuse	• In terms of the organisation, staff may not be adequately trained in good care standards and may not be supervised. • Insufficient staff on a regular basis, a lack of management and low staff morale may also lead to this type of abuse. • Poor **policies and procedures** may result in the denial of individuals' rights through rigid routines and complaints not being taken seriously. • Individuals may appear angry, fearful, frustrated, anxious, upset or withdrawn.
Modern slavery	• Individuals may appear to be unkempt or malnourished. • Individuals may be living in dirty and overcrowded conditions. • Individuals may not have any personal possessions or identification documents. • Signs and symptoms associated with physical and emotional abuse.
Discrimination and hate crime	• Individuals may be denied their rights to access services and information that meet their needs. • Care, support and services offered may not meet individuals' needs or be respectful of their preferences. • Individuals may not be supported to understand what discrimination is and how concerns are reported and responded to. • Individuals may become angry, frustrated and anxious. • Discrimination and hate crime may also result (like other types of abuse) in low self-esteem, depression or withdrawal.
Domestic violence or domestic abuse	• Signs and symptoms associated with financial, physical, sexual, emotional/psychological abuse. • The individual being controlled, verbally abused or humiliated in front of others. • Increasingly becoming isolated from family and friends and low self-esteem may be further indicators.
Abuse by a stranger	Signs and symptoms associated with financial, physical, sexual, emotional/psychological abuse.
Neglect by others	• Malnutrition, dehydration, living in dirty, unsafe conditions. • Changes in the individual's personal appearance, such as looking unkempt, wearing old or dirty clothing, wearing inappropriate clothing for the weather conditions. • The individual may also have pressure sores, rashes and skin infections, untreated injuries and medical conditions. • The individual may unusually not want to interact with others, including care and support services, and may therefore become increasingly isolated, lonely and withdrawn. • A child or young person may also become more isolated from others and not attend school or college or work.
Self-neglect	• Signs and symptoms associated with neglect by others. • The individual may have general apathy for their own well-being.

▲ Table 5.1 Common signs and symptoms associated with harm, abuse and neglect *(continued)*

CASE STUDY

Abuse at home

Charlotte lives at home with her mother and older sister, Zoe. Charlotte is a young carer for her mother who has a physical disability and uses a wheelchair. Charlotte's sister, Zoe, works long hours, and wants Charlotte and her mother to do more tasks around the house.

One evening, Zoe returns home from a long work shift and finds Charlotte and her mother watching television together having a cup of tea. Zoe starts screaming at them both,

telling them that they are both lazy and selfish, and that she is the only one that works hard. Zoe then grabs their cups of tea, smashes them against the wall behind where they are sitting down, and shouts at them that they can cook their own evening meal as she's had enough.

Discussion points:

• Is abuse taking place? Why?
• Does anyone need safeguarding? Why?

KEY TERMS

Policies and procedures: policies describes how an organisation plans to carry out its services. Procedures set out how an organisation expects its employees to put their policies into action on a day-to-day basis.

AC1.4 Legislation, national policies and codes of conduct and professional practice that relate to the safeguarding of individuals – both adults and children and young people and what these mean in practice

AC1.5 How legislative frameworks support the rights of individuals to be protected from harm, abuse and neglect

Legislation

Safeguarding adults, children and young people also involves learning about the legislation that is in place in the UK, and ensuring that your knowledge is current so that your work practices are also current and reflect good practice.

Make sure you are up to date by

- attending training and reading information updates provided by your employer
- referring to the Government's websites:

www.gov.wales

www.legislation.gov.uk

Below is some useful information about the current legislation that exists and what it means in practice for safeguarding adults, children and young people.

You can also refer back to Units 001/002, LO2 for information on this topic.

Social Services and Well-Being (Wales) Act 2014

This Act aims to safeguard and improve the well-being of adults (people aged 18 or over), children (people under the age of 18) and carers (adults or children who provide or intend to provide care and support) in Wales. We have looked at this Act several times in this book. See Figure 1.3 in Units 001/002 for its five key principles.

This Act is set out in 11 parts and explains what local authorities need to do to help people who require care and support. In relation to safeguarding, part 7 is very important because it:

- sets out the main categories of abuse and neglect of adults, children and young people
- defines the meaning of an adult at risk as an adult who is experiencing, or is at risk of, abuse or neglect, has needs for care and as a result of those needs is unable to protect himself or herself against the abuse or neglect or the risk of it
- defines the meaning of a child at risk as a child who is experiencing, or is at risk of, abuse, neglect or other kinds of harm and has needs for care and support
- defines abuse as meaning physical, sexual, psychological, emotional or financial abuse and includes abuse taking place in any setting i.e. in a private dwelling, an institution or any other place
- defines neglect as a failure to meet a person's basic physical, emotional, social or psychological needs, which is likely to result in an impairment of the person's well-being
- explains the roles and responsibilities in safeguarding individuals including knowing about the signs and symptoms of abuse and neglect to look out for, knowing the actions to take when responding to suspicions, allegations or disclosures of abuse including reporting, recording and referral requirements

- places duties on local authorities to report if an adult or child is at risk, make enquiries if an adult or child is suspected of being at risk, set up separate safeguarding boards for adults and children that are responsible for working with agencies in each local authority to ensure they develop effective systems for safeguarding and protecting individuals from abuse, harm and neglect
- introduced a National Independent Safeguarding Board that provides support and advice to children and adults safeguarding boards, to report on the effectiveness of safeguarding arrangements in place for children and adults and make recommendations to the Welsh Government to improve the arrangements in place.

www.legislation.gov.uk, Social Services and Well-being (Wales) Act 2014.

Children Act (1989 and 2004)

- The Children Act 1989 was introduced to ensure children were safeguarded and protected from harm and their welfare promoted. The Act was based on the welfare principle which meant that the welfare of a child must be at the centre of any decision made in relation to the child.
- In 2004, another Act was introduced to strengthen the Children Act 1989. It established a Children's Commissioner for England to champion the views and interests of children and young people. It also encouraged partnership working between agencies such as local authorities, health and social care providers and the police to promote children's well-being.

Data Protection Act (1998 and 2018)

This Act is the main piece of legislation that protects the rights of people who have personal information recorded, used, stored and shared by organisations. It established:

- the rights of adults, children and young people to know what information is being collected about them
- how personal information is used to safeguard people from harm
- that personal information must be kept safe, secure and accessed only by those who have permission to do so.

GDPR 2018

In 2018 a further Act was introduced to strengthen the Data Protection Act 1998 and bring the European Union's GDPR 2018 into UK law. It aimed to:

- safeguard people's personal information online
- give people more control over use of their data
- provide them with new rights to move or delete personal data.

The GDPR is a set of EU-wide data protection rules that have been brought into UK law as the Data Protection Act 2018.

The GDPR gives people greater rights over their personal information. For example:

- People have the right to give and to withdraw their consent for **processing information**.
- Organisations have to demonstrate how they have obtained consent when handling information.
- People's rights and interests must also be safeguarded when information is processed.

Human Rights Act 1998

The Act is a set of rights contained within the European Convention on Human Rights that have been brought into UK law, and include, for example, the right to:

- respect for private and family life
- personal liberty
- not be tortured or treated in an inhuman way
- non-discrimination
- freedom of religion and belief.

The Act protects the human rights of everyone who lives in the UK. This means that action in the UK courts can be taken if a person's human rights have been breached.

Mental Health Act revision 2007

This Act amended the Mental Health Act 1983 and the Mental Capacity Act 2005 (see below). It applies to England and Wales.

It strengthens and promotes the rights of individuals with a mental disorder. For example, an individual can no longer be **compulsorily detained** or have their detention extended if they do not have access to appropriate medical treatment.

Mental Capacity Act 2005

The Act safeguards individuals who are unable to make choices and decisions for themselves because they lack the capacity to do so due to an illness or a disability.

It is based on five principles:

1 Always assume that individuals are able to make their own decisions; never assume that they do not have the capacity to do so.
2 Support individuals so that they can make their own choices and decisions.
3 Respect individuals' rights to make decisions that others may not agree with.
4 All decisions made on an individual's behalf, when they lack capacity, must always be in their best interests.
5 Decisions made on an individual's behalf must be the least restrictive option – the option that promotes the individual's rights as much as possible.

Equality Act 2010

This Act safeguards everyone from unfair treatment and discrimination. It makes it unlawful to discriminate against a person based on one of the following protected characteristics:

- age, disability, gender reassignment, marriage and civil partnership, pregnancy and maternity, race, religion or belief, sex and sexual orientation.

Safeguarding of Vulnerable Groups Act 2006

This Act safeguards vulnerable adults, children and young people from harm, abuse and neglect. It established:

- the **vetting and barring scheme**, which prevents people who are not suitable to work with individuals with care or support needs from doing so
- the Independent Safeguarding Authority, which later merged with the Criminal Records Bureau to become the **Disclosure and Barring Service (DBS)**.

Violence against Women, Domestic Abuse and Sexual Violence (Wales) 2015

This Act requires local authorities and local health boards in Wales to work together to tackle violence against women, domestic abuse and sexual violence, through establishing joint strategies around prevention, protection and support.

The Act also covers:

- all forms of gender-based violence (recognising that both men and women are victims of violence)
- threats of violence or harassment relating to gender or sexual orientation
- forced marriage.

KEY TERMS

Processing information: recording, using, storing and sharing information.

Compulsorily detained: this means being held in hospital and given treatment, whether or not you agree with it, because of concerns for own safety and/or that of others.

Vetting and barring scheme: this ensures that any person who is not fit or appropriate to work with adults, children and young people does not do so.

Disclosure and Barring Service (DBS): the Government service that makes background checks, for organisations, on people who want to work with adults, children and young people with care or support needs.

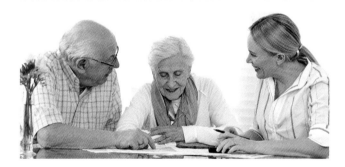

▲ Figure 5.1 How can you uphold individuals' rights to be safeguarded?

CASE STUDY

Safeguarding legislation

Read through again the three scenarios described in the 'Types of abuse' case study on page 44 and discuss which pieces of legislation would be relevant for safeguarding Cadwallen, Charlie and Beca.

National policies

As well as legislation for safeguarding individuals, there are also national policies that have been developed by the Government and provide guidance. These are used by local agencies such as the NHS and local authorities to develop their own policies. Table 5.2 shows some examples of national policies that exist for safeguarding adults, children and young people. Refresh your learning by reviewing Units 001/002/002, LO2.

National policy	Explanation
In Safe Hands 2000: Implementing Adult Protection Procedures in Wales	This policy places a duty on local authorities in Wales to take the lead role in co-ordinating safeguarding policies and procedures for the protection of adults from abuse in their areas. The policy: • encourages different agencies to work together to prevent, identify and respond to the abuse of adults • provides guidance on how to develop effective procedures for preventing abuse • includes examples of written policies, such as reporting abuse and how to share information. This guidance has now been replaced.
Adults – Deprivation of Liberty Safeguards (DoLS)	The DoLS was replaced in 2020 with the Liberty Protection Standards (LPS), which will come into effect in 2022. It applies in England and Wales and was set up by an amendment to the Mental Capacity Act 2005. • Person-centred care is all about empowering people. However, under LPS there are certain times when it is recognised there is a need to deprive people of their liberty. • LPS protects the rights of people in care homes or hospitals when they **lack capacity** to consent to their care and treatment, by ensuring that it does not inappropriately restrict their freedom. • Under the standards, if **restraint** and **restrictions** are used that will lead to an individual being deprived of their liberty in a care home or hospital, then the care home or hospital must ask the local authority if they can deprive the individual of their liberty; this process is called requesting a standard authorisation. Before a standard authorisation can be given, six assessments must take place that consider a number of factors such as whether any harm could occur if the deprivation of liberty doesn't take place and whether deprivation of liberty could be avoided.
Adults – Wales Interim Policy and Procedures for the Protection of Vulnerable Adults from Abuse 2010 (updated 2013)	These procedures were based on the rights of individuals under the Human Rights Act 1998. In terms of safeguarding, this policy: • promotes individuals' rights to be fully involved throughout all stages of the adult protection process • promotes individuals' rights to make decisions about their safety and well-being unless they lack the capacity to make decisions • ensures that safeguarding becomes everyone's business • places a duty of care on everyone to report concerns or incidents of abuse; you will learn more about how concerns or incidents should be recorded and reported in AC1.6. These regulations have now been replaced.
Wales Safeguarding Procedures 2019	These procedures replace the Wales Interim Policy & Procedures for the Protection of Vulnerable Adults from Abuse 2010 (updated 2013) that you read about and the All Wales Child Protection Policy and Procedures 2008 (you will learn about these in the sections that follow). These procedures are aimed at all those who work with adults and children in Wales and include both those in paid and unpaid roles. These procedures build on the principles of the Social Services and Well-Being (Wales) Act 2014: • They provide clear guidance on the safeguarding procedures to follow when working with both adults and children in Wales. • They explain everyone's roles and responsibilities so that individuals can be protected from harm, abuse and neglect.
Children – United Nations Convention on the Rights of the Child 1989	This is an international set of human rights for all children and young people (aged 17 and under). The Convention came into force in the UK in 1992. It safeguards and protects children and young people by setting out the civil, political, economic, social and cultural rights that all children everywhere are entitled to, such as the right to: • privacy • education • be safe from violence • relax • think and believe what they choose • play. The UNCRC also set out how everyone must work together to ensure children's rights are upheld.

▲ Table 5.2 National policies

National policy	Explanation
Children – All Wales Child Protection Policy and Procedures 2008	These procedures are based on the principle that all the people and agencies working with children and young people have a responsibility to safeguard them from harm, abuse and neglect and promote their welfare. These procedures provide guidance in relation to child protection to each of the **local and regional safeguarding children boards** across Wales.
Children – Working Together under the Children Act 2004	This guidance is aimed at all the people and agencies working with children to safeguard them and promote their welfare. It sets out the actions that must be taken when: • there are concerns about a child • a child is being harmed, abused or neglected • a child may be at risk of being harmed, abused or neglected. It also sets out when information must be shared to safeguard and promote children's welfare, including: • how to obtain consent to share information • what to do when consent to share information has not or cannot be obtained (because doing so may put the child at risk of further harm or abuse).

▲ Table 5.2 National policies *(continued)*

KEY TERMS

Lack capacity: when an individual is unable to make a decision for themselves because of a learning disability or a condition, such as dementia or a mental health need, or because they are unconscious.

Restraint: an intervention when a person is trying to harm themselves or others. It involves preventing, restricting or subduing the movement of the body, or part of the body of another person.

Restrictions: interventions used to prevent a person harming themselves or others such as restricting a person's freedom of movement. They are only used for as long as is necessary and as a last resort.

Local and regional safeguarding children boards: these are set up in every local authority, and consist of a number of agencies that oversee local child protection systems to ensure that all organisations work together to safeguard children and promote their welfare.

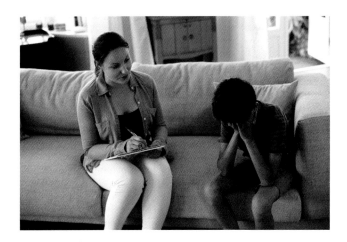

▲ Figure 5.2 How can professionals in Wales safeguard children?

Codes of conduct and professional practice

As well as legislation and national policies there are also codes of conduct that provide guidance and set out the professional conduct and practice expected of those employed in the social care profession in Wales. Table 5.3 shows examples of codes of conduct.

Code of conduct and professional practice	Explanation
Code of Professional Practice for Social Care	This Code sets out seven requirements that social care workers must follow when carrying out their work. Social care workers must ensure that their practice meets these requirements and does not fall below these standards, as doing so may harm an individual's well-being. See Units 001/002, LO2 for a list and descriptions of its seven requirements expected from social care workers.
NHS Wales Code of Conduct for Healthcare Support Workers in Wales	This Code describes the standards of conduct, behaviour and attitude required of all healthcare support workers employed within NHS Wales in both clinical and non-clinical environments. The purpose of the Code is to provide guidance to healthcare support workers within NHS Wales to: • ensure that they are carrying out their work to the required standard • identify areas of their work that they may need to further improve or develop.
Code of Practice for NHS Wales Employers	The Code of Practice for NHS Wales Employers is supported by the Code of Conduct for Healthcare Support Workers employed within NHS Wales that you have learnt about in relation to the standards expected of staff. Both Codes: • support safe working practices • encourage the development of staff so that they feel fulfilled in their work roles and have opportunities to progress in their careers. This Code includes four key areas, as shown in Figure 5.3.

▲ Table 5.3 Codes of conduct and professional guidance

1 Employers must ensure staff are suitable to be employed in their job role and understand their responsibilities and accountabilities, e.g. induction, training, support

2 Employers must have procedures in place so that staff can meet the standards set out in the Code of Conduct, e.g. putting in place and reviewing policies and procedures

3 Employers must provide staff with opportunities to develop and improve their skills and knowledge, e.g. training, education, career progression opportunities

4 Employers must promote the standards set out in this Code and the Code for Healthcare Support workers to staff, individuals and others, and ensure its use, e.g. discussion, leaflets

▲ Figure 5.3 The Code of Practice for NHS Wales Employers

Additional practice guidance issued by NHS Wales or the regulators of health or social care in Wales

Practice guidance	Explanation
The Guide to Consent for Examination or Treatment by NHS Wales	This Guide describes: • how health professionals can obtain **valid consent** from an individual for treatment • what to do if an individual cannot give their valid consent, because the individual is unconscious or has a disability that means they cannot understand or communicate their decision. The guidance is based on the principle that health professionals must respect individuals' rights to make their own decisions about treatment. • This means that a health professional must obtain an individual's valid consent before performing a physical investigation or provide personal care. • Failing to gain valid consent can make an individual feel upset and humiliated. The individual and the health professional's employer could take legal action for failing to ensure the well-being of the individual when providing care and treatment.
Practice Guidance for Residential Child Care for Workers Registered with Social Care Wales	See Units 001/002, AC1.1 for detailed information on this practice guidance. It describes what is expected of residential child care workers who are registered with Social Care Wales, and is aimed at both residential child care workers and their employers to ensure the provision of a professional and safe service to children, young people and their families.

▲ Table 5.4 Examples of other practice guidance

KEY TERM

Valid consent: informed agreement to an action or decision in relation to a person's treatment in an NHS setting. The process of establishing consent will vary according to a person's assessed capacity to consent.

RESEARCH IT

Research the seven areas of guidance set out in the Code of Conduct for Healthcare Support Workers in Wales. You can find the Code using this link: **www.wales.nhs.uk/documents/Code_of_Conduct_ for_Healthcare_Support_Workers_in_Wales.pdf**

CASE STUDY

Professional practice

Morgan has been recruited as a healthcare support worker in Wales and has never worked in the healthcare sector. Morgan would like to find out more about the practice expected in the new job.

Discussion points:

- Which Codes of Conduct might be relevant? Why?
- Which practice guidance might be relevant? Why?

AC1.6 How concerns or incidents should be recorded and reported

Recognising safeguarding concerns or incidents when they occur and knowing how these should be recorded and reported will help you to ensure that your ways of working comply with the legislation and guidance you've learnt about in AC1.4 and AC1.5, as well as maintain the safety and well-being of the individuals, your colleagues and others you work with.

Safeguarding concerns or incidents are when an individual – this could be an individual in receipt of care, a child, a young person, you, a colleague or visitor – is placed in danger or at risk of being injured or harmed. They can include complaints, **allegations** or reported safeguarding incidents. Complaints could be about:

- poor working practices – these may lead to an accident in the care setting, such as not using the correct equipment when moving an individual from one position to another
- insufficient resources – not enough staff may mean that individuals' needs are not met and their well-being is not being safeguarded
- how care settings are managed – poor leadership of workers could result in abuse, harm or neglect taking place and not being recognised.

Allegations or reported safeguarding incidents might:

- relate to one or more types of abuse; you will find it useful to refer back the main categories of abuse and neglect you learnt about in AC1.2
- be made by an individual, you, a work colleague or visitor to your work setting.

It is important to always follow your work setting's safeguarding policy and procedures for the recording and reporting of concerns or incidents. Be open and respectful so that you can build up trust and confidence with the person raising the concern or incident.

You will learn more about the approaches used and the actions to take to respond to suspected, disclosed or alleged harm, abuse or neglect in LO4.

KEY TERM

Allegations: when an individual or another person tells you that they are being abused or that abuse is happening.

How to record concerns or incidents

1 Record the details of the person who the concern or incident relates to – their name, age and address (if you know it) – so they can be safeguarded.
2 Record the concern fully and legibly, using the person's exact words. This will help establish what happened and provide a true and accurate record.
3 Record all information that has been given about the alleged perpetrator so the person can be safeguarded from them.
4 Record any evidence of physical abuse on the individual's body, using a body map to accurately identify where this is. This will be important in terms of evidence of the abuse that has taken place.

5 Record when and where the **disclosure of abuse** happened, including whether anyone else witnessed the disclosure being made.

6 Record all information as soon as possible so that you are less likely to forget the details. This will be important if you are asked to make a statement to the police or court at a later date.

7 Record all information in pen, so that your record cannot be altered or removed at a later date.

8 Record all information with your name printed, your signature, the time the concern was raised or incident happened and a date so that it is auditable and cannot be altered or added to by anyone else.

REFLECT ON IT

Reflect on an occasion when you had to record some important information. For example, you may have had to take down a phone message for someone else.

- What details did you include?
- Why?

How to report concerns or incidents

1 Call 999 if the person is in immediate danger, to safeguard the person and anyone else in the area.

2 Report the information you've recorded to the relevant person so that it can be dealt with; the relevant person will be identified in your work setting's safeguarding policy and procedures, and will have been trained in handling concerns or incidents.

3 Report the concern or incident as quickly as possible, so that you are less likely to forget

any details and the person concerned can be safeguarded from further danger, harm or abuse.

4 Report the actions that have been taken. This information is important so that you can show how you have safeguarded the individual from further danger, harm or abuse.

5 Report the actions that still need to be taken following the concern or incident being reported, so that these can be taken by the relevant person.

6 If the concern or incident is not dealt with seriously by your work setting, report it to the relevant external authority – the police, social services or the CIW. This ensures that all allegations are reported and acted on, and forms part of your work setting's **whistleblowing procedure**. You may find it useful to refer to AC4.5 in relation to more information about whistleblowing.

CIW is the independent regulator of social care and child care in Wales. The inspectorate regulates social care, early years services and local authority care support services. Regulation includes registration, inspection, responding to concerns about regulated services and enforcement.

KEY TERMS

Disclosure of abuse: when a person tells you that abuse has happened or is happening

Whistleblowing: exposing any kind of information or activity that is deemed illegal, unethical or not correct.

CASE STUDY

Recording and reporting concerns

Enzo is 84 years old and lives at home on his own. You are Enzo's home carer and visit Enzo three times a day to support him with personal care and meals. At the end of your morning visit, Enzo discloses to you that one of your colleagues has shouted and upset him for no reason. Enzo adds that he wants the shouting to stop but doesn't want to get your colleague into any trouble.

Discussion points:

- Identify the first three actions you would take in this situation and explain why.
- What information would you record? Why?
- How and when would you report this? Why?

Check your understanding

1 What does the term 'safeguarding' mean?

2 Name two types of abuse and neglect, and their associated signs and symptoms.

3 Name two pieces of legislation/national policies that safeguard children and support their rights.

4 Describe how to record concerns or incidents.

5 Describe how to report concerns or incidents.

Question practice

1 What type of abuse is defined as an organisation having inadequate systems, policies and procedures in place to meet individuals' needs?

   a discrimination

   b institutional

   c hate crime

   d neglect by others

2 Which of these best describes the UNCRC?

   a an international set of human rights for all children and young people (aged 17 and under)

   b a national set of human rights

   c a national set of human rights for all children and young people

   d an international set of human rights for all children and young people (aged 16 and under)

LO2 UNDERSTAND HOW TO WORK IN WAYS THAT SAFEGUARD INDIVIDUALS FROM HARM, ABUSE AND NEGLECT

GETTING STARTED

Think about an occasion or situation where you faced danger or felt unsafe.

- How did you feel afterwards?
- Did you tell anyone about what happened?
- If so, who did you tell and why?

Reflect on what happened:

- Do you think anything else could have been done to prevent this situation from happening?
- If so, who could have helped, and why?
- Review your previous learning in relation to the Social Services and Well-being (Wales) Act 2014 and think about what your responsibilities are in this situation.

AC2.1 The roles and responsibilities of health and social care workers in relation to safeguarding

As you have seen in LO1 of this unit, health and social care workers have a legal responsibility to safeguard the individuals they work with from harm, abuse and neglect, and it is part of their job roles to do this in a way that enables individuals to remain safe.

Health and social care workers will have a job description that sets out the responsibilities they have agreed to with their employer including the work tasks they must carry out and how these must be carried out. Their roles and responsibilities in relation to safeguarding include:

1 **Being knowledgeable**.
- Knowing about the different types of harm, abuse and neglect, and the signs and symptoms associated with these.

255

- Knowing what to do if an individual is at risk of or is being harmed or abused, to prevent any further harm or abuse from taking place.
- Lack of knowledge may mean that incidents of harm, abuse and neglect are not identified, and the individuals continue to be placed in danger.

2 **Following the policies and procedures where they work**.
- Adhering to the requirements of their employer's agreed ways of working when safeguarding individuals.
- Following their employer's procedures for reporting and recording concerns or incidents to maintain the safety and well-being of individuals.
- Not following procedures may mean that health and social care workers do not fulfil their legal responsibilities and duty to safeguard and protect individuals.

3 **Supporting individuals**.
- Supporting individuals to understand their rights to be protected from being placed in danger, abused or neglected so that they are less likely to be abused by others.
- Supporting individuals to understand how they will be supported if they are being harmed, abused or neglected, so that they feel confident in saying when this is happening.
- Not supporting individuals may mean that they continue to be abused by others.

- You will learn more about the different ways to make individuals aware of how to keep themselves safe in AC2.7.

AC2.2 The role of *advocacy* in relation to safeguarding

We have already looked at advocacy in Units 001/002 AC2.4, but here we will go into more details about the different kinds of advocacy available to support individuals.

Advocacy services support individuals during the safeguarding process to make their views known and represent their interests when they have difficulties doing so; this might be, for example, for an individual who has an illness or disability. This involves:

- supporting individuals to express their views, preferences and opinions
- enabling individuals to make informed choices and decisions.

Advocacy is important because it enables individuals to:

- be listened to
- receive information, advice and support
- have the opportunity to explore their options and rights.

Table 5.5 shows some examples of the different types of advocacy and how they can benefit individuals in relation to safeguarding.

Type of advocacy	Explanation
Self-advocacy	Supporting an individual to develop the skills to speak up for themselves and what is important in their life and for their well-being.
	Self-advocacy can increase an individual's confidence when speaking up about a difficult issue.
Informal advocacy	Supporting an individual to speak up and represent themselves by others who know the individual, such as the individual's family and friends.
	Informal advocacy can maintain an individual's best interests.
Collective advocacy	Supporting a group of individuals who have shared interests to represent their views, preferences and experiences.
	Collective advocacy can help an individual to feel less anxious or alone when raising a safeguarding issue.
Peer advocacy	Supporting an individual to speak up for themselves by an advocate who shares similar experiences or is of the same age or gender to that of the individual.
	Peer advocacy can help an individual to increase their self-awareness by sharing how they are feeling with someone else who understands their situation.
Citizen advocacy	Supporting an individual to speak up for themselves by an advocate who is an ordinary citizen of their community and develops a relationship with the individual over a long period of time.
	Citizen advocacy can help an individual to develop a long-term one-to-one relationship with a person who they feel they can trust and confide in.

▲ Table 5.5 Types of advocacy

Type of advocacy	Explanation
Independent volunteer advocacy	Supporting an individual to speak up for themselves by an advocate who is trained and supported by an organisation and is a volunteer.
	Independent volunteer advocacy can provide individuals with information about the safeguarding process.
Formal advocacy	Supporting an individual or a group of individuals to speak up and represent themselves by others who are trained and paid by an organisation.
	Formal advocacy can ensure that individuals access advocates' specific knowledge and expertise about the safeguarding process or in relation to a specific situation.
Independent professional advocacy	Supporting an individual to speak up for themselves by an advocate who is trained by an organisation and paid to carry out their role.
	Independent professional advocacy can support individuals with specific issues in relation to the safeguarding process.

▲ Table 5.5 Types of advocacy *(continued)*

CASE STUDY

Types of advocacy

Read the following three scenarios. Which types of advocacy would these individuals benefit from and why?

1 Caitrin is 10 years old and, after a safeguarding concern at home, is living with a foster carer. Caitrin needs support to speak about her well-being.
2 Aderyn is 19 years old, has mental health needs and is living with a partner who, it has been alleged, has been physically abusive.
3 Tom is 54 years old and has the onset of dementia. Tom was recently targeted by a stranger who tried to obtain money from him fraudulently. Tom needs support to understand the safeguarding process.

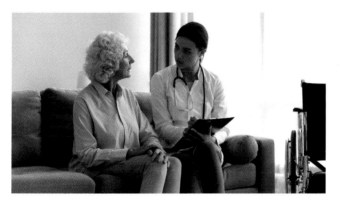

▲ Figure 5.4 How can an advocate support an individual during the safeguarding process?

AC2.3 The importance of establishing relationships that support trust and rapport with individuals

Establishing relationships with individuals that support trust and rapport is very important because individuals will feel at ease with you and therefore be more likely to confide in you if they or someone they know have experienced abuse or neglect from others.

Supportive and trusting relationships will also enable individuals to feel more confident in themselves, and therefore make them more likely to recognise, challenge and report abuse when this occurs.

By not establishing working relationships that support these principles of trust and respect will mean that you will be failing in your duty to care for individuals in a way that promotes their well-being. Individuals will not feel that they can confide in you or trust you, and therefore their abuse and neglect by others may continue unreported.

Do	Don't
Be patient and understanding with individuals so that they can approach you and build trust in you.	Don't rush individuals during communications, as this will make it more difficult for them to confide in you and may lead to inaccurate or incomplete information being shared with you.
Be open and honest when working with individuals so that they can build trust and rapport with you.	Don't look disinterested or distracted when communicating with individuals, as it will be more difficult to build up a rapport with them.
Listen to individuals so that you can get to know who they are and understand their views, needs and preferences.	Don't impose your views and preferences on individuals as this may mean that they will not trust you to share what they think.
Show empathy by understanding the situation from the individual's point of view.	Don't ignore what an individual is telling you or expressing, as they will not feel respected or want to build a working relationship with you.

▲ Table 5.6 Dos and don'ts for establishing relationships that support trust and rapport with individuals

REFLECT ON IT

Reflect on someone that you have a close relationship with. This may be with a family member or a friend you've known for a long time.

- What makes this relationship different from others?
- Why do you trust this person?
- How would you feel if you couldn't trust this person?

AC2.4 The importance of person/child-centred practice in safeguarding

What is person/child-centred practice?

Person/child-centred practice in safeguarding involves supporting individuals in a way that keeps individuals as the focus and takes account of their unique needs, views and preferences. This kind of practice also enables individuals to contribute to the decisions they make, including the care and support they require.

The care and support provided to individuals by workers is underpinned by a set of values commonly referred to as 'person-centred values'. See Table 1.4 in Units 001/002 for a full description of these **values** and what they mean in relation to providing care and support.

Person/child-centred values can include supporting individuality, showing respect for individuals' privacy and their right to make their own choices, and treating individuals with dignity and respect. These values can be applied when safeguarding individuals when you:

- ask individuals how they want to be supported during the safeguarding process (individuality)
- do not question individuals when they disclose abuse (privacy)
- provide individuals with different options when making decisions about their well-being so that they can choose the option that is best for them (right to make their own choices)
- show understanding and respect for individuals' views, including when different to your own (dignity and respect).

KEY TERM

Values: ideas that form the system by which a person lives their life; often a person's beliefs can develop into their values.

Why is person/child-centred practice important?

As you will have learnt, person/child-centred practice in safeguarding provides care and support so the individual remains the focus. Person/child-centred practice is important and benefits both individuals and workers because:

- enabling individuals to make their own choices and decisions will mean that they feel more confident and more in control of their lives
- taking into account individuals' needs, views and preferences will have a positive impact on individuals by enabling them to live how they want to
- supporting individuals to understand what their rights are will show them that you respect and value them, and genuinely care
- you will be carrying out your job role to the required standards
- this will enable you to follow good practice, and provide safe and effective care and support
- promoting partnership working will mean that you will learn how to work together with individuals and others who are involved in their lives, such as their families, friends and other professionals.

Not following person/child-centred practice in safeguarding must be avoided as this can have negative consequences:

- You would not be carrying out your job role to the required standard, which can result in unsafe practices. This could end your career in health and social care.
- Safeguarding concerns could be missed if you don't work in partnership, and individuals could be placed in danger of harm, abuse and neglect.
- Individuals would not feel valued or respected. They may become angry or upset that their needs, views and preferences have not been taken into account, which would make it difficult to build up rapport and trust with them.

AC2.5 The importance of working in ways that uphold the rights of individuals

As you will have learnt in ACs 1.4 and 1.5, the rights of individuals are set out and supported by legislation such as the Children Act 1989 and 2004, Human Rights Act 1998, the Equality Act 2010 and Social Services and Well-Being (Wales) Act 2014. You may find it useful to review your previous learning about legislation and how it safeguards individuals. Everyone is legally entitled to have their rights respected and upheld.

It is important to work in person-centred ways that support individuals to understand their rights and how these can be met, because this helps to safeguard individuals from harm, abuse and neglect by:

- raising their awareness about what is or what is not safe and effective care or support
- supporting them to understand what good care and support looks like and how they can be supported to live safely and well
- being more confident and assertive, therefore more likely to report any harm, abuse and neglect when it occurs
- promoting their safety, security and therefore their well-being
- instilling trust and confidence between individuals and workers
- meeting individuals' needs.

AC2.6 Ways to promote an environment where individuals can express fears, anxieties, feelings and concerns without worry of ridicule, rejection, retribution or not being believed

Individuals may experience a range of feelings and emotions when they have suffered from harm, abuse or neglect. This can include fear and anxiety, worry about being able to continue to live where they are if they report abuse, being laughed at, having their concerns rejected or not being believed.

These feelings can arise whether the abuse is fairly recent, has only occurred once or has been going on for a long period of time. Abuse can have a detrimental impact on an individual, including how they view and relate to others. It is therefore essential to create an environment where individuals feel comfortable and are able to raise and express any fears, anxieties or concerns without worrying about not being believed.

The two diagrams in Figure 5.5 provide examples of ways to promote an environment that encourages well-being, where individuals feel they can openly express their feelings and concerns. The first diagram refers to the physical environment, which includes the actual work setting and its contents, and the second diagram refers to the social environment, which includes the atmosphere within the work setting and the working relationships that exist between individuals, you and other workers.

Ensuring the work setting is clean and uncluttered will make the individual feel relaxed and more likely to want to express their feelings and anxieties.

Ensuring the layout in the work setting is open and easy to move around in will make the individual feel at ease and more likely to share their feelings and concerns.

Ensuring the individual is in a room where they have some of their personal belongings around them will make them feel at home and more likely to express how they feel.

1
THE PHYSICAL ENVIRONMENT

Ensuring the work setting is well maintained and does not contain broken furniture and fixtures will make the individual feel safe and more likely to express their fears.

Ensuring the temperature of the room is neither too hot or too cold will make the individual feel comfortable and more likely to say if they have any concerns.

Ensuring the room is calm and free from distractions will make the individual feel they are the focus and more likely to express their anxieties and feelings.

▲ Figure 5.5(1) Ways to promote an environment where individuals can express their feelings and concerns: the physical environment

A welcoming and inviting work setting will make the individual feel relaxed and more likely to feel able to express their feelings without worrying about not being believed.

A work setting where workers are caring and understanding when supporting individuals will make them feel comfortable, and more likely to express their feelings without worry of ridicule.

A stimulating environment where the individual's needs are met will make them feel valued and more likely to express their concerns without worrying about retribution.

2
THE SOCIAL ENVIRONMENT

A work setting that is representative of individuals' diverse backgrounds (age, gender, culture) will provide individuals with a sense of belonging and make them more likely to share their feelings and concerns.

A work setting where workers respect individuals will build up their trust, and an individual will be more likely to express their fears and anxieties without worry of rejection.

A work setting where policies and procedures are complied with will reduce the likelihood of an individual being harmed, abused or neglected. The individual will feel secure and more likely to share their fears.

▲ Figure 5.5(2) Ways to promote an environment where individuals can express their feelings and concerns: the social environment

AC2.7 Ways to make individuals aware of how to keep themselves safe

Raising individuals' awareness of how to keep themselves safe can be a very effective way to safeguard them from harm, abuse and neglect because it places individuals in control of their own personal safety. This means that they are less likely to be targeted by others because they will not be perceived as vulnerable. Below are some examples of how to make individuals aware of how to keep themselves safe.

Provide information

Information in the form of leaflets, videos, photographs, discussions about the dangers that exist can be provided to individuals. Individuals can be warned about the dangers that exist at home, such as:

- Do not open the door without checking who it is first, to avoid people with no authorisation from entering.
- Do not overload electrical sockets so that electrical fires are prevented.
- Do not block fire escape routes with personal belongings or furniture in case of the outbreak of a fire.

Individuals can also be warned about the dangers that exist in the community. For example:

- Keep safe, by not walking on their own late at night.
- Do not meet someone they've met online on their own or in an isolated location, in case they are not who they say they are.
- Do not engage in activities without first **assessing the risks** of doing so, to avoid injuries.

Involve individuals

Working with individuals to promote their own personal safety will encourage them to think about and make decisions that put their own safety first. For example:

- Discuss with individuals the dangers involved in developing their independent cooking skills, such as using sharp knives and operating the oven safely.
- Explain the precautions that they can take to reduce the potential risks, such as developing safe cutting techniques when using knives and using reminders to ensure the oven is switched off after use.

You will learn more about ways of working that keep everyone safe later in this unit in AC2.9.

KEY TERM

Assessing the risks: identifying dangers with the potential to cause harm, deciding on the level of risk and putting in place processes for reducing or controlling these risks.

CASE STUDY

Child-centred practice

Kamile works in an after-school club and has noticed how one of the children who attends regularly seems withdrawn and at times untidy in their appearance. Kamile is very concerned about this child and wants to provide support and promote their well-being.

Discussion points:
- How can Kamile ensure the child remains the focus when supporting them?
- What can Kamile do to ensure the child feels comfortable in expressing their feelings and any concerns they may have?
- How can Kamile work with the child to make them aware of how to keep themselves safe?

AC2.8 Ways to make individuals aware of the risks associated with the use of social media, internet use and phones

As you have learnt, you have a duty of care to maintain the safety of individuals you support, and to promote their well-being. It is therefore important that you know about the risks associated with the use of social media, internet use and phones so that you can inform individuals.

Risks associated with the use of social media, internet use and phones

Social media

Social media and social networking sites such as Facebook and Twitter are a popular way to keep in touch with family and friends and make new friends, but they also have the potential to pose risks to individuals' safety and well-being:

- Individuals may feel upset if excluded from chats and videos that have not been sent to them but have been sent to some of their friends.
- When making new friends, it is important for individuals to be made aware that not all information people share about themselves is true.

The internet

Using the internet can also be a good way of individuals keeping in touch with family and friends through the sharing of photographs, messages and videos. However, sharing this kind of personal information can put individuals in danger if the information is abused or used dishonestly.

- Individuals need to be made aware of the risks of searching for information on unofficial websites that may contain offensive, racist or sexually explicit language.
- Sometimes individuals may use search engines such as Google and Bing to find information about what is happening in their local community. This sometimes means sharing their location, which is then made public to others who could exploit this.

Mobile phones

These can be used by individuals to access websites and download apps such as Instagram and Snapchat, to comment on and share images with others.

- Although these are good ways to keep in touch with others, these kind of apps send out information about individuals' locations. This could make them the target for abuse such as online bullying and emotional abuse.
- Using phones when out of the setting puts individuals at risk of being targeted, having their phone stolen and/or their security passwords on their phones compromised. This would leave them open to fraud.

Making individuals aware of the risks of social media, internet use and phones

Making individuals aware of the risks of social media, internet use and phones involves:

- educating individuals about online safety
- discussing the risks with them
- making suggestions for how they can safeguard themselves online.

Ensuring that individuals can share their concerns with workers if they are made to feel uncomfortable during any type of online activity is also extremely important, and an effective way of preventing any harm or abuse from taking place and/or continuing.

Table 5.7 includes some suggestions for raising individuals' awareness of the risks that exist with these types of online activity.

Online activities	How to make individuals aware of the risks
The use of social media	• Show individuals how to check if a social networking site is official and secure, and understand why this is important, so that they avoid chats or transactions with people who may not be who they say they are. • Discuss the dangers of sharing personal information and photographs, as they may be shared publicly with other people without the individual's agreement. • Emphasise that individuals do not have to accept requests and invitations from people they do not know, so that they stay in control of who they are friends with.
The use of the internet	• Make individuals aware of the dangers of using the internet, and meeting people or receiving emails/messages from people who are not who they claim to be. • Reassure individuals that when this happens that they can report these people. Show them how to block these people so they cannot make unwanted contact again. • Make individuals aware of safe ways of using the internet: only use official sites to make transactions to avoid fraud, and complete all transactions in private to avoid others seeing their personal information.
The use of phones	• Make individuals aware of how they can minimise the risk of other people accessing their phone and the personal information it contains. Show them how to use passwords or face ID to prevent others accessing their personal information. • Make individuals aware of why phones have privacy settings, so that their privacy is protected and their information cannot be accessed by others. • Show individuals how to switch on these privacy settings, so that other people are unable to access their phone or contact them.

▲ Table 5.7 Promoting online safety and raising individuals' awareness

RESEARCH IT

Research a news story that involved an individual being abused or harmed online.

- What type of abuse happened?
- What could have been done to make this individual aware of the risks? Why?

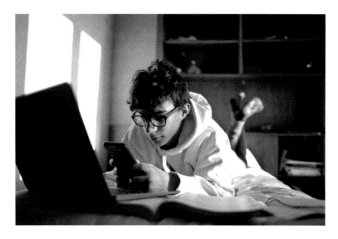

▲ Figure 5.6 What can you do to promote online safety?

AC2.9 Ways of working that keep both the worker and the individual safe

To keep yourself and the individual safe, you need to work in person-centred ways that keep their safety and well-being at the centre of your work and that follow safe and legal work practices.

You may find it useful to review your previous learning around person/child-centred practice in safeguarding (AC2.4), working in ways that uphold individuals' rights (AC2.5) and ways to make individuals aware of how to keep themselves safe (AC2.7).

Below are some additional examples of working that promote the safety of both the worker and the individual. Can you think of any others?

- **Stay up to date** – you can achieve this by attending training in your work setting, reading about good working practices and learning from more experienced colleagues at work. In this way you can ensure that your work practices are meeting legal requirements. Not doing so may mean that you are placing yourself and individuals unnecessarily in danger.
- **Learn new skills** – online safety is an important area that both you and individuals need to be aware of. Learning new IT skills and improving your knowledge of online safety will help you to support and advise individuals how to stay safe when carrying out online activities and keeping personal information secure, as online processes can change very rapidly.
- **Follow policies and procedures** – your employer's safeguarding policies and procedures are based on laws and regulations, so complying with these will keep both you and the individual safe. This may be in relation to health and safety, infection control and/or safeguarding work practices. Not doing so will mean that you are practising unlawfully and unsafely; thus placing your career at risk as well as the safety and well-being of individuals.

Now read the case study below that focuses on an individual's well-being, and consider how safe ways of working could be promoted.

CASE STUDY

Personal safety

Alan's mental health has recently deteriorated: his mother, who he was living with, has died, and he has lost his job after being **furloughed** during the **COVID-19 pandemic**. Alan feels very isolated living on his own in his two-bedroom flat, and has been thinking about getting a lodger. He thinks this will help with paying the bills, and also provide some company at home so he will not feel alone.

Alan has never had a lodger living with him before and does not know how to go about this. He asks you for some advice.

Discussion points:

- What advice would you give Alan in relation to his mental health? Why?
- What advice would you give Alan in relation to having a lodger? Why?
- How would you ensure that the advice you gave to Alan complied with safe ways of working?
- How would you support Alan to make his own decisions and keep himself safe?

KEY TERMS

Furloughed: when employers tell their staff not to come into work for a fixed period of time because there is not sufficient work for them to do.

COVID-19 pandemic: also known as the coronavirus disease pandemic. It is caused by a virus that was first identified in 2019 and spread globally around the world.

Check your understanding

1 What does the term 'advocacy' mean in relation to safeguarding?

2 State why it is important to establish relationships that support trust and rapport with individuals.

3 Describe one way to make individuals aware of how to keep themselves safe online.

4 Name two ways of making individuals aware of the risks of using the internet.

Question practice

1 Person/child-centred practice in safeguarding is important because it:

  a enables workers to make choices and decisions

  b supports individuals to understand their rights

  c allows workers to work with individuals only

  d does not take into account individuals' needs and preferences

2 Which of the following ways of working will keep both the worker and the individual safe?

  a attending safeguarding training

  b not keeping IT skills up to date

  c not complying with the employer's safeguarding procedures

  d complying with some safeguarding work practices

LO3 UNDERSTAND THE FACTORS, SITUATIONS AND ACTIONS THAT COULD LEAD OR CONTRIBUTE TO HARM, ABUSE OR NEGLECT

GETTING STARTED

Think about a work setting such as a residential care home or hospital that you've heard or read about that failed to protect individuals from harm, abuse or neglect.

- How long did the abuse, harm or neglect go on for?
- Why was it not reported earlier?
- Why do you think these individuals were not protected?

AC3.1 Why some individuals could be more at risk from harm, abuse or neglect

You have already learnt about different ways of working that can safeguard individuals from harm, abuse and neglect, including the safeguarding requirements set out in part 7 of the Social Services and Well-being (Wales) Act 2014. It is also important to know about what makes some individuals more at risk from being harmed, abused or neglected so that you can be extra vigilant. For example:

- **Individuals who require care or support from others** will be dependent on others to have their physical, emotional and social needs met, and therefore less likely to report the abuser because they may fear they will lose their care or support or that the abuser may lose their job.

- **Individuals who have high care or support needs** may be more at risk from abuse, harm or neglect, because meeting their needs may place significantly more demands and strain on workers, which can lead to abuse occurring.

- **Individuals who have specific communication difficulties** because of a disability such as a learning disability or an illness such as a stroke may find it difficult to communicate that abuse is happening, and therefore be more at risk from harm, abuse or neglect.

- **Individuals who have specific conditions such as dementia** may have memory and speech difficulties associated with their condition, and therefore may not be able to communicate and/or recall that abuse has taken place. This makes them more vulnerable to abuse.

- **Individuals who are frail** because of age may have poor mobility, and will be less likely to defend themselves or get away from an abuser who may be physically stronger than they are.
- **Individuals who experience anxiety or depression** may also experience a loss in confidence and low **self-esteem**. They are therefore more at risk of being abused because they will be less likely to challenge abuse.
- **Individuals with mental ill-health** may have experienced **hallucinations** and false beliefs as part of their illness. They could be targeted by an abuser because they will be less likely to be believed by others if they report abuse.
- **Individuals with a history of substance misuse** such as alcohol and/or drugs may be more at risk because they may be taken advantage of by an abuser while they are misusing substances.
- **Individuals with a history of violent behaviour** because of a condition such as dementia or as a result of substance misuse may be at risk from abuse, as they may become violent towards workers and may make it difficult to provide care or support.

Children and young people may be at risk from abuse, for example:

- they may be more likely to be exploited if they are living in a household where abuse takes place
- if they are living away from home such as in residential care, or
- if they are homeless.

Other factors that may make children and young people more vulnerable could include having friends and families involved in criminality, experiencing a bereavement or having low self-esteem.

KEY TERM

Hallucinations: a person experiencing something that isn't really there but feels real to the person. Hallucinations could be visual and involve seeing something such as a fire, or auditory and involve hearing something that isn't really there, such as a voice.

REFLECT ON IT

Reflect on an individual who you know about and has care or support needs.

- How do you know about them?
- Where do they live?
- Why might they be more at risk from harm, abuse or neglect?

AC3.2 Why abuse may not be disclosed by adults, children and young people, family, friends, workers and volunteers

You will probably have heard about tragic situations where abuse happened over many years without being reported, and you may have wondered why and how this could have happened.

It takes courage to disclose abuse, and for this reason disclosures of abuse may not be made. Understanding why abuse may not be disclosed by different parties will give you a better insight into how abuse can continue to happen:

- **Adults** – might not disclose because they do not realise that what is happening to them is abuse. Refer back to AC3.1 for reasons why some individuals may be more at risk from abuse. It may also be difficult for adults to disclose abuse if the abuser is someone they like or have known for many years, because they may feel that they have a duty to protect this person and say nothing. Adults may also be anxious about what will happen to them and to their abuser if they disclose abuse – will they lose their care/support, and will the abuser be prosecuted?
- **Children and young people** – may be afraid of their abuser, who might have threatened them or their family if they do tell anyone about the abuse. Children and young people may also worry that they will not be believed, particularly when their abuser is in a position of responsibility such as a worker providing care or support. They may also worry about what will happen to them if they

disclose abuse – will they be blamed for what has happened?

- **Family and friends** – may worry about the repercussions for their relative's care or support if the abuser is a worker. If the abuser is a family member or a close friend of the family, they may worry that disclosing abuse will be an act of betrayal and be pressurised by the abuser and also by other family and friends. A family member or friend may be reluctant to disclose abuse as they may worry about how this will be dealt with and perceived by others.
- **Workers and volunteers** – when the abuser is another worker or volunteer, they may find it difficult to accept that someone they work with could be capable of abuse, or they may worry that their concerns are incorrect and could result in a work colleague losing their job. Similarly, a worker or volunteer may find it difficult to disclose that abuse is happening when the abuser is in a more senior position; they may worry that they will not be believed or that doing so may have repercussions for their job.

CASE STUDY

Living at home

Amira is 70 years old, has osteoarthritis (a condition that causes pain, stiffness and inflammation in joints such as in the hands, feet, knees and hips), and needs support when walking and doing everyday activities such as washing, dressing, eating and drinking. Amira lives at home with her son who works part-time and cares for her.

Amira speaks to her daughter, who lives abroad, every day on the telephone and has told her several times that she is unhappy living at home because she's not being looked after properly. Amira's daughter is very worried about her mother, but whenever she suggests discussing how Amira feels together as a family, Amira refuses and asks her not to say anything.

Discussion points:

- Why may Amira be at risk of harm, abuse or neglect?
- Why may Amira not want to discuss what is happening?
- If you were Amira's daughter, what would you do?

AC3.3 Actions, behaviours or situations that increase the risk of harm or abuse

Being aware of the actions, behaviours and situations that can also contribute to harm and abuse happening will make you more alert at recognising when these can present risks to individuals' well-being. Some examples of these actions, behaviours and situations are detailed below, including how they can increase the risk of harm or abuse.

Asylum seeking

For the year ending June 2020, the UK Government's statistics indicate that:

- 32,423 applications for asylum were made in the previous 12 months.
- 2,868 applications were made by unaccompanied children.
- The top five countries of origin of people seeking asylum were Iran, Albania, Iraq, Eritrea and Pakistan.
- 3,000 people seeking asylum are in receipt of support in Wales (1,503 in Cardiff, 863 in Swansea, 467 in Newport, 141 in Wrexham).

(www.gov.uk, *Immigration statistics, year ending June 2020*, second edition)

KEY TERM

Asylum seeker: a person who escapes from their home country because of fear or danger and seeks refuge and safety in another country.

Asylum seekers are at risk of harm or abuse because they are not allowed to work and are provided with just over £5 per day by the UK Government to live on.

This means that they may be more likely to end up homeless and unable to support themselves. They are vulnerable to exploitation by others who tempt them with offers of work, good pay and accommodation, but end up giving them harsh conditions to work and live in, and in some cases treating them like slaves.

In addition, people seeking asylum and waiting to have their claims processed can experience abuse from others. For example, in Penally, West Wales there is a camp where people seeking asylum live. Protesters who object to it being there have gathered outside and shouted abuse – they do not want the camp there as they believe that the people living there pose a danger to their community.

Criminalisation

People who receive prison sentences after being convicted of illegal activities can be harmed or abused by others in prison.

Criminalisation may also result in these people being excluded from their families and/or communities because of the crimes. Feelings of rejection and not being wanted can increase the risk of self-harm and/or may lead to these people becoming a member of a gang where they feel they belong.

Having a history of offending and a criminal record may also make it difficult to find employment. This increases the risk of people of being homeless and not being able to support themselves, which again can make them more vulnerable to being harmed or abused by others.

Different types of bullying

There are many different types of bullying that can be experienced by individuals that can increase the risk of harm or abuse. For example:

- physical bullying, such as hitting or pushing
- verbal bullying, such as name calling and intimidation
- **social bullying**, such as spreading rumours about an individual and encouraging others to exclude an individual
- **cyber bullying**, such as hurtful texts and pretending to be the individual online.

All these different types of bullying are deliberately aimed at causing harm and humiliation to individuals. They can have both short-term and long-term detrimental effects.

KEY TERMS

Social bullying: bullying carried out without the individual knowing, designed to harm the individual's reputation.

Cyber bullying: bullying carried out through computers, phones and other electronic devices.

Domestic abuse

Read ACs 1.2 and 1.3 for information about this type of abuse.

The risk of harm or abuse is increased because individuals will have become both physically and emotionally isolated from others who know them. They may feel they are unable to leave their domestic situation.

Female genital mutilation

Read AC1.2 for information about FGM.

It is very difficult for girls and women experiencing this abuse to recognise it as abuse, as it may be part of their culture and beliefs.

In addition, as this practice involves physically harming girls and women, individuals will experience severe pain, and some even suffer from excessive bleeding which can result in death.

This will also have an emotional impact on individuals. This could cause them to become withdrawn and anxious, and develop depression.

Forced marriages

Forced marriages are those where either one or both people involved don't consent to the marriage. Forced marriage is usually due to cultural or religious beliefs so the individual is brought up to believe that this is what should happen.

People in forced marriages could be at increased risk of harm or abuse. It is possible that they were forced into the marriage through either emotional abuse, by their family making them feel they will bring shame to the family if they don't agree, or financial abuse, with their family threatening to disown them or take away financial support.

Hate crime

Read AC1.2 for information about hate crime.

Hate crime leads to individuals being targeted by others because of their differences, such as a disability or their sexual orientation, and being physically or emotionally harmed and abused.

Homelessness

Being homeless makes individuals vulnerable and more likely to be harmed or abused by others, because not having somewhere to live will mean individuals live in unsafe environments such as on the streets.

Homelessness will also mean that individuals have to depend on others to help them survive. They might meet dishonest people who engage them in illegal activities that they may feel that they have no choice but to do.

Homelessness can also lead to individuals feeling unworthy and having low self-esteem. This could lead to individuals self-harming or misusing substances.

Human trafficking/modern slavery

Victims of human trafficking and modern slavery are commonly trafficked from outside the UK, but there are some that also live in the UK and are targeted.

These individuals' vulnerability – such as having fled a war-torn country, becoming unemployed and subsequently homeless, or due to having a learning disability – makes them more likely to be exploited by being falsely promised work, money, a home and education.

The impact on these individuals can be detrimental to their lives.

Learning disability

Individuals who have a learning disability may be more likely to be harmed or abused, because their disability may mean that they may not understand what abuse is and/or that they are being abused.

Individuals with a learning disability may also be targeted by those who falsely claim to be their friend but in fact end up being their abuser.

Mental ill-health

Individuals who experience mental ill-health may be at great risk of harm or abuse because their condition might cause them to be physically or verbally abusive towards others. This can lead to people ignoring, neglecting or abusing them.

Individuals with mental ill-health can also experience depression. They may become withdrawn and unable to care for themselves or say when they need support from others, which could lead to self-neglect and also neglect by others.

Radicalisation

Radicalisation is a process by which people start to believe and support extremist ideologies and terrorism.

People that have been radicalised will be encouraged to carry out violence and acts of terrorism, and may therefore be harmed themselves when doing so.

People that have been radicalised are at risk of emotional abuse by those who want to lure them into terrorism because their vulnerability will be exploited – for example, due to being rejected or excluded by their family and friends, or because they have experienced a trauma in their lives.

Self-neglect

Read ACs 1.2 and 1.3 for information about this type of abuse.

The risk of harm or abuse is increased when individuals have low self-esteem and have become withdrawn. They are more likely to be targeted by people who want to harm or abuse them.

Sexual exploitation

Sexual exploitation is a form of sexual abuse (read ACs 1.2 and 1.3 for information about this type of abuse). This occurs when an individual is exploited for sexual purposes in exchange for affection, gifts or money.

Sexual exploitation can increase the risk of harm or abuse, because the individual is being manipulated and falsely led to believe that this is all part of being in a loving relationship.

As a result, the individual may not realise that this is a form of abuse, and may also feel ashamed about their behaviour.

Substance misuse

Misuse of substances can lead to mental ill-health, physical and emotional difficulties.

Individuals may experience anxiety and depression. This puts them at risk of self-neglect and neglect by others, if their misuse of substances leads to illegal activities and criminalisation.

Exploitation of individuals may also occur because they will have to obtain money and substances. As a result, they may be forced to carry out illegal activities or they may be sexually exploited.

CASE STUDY

At risk of abuse

Read the following three scenarios. Discuss the factors that may make these individuals at more risk of abuse.

1　Rhoswen has lost their job and is now homeless. This is making Rhoswen feel very anxious.
2　Mackenzie has a criminal record and is moving to a new area to live.
3　George has a learning disability and has experienced cyber bullying.

AC3.4 Features of perpetrator behaviour and grooming

Knowing about some of the features of perpetrator behaviour and grooming is important, as it can help you to recognise when individuals are being manipulated and groomed so that they become isolated, dependent and therefore vulnerable to being harmed and abused. This is very important, particularly as you will have learnt that some individuals may not have the capacity to understand that they are being groomed or be too afraid to tell anyone as a result of their personal situation. Children and adults are therefore vulnerable to grooming.

Some of the features of perpetrator behaviour and grooming children can include:

- forming a relationship with a child and making the child feel 'special', or taking an extra interest in them by giving them expensive gifts and taking photographs of them together to gain their trust
- encouraging the child to keep their communications/meetings a secret to exploit the child and prolong the abuse
- telling sexualised jokes or stories to see how the child responds
- touching the child, at first through hugs and then through inappropriate touching such as kissing to see how the child responds

- intimidating the child by threatening them or their family if the child tells anyone about the abuse, to instil fear and to avoid being reported.

Some of the features of perpetrator behaviour and grooming adults can include:

- preventing the individual from seeing their family and friends so that they become isolated and dependent on them
- encouraging the individual to spend all their time with them, so that the individual gives up their education or job
- making the individual believe that the perpetrator is their friend or partner, although the individual does not really know anything about them
- giving the individual gifts, such as expensive jewellery or items of clothing, that the individual would not usually buy for themselves
- placing pressure on the individual to hand over money or carry out sexual acts. This may result in the individual being worried about having sufficient funds to pay for day-to-day items, or becoming unusually withdrawn or angry.

AC3.5 The value of learning from reviews and reports into serious failures to protect individuals from harm, abuse or neglect

Everyone has a responsibility to safeguard and protect individuals from harm, abuse or neglect. Sometimes, however, serious failures to safeguard individuals occur. For example, in 2016 an adult care home manager, Mr Ashley Bowen, who managed the St James Care Home in Swansea, failed in his duty to protect the individuals of the care home from harm, abuse and neglect by allowing them to be ill-treated and abused. The abuse experienced by the individuals included:

- sleeping in cold, damp bedrooms
- having no blinds in their bedrooms to enable privacy
- living in a poorly maintained home which had trip hazards
- not being allowed to go outdoors or leave the care home.

After a serious failure to protect individuals has occurred, the local and regional safeguarding boards undertake an Adult Practice Review (APR) or Child Practice Review (CPR) that considers if harm, abuse or neglect could have been predicted or prevented from taking place. Once completed, a report into its findings is published so that services can be improved and that situation is prevented from happening again.

Between 1 April 2017 and 31 March 2018, there were five CPRs and five APRs in Wales. Some of the suggested improvements included:

- clearer communication and information sharing between different agencies, professionals and families when safeguarding individuals

- more training required on how to identify potential signs and symptoms of abuse in individuals earlier
- improvement of professionals' understanding of safeguarding legislation and guidance
- ensuring that individuals are involved in the safeguarding process, so that their needs are maintained as the focus and not overlooked.

(Public Health Wales, *Learning from Reviews 1 April 2017 to 31 March 2018*)

RESEARCH IT

- Research a report completed and published for an APR or CPR undertaken in Wales.
- Produce a leaflet that describes the value of learning from this report and improving services.

Check your understanding

1 Name two features of perpetrator behaviour and grooming.

2 Why are reviews and reports into serious failures to protect individuals from abuse important?

Question practice

1 Which of the following statements is FALSE?

Abuse is sometimes not disclosed by children and young people because:

a they think they will not be believed

b they think they will not be blamed

c they may be afraid of their abuser

d they may worry about their family

2 Which of the following statements is TRUE:

The risk of harm or abuse:

a only asylum seekers are at risk of abuse

b does not increase if you are homeless

c increases if you misuse substances

d only if you experience mental ill-health are you at risk of abuse

LO4 UNDERSTAND HOW TO RESPOND, RECORD AND REPORT CONCERNS, DISCLOSURES OR ALLEGATIONS RELATED TO SAFEGUARDING

AC4.1 Approaches used to respond to suspected, disclosed or alleged harm, abuse or neglect

Recognising the main types of harm, abuse and neglect and their associated signs is essential for safeguarding individuals and promoting their well-being. Responding straight away and in line with your employer's agreed ways of working when abuse is **suspected**, disclosed or **alleged** is also very important for ensuring that individuals are kept safe and protected from being harmed, abused or neglected.

Responding to suspected harm, abuse or neglect

Below are some examples of approaches that can be used to respond to suspicions of harm, abuse or neglect:

● **Trust your instincts** – if you have suspicions that abuse may be happening, trust your instincts and act on them. Don't ignore what you suspect, or the suspicions someone else has and has told you about.
● **Raise your concerns** – don't worry about being incorrect, particularly if the alleged perpetrator is a colleague or in a position of authority such as your manager. It is better you raise your suspicions so that they can be looked into, and in this way the individual can be protected.
● **Support the individual** – reassuring the individual that they are not to blame and explaining that you will do everything you can to help and protect them is also very important. This could involve ensuring

individuals have access to independent support during the safeguarding process when they require it, such as an advocate. If you notice the individual is bleeding or is in pain, support the individual by asking them if they would like any treatment. If the injury is of a more serious nature, this must be reported and medical help accessed immediately.

Responding to disclosed or alleged harm, abuse or neglect

Below are some approaches that can be used to respond to disclosures or allegations of harm, abuse or neglect:

● **Take the disclosure or allegation seriously** – if an individual discloses or alleges abuse, show that you believe what an individual is saying by reassuring them that they have done the right thing by telling you. An individual will be more likely to trust you with sensitive information if they feel you believe them and understand how they are feeling.
● **Actively listen** – you can also show the individual you are taking what they are telling you seriously by **actively listening** to what they are saying – by looking interested, not looking shocked, and not rushing them.
● **Do not question the individual** – let the individual speak and do not interrupt them so that they can say what they want to. Remember not to ask the individual too many questions, as it is not your job to question them.

REFLECT ON IT

Responses to suspected, disclosed or alleged harm, abuse or neglect should be calm and constructive. It is also important that any information you give to individuals, in response to their questions about what will happen next, is honest. This will maintain trust and confidence in your working relationship with the individual and the safeguarding process.

- What skills do you have that would help you to do this?

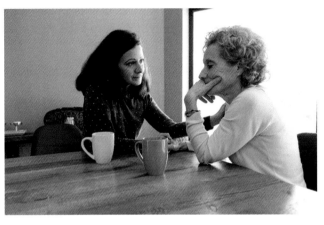

▲ Figure 5.7 Can you recognise if an individual is being harmed, abused or neglected?

AC4.2 Actions to take if harm, abuse or neglect is suspected, disclosed or alleged

AC4.3 Actions to avoid if harm, abuse or neglect is suspected, disclosed or alleged, taking account of any future investigations that may take place

Responding to harm, abuse or neglect must always be followed through with taking action. Table 5.8 provides tips on actions to take and to avoid if harm, abuse or neglect is suspected, disclosed or alleged. Remember that every work setting will have their own agreed procedures to follow, so always check that you know what these are.

Do	Don't
Follow your employer's safeguarding procedures to protect the individual and prevent the harm, abuse or neglect from continuing.	Don't delay in raising your concerns immediately. Delay might prolong an individual's distress and pain.
Ensure the individual is safe and receives medical help as soon as possible, to prevent them from further harm or abuse, or to prevent their condition from deteriorating.	Don't approach or challenge the perpetrator of the harm, abuse or neglect. You may place the individual at further risk of abuse.
Preserve all evidence related to a suspicion or allegation of abuse so that an investigation into what happened can take place. This evidence may support suspicions and allegations so that the person carrying out the abuse can be prosecuted and brought to justice.	Do not move, wash or touch any items that have been used in the abuse so that they can be preserved as evidence of abuse.
Discuss your concerns with the named person in your work setting. This may be your manager or a designated person that safeguarding concerns are reported to, so that action can be taken as soon as possible.	Don't rush when recording your concerns; you might record inaccurate or incomplete information that will jeopardise any future investigations that take place, and therefore fail to protect the individual from further harm, abuse or neglect.
Follow the advice or guidance given by the person you report your concerns to, because they will be experienced in this area and will ensure that you are following your employer's procedures.	Don't report or record your concerns in a public area where others may hear or see, so that the individual's privacy and dignity can be upheld.
Record your concerns fully and accurately so that there is a permanent record. This record shows the actions you have taken, and will be useful if at a later stage there is an investigation into what happened and improvements to services that could be made.	Don't destroy any evidence that there may be of abuse, so that it can be preserved for any future investigations that may take place.

▲ Table 5.8 Actions to take or avoid if harm, abuse or neglect is suspected, disclosed or alleged

CASE STUDY

Responding to abuse

You are a mental health support worker. Cadell, one of the young people you provide support to, tells you that he does not feel comfortable when he's alone with his uncle who visits him at the weekends.

Discussion points:
- What approaches would you use when responding to Cadell? Why?
- What actions would you take? Why?
- What actions would you avoid? Why?

AC4.4 Boundaries of confidentiality in relation to safeguarding and information that must be shared

Confidentiality in relation to safeguarding means keeping safe and private all personal information that is held about individuals, including information in written and spoken form. It is important that all information is protected so that individuals' privacy is respected.

At times you may have to share what you have been told, heard or observed with your manager or an external professional or organisation. In certain situations, this may occur even if an individual, colleague or another person has told you not to do so. These situations include:

- when the individual is being or is at risk of being harmed, abused or neglected
- when female genital mutilation of a girl under the age of 18 has taken place
- when the individual poses a risk of harm to someone else
- when a serious crime has taken place
- when an infectious disease needs to be notified
- to prevent terrorism
- when an allegation of abuse that is not dealt with seriously by the care setting may need to be referred to the police, adult social care services or CQC so that the allegation is reported and acted on

(you will learn more about this process, referred to as whistleblowing, in AC4.5).

In these situations, it is important to explain in confidence to the individual that you need to share this information, to protect them before you do so.

If you are unsure about sharing confidential information, seek advice from your manager or another colleague before sharing the information. For example, this may be necessary when an individual's family asks for some information about the individual's well-being, or an individual does not give their permission to share an allegation of abuse.

AC4.5 The term 'whistleblowing'

Whistleblowing means reporting any unsafe or illegal working practices used in a work setting.

If you believe that there are failures within a work setting that place individuals in danger of abuse, harm or neglect, and that they are not being responded to or taken seriously within the work setting, you can report these practices and your concerns to external organisations such as the independent regulator CIW, **Health Inspectorate Wales (HIW)**, the police or local authority. Your work setting will have a whistleblowing procedure in place.

We looked at whistleblowing in Unit 002, AC1.6, which might be helpful for you to review.

KEY TERM

Health Inspectorate Wales (HIW): reviews and inspects NHS and independent healthcare organisations.

You can report your concerns directly to CIW by telephoning or emailing them. The information you share with them will be treated as confidential, and if you prefer, you do not have to leave your name or contact details.

All whistleblowers receive protection. This means that their employment rights or career will not be affected as a result of them reporting their concerns. Remember too, it is your duty of care to promote individuals' safety, well-being and prevent them from being harmed, abused or neglected.

RESEARCH IT
- Research the CIW website and read their guidance on how to report concerns of harm, abuse or neglect to them.
- Share this information with someone you know.

AC4.6 The importance of reporting any concerns about possible harm, abuse or neglect and the duty that everyone has to do this

Reporting any concerns about possible harm, abuse or neglect is important because it:

- prevents individuals from continuing to be harmed, abused or neglected
- upholds individuals' rights to live safely, free from harm, abuse or neglect
- promotes individuals' well-being
- shows individuals that you will not tolerate any type of harm, abuse or neglect
- instils trust and confidence in the safeguarding process.

As you have read in ACs 1.4 and 1.5 earlier on in this unit, all workers are legally required to have a duty of care towards the individuals they support and care for. Similarly, everyone has a duty to report any concerns about possible harm or abuse or neglect, because doing so means that you are:

- acting in the best interests of individuals and therefore making sure that they are kept safe and free from harm, abuse or neglect
- taking action to prevent further harm, abuse or neglect of individuals
- promoting individuals' well-being by supporting their rights to live with dignity and in safety, free from harm, abuse or neglect.

AC4.7 Potential barriers to reporting or raising concerns

Reporting or raising concerns takes courage and can be difficult to do for different reasons. For example, a worker may have experienced harm, abuse or neglect themselves; they might find it difficult to discuss abuse and so may ignore the possible signs that it is happening. Remember that:

- support is always available if this is the case
- taking care of yourself is important.

Sometimes, reporting or raising concerns may be difficult where the alleged perpetrator is a friend, an experienced work colleague or a supportive manager:

- You might feel conflicted between your legal duty to protect the individual and your moral duty to stand by your friend, work colleague or manager.
- In addition, you might find it very difficult to accept that someone you know would be capable of causing harm to others, and may convince yourself that they are mistaken.
- Fear of making a mistake and of upsetting others at work may mean that concerns are not reported.

Having a clear safeguarding procedure that sets out how to report or raise concerns is important. Not having a procedure in place can be a barrier to reporting or raising concerns, which could place individuals at risk of further danger or harm.

You may also find it useful to read AC3.2 in this unit that contains additional information about why abuse may not be disclosed by adults, children and young people, family, friends, workers and volunteers.

AC4.8 Actions to be taken where there are ongoing concerns about harm, abuse or neglect, or where concerns have not been addressed after reporting

It is part of your duty of care towards individuals to make sure that your concerns about harm, abuse or neglect are fully addressed after reporting them. You should take the following actions if you continue to have ongoing concerns about harm, abuse or neglect:

1 Discuss your concerns with the designated safeguarding person in the work setting. If you believe that your reported concerns have not been

addressed, tell the designated safeguarding person this and ask them to tell you what has been done.

2 If you are still not satisfied after discussing your concerns with the designated safeguarding person, report your concerns to the next level of management in the work setting.

3 If you are still not satisfied after reporting your concerns to the next level of management, contact an outside agency such as CIW, HIW, the police or local authority to report them.

CASE STUDY

Emiliano works in a day care centre providing support to older individuals. Yesterday he noticed that after a family member visited at lunch time, their relative was upset. This individual later disclosed to Emiliano that her sister had shouted at her. Emiliano raised this immediately with his manager who thanked him for doing so. Today Emiliano has noticed that this individual's sister is due to visit again at lunchtime. Emiliano is very worried about this.

Discussion points:
- What actions must be taken by Emiliano? Why?
- Why is it important that Emiliano follows his employer's safeguarding procedure?

AC4.9 Key information that must be reported and recorded, when this should happen and how this information is stored

You will find it useful to review your learning from AC1.6 in relation to how concerns or incidents should be recorded and reported.

Key information that must be recorded and reported and when this should happen

1 Record and report what you have been told, using the person's exact words or exactly what you observed. This will help to preserve the evidence and ensure a true and accurate record of what happened.

2 Key information to record and report will include:
- your name and details
- your signature
- the date and time
- who you are and how you are related to the individual (such as a care worker)
- the actions you have taken
- whether you've shared your concern, and if so with whom and when
- whether your concern has been responded to, and if so when
- details about your concern (avoid using abbreviations), including who your concern is about, why you are concerned, and how this has affected you and others.

3 Record and report information at the earliest opportunity so that you do not forget what you've been told or observed. This will also be important if there is a future investigation and you need to make a statement to the police or court.

CASE STUDY

Reporting and recording key information

You are an experienced residential care worker and your manager has asked you to develop a good practice guide for new members of staff when reporting and recording safeguarding concerns or incidents.

Discussion points:
- What key information must be reported and why?
- What key information must be recorded and why?
- What are the consequences of not reporting and recording this key information?

How key information is stored

All work settings have procedures in place for storing key information, both manually and electronically. It is important that you know these procedures so that your work practices are correct and comply with your employer's procedures and legislation.

Secure systems for storing key information must be in place, to prevent access for unauthorised people and to uphold individuals' rights to privacy of information.

See Unit 005, AC4.3 for guidance on keeping paper-based and electronic files safe.

AC4.10 The process used to record written information with accuracy, clarity, relevance and an appropriate level of detail

See also Unit 005, AC4.5 for guidance on recording information.

All records that are accessed and completed at work are legal documents. Because written information may be referred to in the future and accessed by others who provide care or support to individuals, it is important that they are written accurately, clearly and contain information that is relevant and includes an appropriate level of detail.

Your employer's procedures will set out the process to follow when recording written information. Here are some tips:

- **Accuracy** – record written information accurately by completing your written record as soon as possible. For example, if you observe an individual being harmed, record this information as soon as possible after you've observed it, as you will be less likely to forget what you have observed. Information recorded about a safeguarding concern must be based on what you have seen or observed (fact) and not on what you think (opinion) or feel (judgement) has happened.
- **Clarity** – record written information with clarity, by using legible handwriting which can be read easily by others and permanent ink that cannot be erased or altered. Information must also be written using the correct spelling and grammar so that it can be easily understood by others.
- **Relevance** – only include the necessary details and required information in your record. The information should only relate to the individual, so it is clear who the record is about.

- **Appropriate level of detail** – only record the necessary and important details. You will find AC4.9 in this unit useful for the key information that must be recorded. Your record must include the date, time and your signature, so that it is clear that you wrote this record and to prevent anyone else adding to it or amending it at a later stage.

AC4.11 The differences between fact, opinion and judgement and why understanding this is important when recording and reporting information.

You can refer back to Unit 005, AC4.7 and AC4.8 for more information on the differences between fact, opinion and judgement.

As you will have learnt, safeguarding records and reports are legal documents. It is important therefore that all records and reports provide a true picture of what really happened, as not doing so may mean that the individual is not protected from harm, abuse or neglect or that their condition worsens. Not recording and reporting the facts can also mean that you risk putting your own job and career at risk.

- Factual information refers to what has actually happened.
- Information based on opinion refers to what you think has happened.
- Information based on judgement refers to what you feel has happened, your gut instinct.

It is very important to understand the differences between these so that the correct decisions can be made and the necessary actions taken. For example:

- Recording that an individual told you that he was worried about his money being taken, by using the individual's exact words, when and where he told you, is a **fact**. This would lead to further action being taken when you reported this to your manager.

277

- Recording and reporting that the individual was worried about his money is not factual – it is your **opinion**. This could mean that no further action is taken.
- Recording and reporting that you feel that the individual does not have sufficient money is not factual – it is your **judgement**, and may not lead to further actions being taken.

Remember to be aware of what you record and report and how you do it.

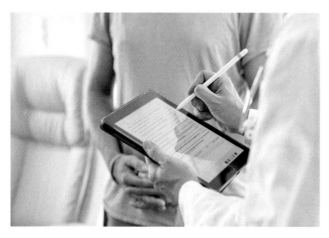

▲ Figure 5.8 Do you know your responsibilities when recording and reporting safeguarding information?

Check your understanding

1 Describe two actions to take if abuse is suspected, disclosed or alleged.
2 Describe in one sentence what whistleblowing means.
3 Name two barriers to reporting or raising concerns about abuse.

Question practice

1 If harm, abuse or neglect is suspected, disclosed or alleged, you must not:
   a follow your employer's safeguarding procedures
   b ensure the individual is safe
   c record your concerns fully
   d delay in raising your concerns

2 The actions that can be taken when there are ongoing concerns about harm, abuse or neglect are:
   a Discuss your concerns again with the designated person only.
   b Report your concerns to the next level of management only.
   c Contact an outside agency such as CIW only.
   d All of the above.

FURTHER READING AND RESEARCH

Books and booklets

Age UK, Cymru (2020), *Safeguarding older people in Wales from abuse and neglect*.

NHS Wales (2008, as amended 2016), *Code of Conduct for Healthcare Support Workers in Wales*.

NHS Wales (2008, as amended 2016), *Code of Practice for NHS Wales Employers*.

Social Care Wales (2017), *Code of Professional Practice for Social Care*.

Social Care Wales (2019), *The residential child care worker: Practice guidance for residential child care workers registered with Social Care Wales*.

Welsh Government (2017), *Guide to Consent for Examination or Treatment*.

Weblinks

Age UK, Cymru's website for information for older people in Wales including factsheets and guides on health and well-being:
www.ageuk.org.uk/cymru/

Bullying UK's website for information, guidance and factsheets about different types of bullying:
www.bullying.co.uk

CIW website for information about the quality and safety of services for the well-being of the people of Wales:
www.careinspectorate.wales

The Welsh Government's website for information about current and relevant legislation for safeguarding children, young people and adults:
https://gov.wales/safeguarding-guidance

The National Crime Agency's website for information and statistics about human trafficking and modern slavery:
www.nationalcrimeagency.gov.uk

NSPCC's website for information about different types of abuse:
www.nspcc.org.uk

NHS Wales' website for information about the Code of Conduct for Healthcare Support Workers in Wales, and the Code of Practice for NHS Wales Employers:
www.wales.nhs.uk

Welsh Refugee Council's website for information and articles about people seeking asylum in the UK:
www.wrc.wales

HEALTH AND SAFETY IN HEALTH AND SOCIAL CARE

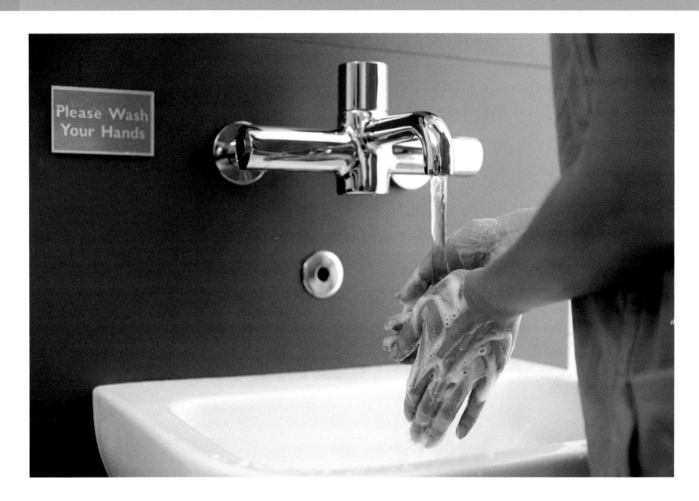

ABOUT THIS UNIT

Guided learning hours: 30

Health and safety is everyone's responsibility in health and social care. In this unit you will explore how health and safety, infection prevention and control, fire safety and food safety legislation influence employers', workers' and other people's roles and responsibilities in the workplace.

You will learn about the use of risk assessment in relation to health and safety, as well as how to promote fire safety and safe moving and handling practices. This unit will also equip you with knowledge of good practices to follow in relation to infection prevention and control, food safety, handling hazardous substances, maintaining security and managing stress in the workplace.

Learning outcomes

LO1: Know how to meet legislative requirements for health and safety in the workplace

LO2: Know how risk assessments are used to support health and safety in the workplace

LO3: Know how to promote fire safety in work settings

LO4: Know the key principles of moving and handling and moving and positioning

LO5: Know the main routes of infection and how to prevent the spread of infections in the workplace

LO6: Know how to implement food safety measures

LO7: Know how to store, use and dispose of hazardous substances safely

LO8: Know how to maintain security in the work setting

LO9: Know how to manage stress

LO1 KNOW HOW TO MEET LEGISLATIVE REQUIREMENTS FOR HEALTH AND SAFETY IN THE WORKPLACE

GETTING STARTED

Think about the meaning of the term 'health and safety', and how this relates to you, your family and friends.

- How do you maintain your own health?
- How do you keep others you know safe?
- Why is this important? What are the consequences of not doing so?

AC1.1 Key relevant legislation that relates to health and safety in the workplace and what this means in practice

Why health and safety legislation is important

Care and support are provided across a range of health and social care settings that can include day care facilities, residential homes for adults and children, supported living facilities where 24-hour care is provided, individuals' own homes and foster care. These health and social care settings are environments where accidents, injuries and illnesses can occur, as the statistics below from the **Health and Safety Executive (HSE)** show. In 2019/2020:

- 1.6 million workers were suffering from work-related ill-health (new or longstanding).
- 828,000 workers were suffering from work-related stress, depression or anxiety (new or longstanding).
- 480,000 workers were suffering from work-related **musculoskeletal disorders** (new or longstanding).
- Most common **accident** types reported by employers included: slips, trips or falls on same level (29 per cent), handling, lifting or carrying (19 per cent), struck by moving object (11 per cent), acts of violence (9 per cent) and falls from a height (8 per cent).

(HSE, November 2020, *Health and safety at work, Summary statistics for Great Britain 2020*)

KEY TERMS

Health and Safety Executive (HSE): the regulator for workers in England, Scotland and Wales. Its role and responsibilities include enforcing the law, reviewing regulations, producing research and statistics.

Musculoskeletal disorders: injuries, damage or disorders of the joints or other tissues in the upper and lower limbs or the back.

Accidents: unexpected and unintentional events that cause damage or personal injury, such as a fall.

Knowing about the health and safety legislation that exists in the **workplace** and understanding what this means in practice is important for safeguarding individuals, workers and visitors to health and social care settings.

Individuals accessing care and support may be more at risk of having accidents, injuries and illnesses, because they may have health conditions that make them more vulnerable. For example, an individual who has:

● had a **stroke** may have difficulties walking that may result in them tripping
● **vision loss** may be more likely to have a fall
● a respiratory condition such as **COPD (chronic obstructive pulmonary disease)** and contracts coronavirus may become very ill.

Workers may also be more susceptible to having accidents, injuries and illnesses, for example, because their work involves:

● carrying out high risk tasks such as moving and positioning individuals
● providing intimate care or supporting individuals who may be unwell and show **aggressive behaviour**
● supporting children and young people with high risk activities, for example, using play equipment such as climbing frames that may be slippery or damaged, going on walks to the park which may lead to falls, or painting and modelling using materials such as scissors and paint that may pose a risk if not used correctly.

Others, such as individuals' families and friends, who visit health and social care settings may also be at risk of having accidents if, for example, they do not follow the workplace's arrangements for their own personal safety such as only accessing areas of the building they have permission to access and having workers present when children and young people are around.

KEY TERMS

Workplace: a setting in which care and support is provided, such as residential child care, individuals' own homes, foster care.

Stroke: a life-threatening medical condition that occurs when the blood supply to part of the brain is interrupted.

Vision loss: severely or partially impaired vision.

COPD (chronic obstructive pulmonary disease): a group of lung conditions that result in long-term breathing difficulties.

Aggressive behaviour: may range from verbal to physical abuse, threatening behaviour can cause physical or emotional harm to others.

Regulator: an organisation that supervises a particular sector.

Key relevant health and safety legislation

Legislation is in place to ensure that everyone who lives, works in or visits workplaces such as health and social care settings is safeguarded. Table 6.1 below provides you with information about the key and relevant pieces of health and safety legislation that must underpin every employer's agreed ways of working.

Health and safety legislation	What this means in practice
The Health and Safety at Work Act (HASAWA)1974	This key Act forms the basis of all other health and safety regulations and guidelines in the workplace. ● It protects the health and safety of everyone in the workplace. In health and social care settings this includes individuals, workers and visitors such as individuals' families, advocates and other professionals, such as GPs, social workers, contractors. ● It established the HSE as the regulator for the health and safety of people in the workplace in the UK. ● It established the responsibilities of employers and employees for health and safety at work (you will learn more about these in AC1.2).

▲ Table 6.1 Health and safety legislation, and what it means in practice

Health and safety legislation	What this means in practice
The Management of Health and Safety at Work Regulations (MHSWR) 1999	• Employers and managers must assess and manage actual and potential dangers in the workplace by carrying out **risk assessments** (you will learn more about this in LO2). • Employers must provide health and safety information, training and supervision. • Workplaces should appoint competent people to be responsible for managing health and safety. In a health or social care setting this could be the manager. • Workplaces must have procedures in place for **emergency** situations, such as for fire safety (see LO3 for more information) and security (see LO8 for more information).
Workplace (Health, Safety and Welfare) Regulations 1992	Workplaces must be safe and comfortable environments to work in. They must: • not be too hold or cold • avoid having poorly lit areas that may lead to accidents • have well-ventilated areas • have flooring that is safe, not worn and non-slippery • have windows and doors that can be closed securely. These regulations also require: • welfare facilities to be available to all employees – separate areas for employees to eat and drink in, well-lit toilets with hot and cold water, soap, wash basins and hand drying facilities. • workplaces to be maintained – regularly cleaned, spillages removed immediately and waste disposed of safely (see LO5, LO6 and LO7 for more information).
Manual Handling Operations Regulations 1992 (as amended) (MHOR)	These require employers to: • eliminate or minimise risks associated with manual handling activities, such as avoiding lifting heavy equipment where possible and using risk assessments to manage all manual handling tasks safely • provide information, training and supervision about safe manual handling.
Provision and Use of Work Equipment Regulations 1998 (PUWER)	These require employers to ensure that all equipment: • is used safely in the workplace – employees must receive training on how to use it safely including taking precautions • has visible warning signs and that employees understand what these mean.
Lifting Operations and Lifting Equipment Regulations 1998 (LOLER)	These require employers to ensure that: • all lifting equipment used in the workplace is safe to use. For example, maintaining **hoists** as per the manufacturers' instructions. • all those using lifting equipment as part of their work activities have been trained and are competent to do so.
Reporting of Injuries, Diseases and Dangerous Occurrences Regulations 2013	These require employers to: • report and keep records for three years of work-related accidents that cause death and serious injuries (referred to as reportable injuries), diseases and dangerous occurrences (**incidents** with the potential to cause harm) • have procedures for reporting injuries, diseases and incidents • provide information and training on reporting injuries, diseases and incidents.
Personal Protective Equipment (PPE) at Work Regulations 1992	These require employers to: • provide free PPE such as gloves, aprons and face masks for protection against infections (for more information, see AC5.12) • maintain PPE in good condition so that it is effective when being used • provide training in the use of PPE – when, why and how to put it on and dispose of it safely.
COSHH Regulations 2002	These classify hazardous substances (such as cleaning materials) under the following types: very toxic, toxic, harmful, corrosive and irritant (see LO7 for more information). The regulations require employers to: • prevent or control exposure to hazardous substances by carrying out risk assessments and having safe working procedures in place for employees when using them • provide information, training and supervision so that work activities can be carried out safely.

▲ Table 6.1 Health and safety legislation, and what it means in practice *(continued)*

KEY TERMS

Risk assessment: a process used in workplaces for identifying hazards, assessing the level of risk and reducing or controlling the risks identified.

Emergency: a situation that causes immediate danger, such as a first aid emergency.

Hoist: equipment used to support and carry an individual as they are moved from one place or position to another.

Incidents: unexpected events that cause damage to property, such as a broken window.

RESEARCH IT

- Using the www.hse.gov.uk website for up-to-date information on current legislation, research two of the pieces of health and safety legislation you learnt about in Table 6.1.
- Produce a leaflet about these pieces of legislation and include details of why they are important in the workplace.

AC1.2 Responsibilities of employers, the worker and others for health and safety at work

The health and safety legislation you read about in AC1.1 requires every workplace to have in place policies and procedures that set out the health and safety responsibilities for **employers**, **workers** and others such as individuals' families and outside professionals who may visit health and social care settings such as advocates, social workers and nurses.

These policies and procedures should ensure that all work activities are carried out safely and in line with current health and safety legislation. Table 6.2 details how health and safety responsibilities are shared by all three of these groups. Remember that health and safety is everyone's responsibility.

Employers' health and safety responsibilities	Workers' health and safety responsibilities	Other people's health and safety responsibilities
To provide a safe workplace and have health and safety procedures in place: for example, by ensuring that the workplace is cleaned and maintained regularly.	To take reasonable care of their own and others' health and safety: for example, by reporting a spillage on the floor so that it no longer poses a danger.	To follow the employer's health and safety procedures when visiting: for example, by signing the visitors' book when entering and leaving.
To provide a workplace where risks are assessed, minimised or avoided where possible: for example, by completing risk assessments.	To take reasonable care not to put themselves or others at risk: for example, by staying at home if feeling unwell.	To comply with the employer's health and safety risk assessments: for example, by reporting any dangers they notice such as a broken outside door.
To provide information, training and supervision around health and safety: for example, by organising a health and safety training day.	To comply with the employer's health and safety information, training and supervision: for example, by attending the health and safety training day.	To comply with the employer's health and safety information, training and supervision: for example, by washing their hands when entering the building.
To provide welfare facilities: for example, by providing access to clean and well-lit toilets that include hot and cold water, hand washing and hand drying facilities.	To use the welfare facilities provided by the employer: for example, by washing their hands and drying them before and after their work activities.	To use the welfare facilities provided by the employer: for example, by using the visitors' toilet when visiting.
To provide first aid facilities: for example, by ensuring there is a fully stocked first aid box.	To use first aid facilities for the purpose they were intended for: for example, not misusing the contents of the first aid box for a craft activity.	To access the first aid facilities provided by the employer when required: for example, only accessing these with authorisation.
To provide safety signs: for example, when cleaning is in progress to alert workers and others that the floor is wet and therefore slippery.	To understand the meaning of the safety signs used: for example, to respect the safety sign that the floor may be wet by not entering the room.	To comply with the employer's safety signs: for example, not ignoring a safety sign or moving it.

▲ Table 6.2 Health and safety responsibilities

Employers' health and safety responsibilities	Workers' health and safety responsibilities	Other people's health and safety responsibilities
To provide protective clothing free of charge: for example, providing aprons, gloves, face masks.	To use PPE provided by the employer in accordance with training and instructions; for example, using safe practices when putting on and disposing of aprons and gloves.	To use PPE provided by the employer when visiting: for example, wearing a clean face mask and ensuring it is worn over the nose and mouth.
To provide equipment required for carrying out work activities safely: for example, providing a bed lift for an individual that is unable to mobilise independently.	To use the equipment provided by the employer in accordance with training and instructions: for example, ensuring the equipment is clean and in working order before using it.	To report if equipment is not clean or safe to use: for example, following the employer's reporting procedures.
To report accidents and incidents to the HSE: for example, if a worker slips over and injures their back.	To report accidents and incidents to the employer in line with the employer's health and safety procedures: for example, completing the accident book and/or incident form.	To report accidents and incidents witnessed to the employer: for example, reporting a visibly worn carpet on the stairs.

▲ Table 6.2 Health and safety responsibilities *(continued)*

KEY TERMS

Employer: in the case of foster carers or adult placement/shared lives carers, this is the agency. In the case of personal assistants, this is the person employing them to provide care and support.

Worker: the person providing care and support or services to individuals

CASE STUDY

Health and safety responsibilities

Read the following three scenarios and for each one, discuss whose responsibility it is to address the health and safety concerns, i.e. the employer's, the employee's or someone else's.

1. Adain works in a day centre and notices there is a spillage on the bathroom floor.
2. Marie works in a play group and notices one of armchairs in the seating area is broken.
3. Chris works in a care home and notices that the hoist is not working.

AC1.3 The importance of working within the limits of own role and responsibilities

Most health and social care settings will have a job description for workers that details the responsibilities of their work role.

If the employer is the individual that the worker provides care and support to, the individual may provide the worker with written guidance that is included in their job description, or it may be in the form of a personal plan of work that the individual has prepared. In terms of health and safety, this will include workers' health and safety responsibilities and how they must carry these out. Complying with the job description or personal plan of work involves working within the limits of the job role and its responsibilities. This includes only carrying out health and safety responsibilities that have been agreed with the employer.

If the employer employs less than five employees then there is no legal obligation to provide their employees with a written statement, written guidance or a personal plan of work of their general policy with respect to health and safety at work. Verbal information would suffice legally.

Working within the limits of your job role and responsibilities is important for ensuring that you:

- only carry out the responsibilities that you are trained and qualified to do. Not doing so can mean that you carry out work activities in an unsafe way, and place yourself and others at risk – for example, using a hoist when moving an individual from one position to another when you have not been trained to do so may result in you injuring the individual and/or your back.

- are answerable for carrying out your responsibilities (also referred to as being accountable). Not doing so can mean that you take on tasks that are not your responsibility – for example, if you try to fix a broken wheelchair when this is not in your area of expertise, you may place those who use it at risk of being injured by it. Your responsibility would be to report that it is not working to your employer, so that it can be removed and fixed by someone who is trained and qualified to do so.

- carry out your work activities as required by your employer. Not doing so may mean that you cannot show your employer that you are carrying out your responsibilities as expected of you, or that you are doing these to a high standard.

- carry out your duty to ensure the safety of yourself, individuals and others in the health and social care setting you work in. Not doing so can have serious consequences and can mean that you lose your job for not carrying out your health and safety responsibilities – for example, supporting an individual to go for a walk on your own when the procedures state that two people must support the individual may result in you injuring your back, and the individual falling and sustaining a serious head injury.

CASE STUDY

Marie is a support worker employed by an agency to assist Sian, who has a learning disability, with household tasks including cooking, shopping and cleaning.

This afternoon, Marie arrives as usual to assist Sian with making lunch. Marie notices that Sian is not her usual self and looks a little unhappy, and so asks her what's wrong. Sian explains that this morning she was planning on going out with her friend Lucy to the park but didn't because Lucy was feeling unwell, and so feels unhappy about spending all day in the house. Sian tells Marie that she knows she can't take her out because the support she requires hasn't been agreed in her care plan or risk assessment. Marie feels upset for Sian and suggests that she takes her out, as it should be fine providing they don't say anything to anyone.

Discussion points:

- Do you agree with Marie's actions? Why?
- Why is it important for Marie to follow Sian's care plan and risk assessment? What could be the consequences of not doing so?
- What could have Marie done differently in this situation?

AC1.4 The importance of raising concerns about practices or working conditions that are unsafe or risky

Unsafe practices and working conditions

Recognising ways of working or working conditions that are unsafe or risky and knowing about the procedures in place for reporting these is essential for ensuring that you:

- carry out your health and safety responsibilities to the best of your ability
- do not place an individual, worker or others such as visitors in danger or at risk of being injured or harmed.

Figure 6.1 outlines examples of some of these practices that could happen in a health or social care setting.

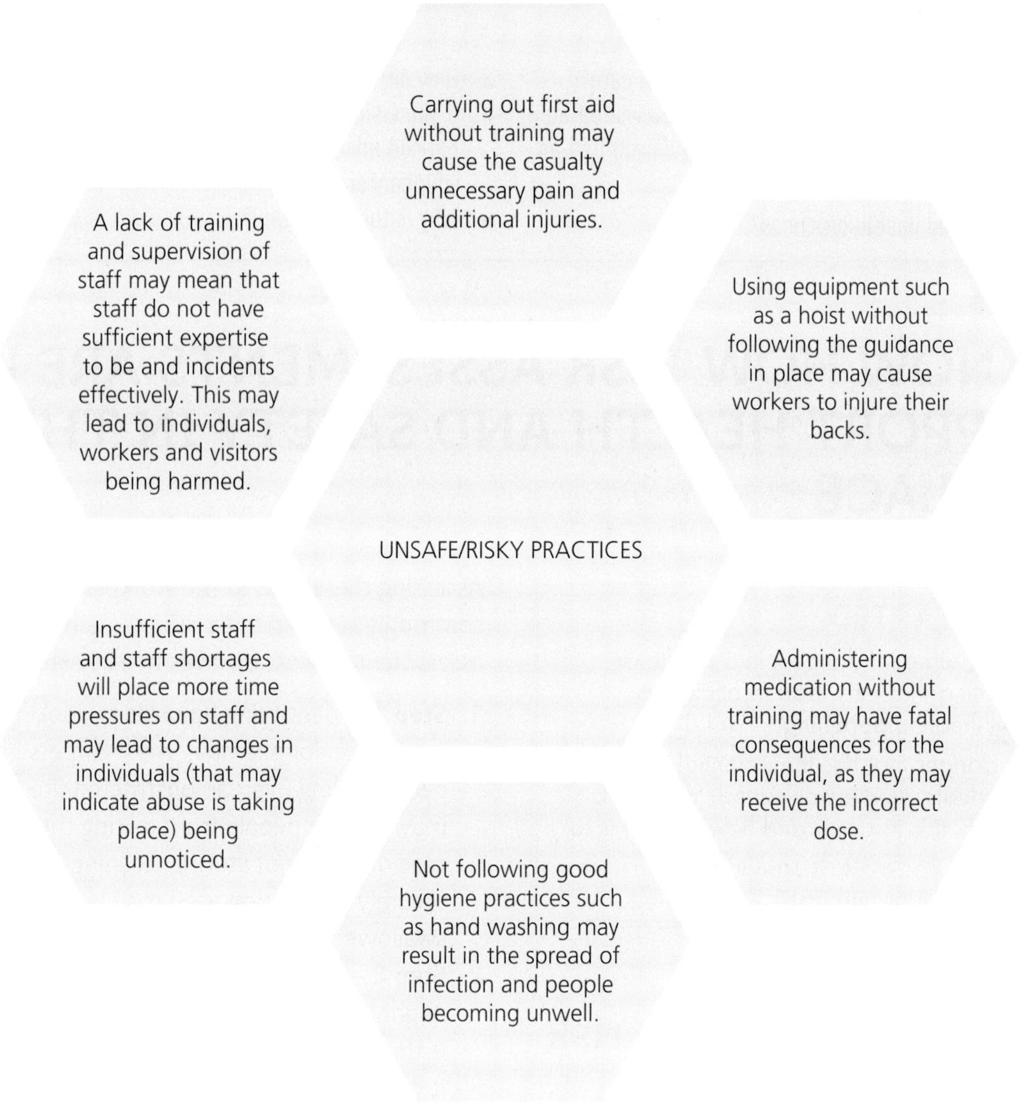

Carrying out first aid without training may cause the casualty unnecessary pain and additional injuries.

A lack of training and supervision of staff may mean that staff do not have sufficient expertise to be and incidents effectively. This may lead to individuals, workers and visitors being harmed.

Using equipment such as a hoist without following the guidance in place may cause workers to injure their backs.

UNSAFE/RISKY PRACTICES

Insufficient staff and staff shortages will place more time pressures on staff and may lead to changes in individuals (that may indicate abuse is taking place) being unnoticed.

Administering medication without training may have fatal consequences for the individual, as they may receive the incorrect dose.

Not following good hygiene practices such as hand washing may result in the spread of infection and people becoming unwell.

▲ Figure 6.1 Unsafe/risky practices and working conditions in health and social care settings

Raising concerns

Raising concerns about unsafe/risky practices or working conditions in health and social care settings by using the employer's procedures is important for:

- maintaining the safety of individuals, workers and others who visit. Not doing so can lead to accidents happening that could have been prevented – for example, not raising concerns about a loose step may result in someone falling over.
- maintaining the well-being of individuals, workers and others who visit. Not doing so can lead to abuse happening – for example, not raising concerns about a worker verbally abusing an individual may lead to the abuse continuing and/or worsening and may place the individual and others at further risk.

- complying with health and safety legislation. Not doing so can lead to unlawful practices continuing – for example, not raising concerns about a heater in an individual's room that is not working may lead to the individual becoming cold.
- complying with the employer's procedures. Not doing so can lead to health and safety responsibilities not being met – for example, not raising concerns about a worker's unsafe practices when handling food may lead to people becoming unwell and could even lead to fatalities.

287

REFLECT ON IT

Reflect on an occasion you visited a health or social care setting. For example, this may have been when you visited an individual in hospital or in their own home or when you had an appointment at the GP's surgery or opticians.

- Did you notice any unsafe practices?

- How did this make you feel?
- If you visited this health or social care setting again and noticed unsafe practices taking place, how could you raise your concerns?
- Why is this important?

LO2 KNOW HOW RISK ASSESSMENTS ARE USED TO SUPPORT HEALTH AND SAFETY IN THE WORKPLACE

GETTING STARTED

Think about the different dangers in a health or social care setting that may lead to accidents, injuries and ill-health happening.

Choose one danger that has the potential to cause harm to individuals, workers or visitors, and think about how likely it is to occur and how likely it is to cause harm.

- Is it low, medium or high risk?
- Why is this?

AC2.1 What is meant by 'risk assessment' in relation to health and safety

In LO1 you learnt about employers, workers and other people's health and safety responsibilities, and how these link to health and safety legislation and policies and procedures in the workplace.

Under the Management of Health and Safety at Work Regulations (MHSWR) 1999, employers are required to reduce and where possible prevent health and safety risks from happening. Similarly, workers and others must also protect themselves and others from any dangers that they see or become aware of.

Assessing these risks in the workplace is a process commonly referred to as risk assessment. The risk assessment process involves five key steps:

1 **Step 1** – identifying **hazards** by looking around the workplace: for example, worn carpets can lead to people falling over; an obstructed fire escape route may prevent people from exiting the building in the case of a fire; not storing cleaning detergents away securely after being used may lead to them being swallowed accidentally by an individual.

2 **Step 2** – assessing the level of risk by assessing who might be harmed and how, deciding how likely it is that someone could be harmed and how serious it could be: for example, there is a high risk that an obstructed fire escape route could harm everyone in the workplace by obstructing people's escape route in the event of a fire.

3 **Step 3** – controlling the risks by looking at the controls that are in place. Have they eliminated the hazard? If not, can the level of risk be reduced to minimise the likelihood of harm? For example, provide additional training to workers on fire safety and prevention so they understand the dangers of obstructing fire escape routes.

4 **Step 4** – recording the findings of your risk assessment by recording the hazards, the risks these

pose (including who might be harmed and how) and what you are doing to control the risks. To comply with health and safety legislation, an employer with five or more employees is required to record their findings. You will learn more about the importance of risk assessment in relation to identifying hazards in AC2.3.

5 **Step 5** – reviewing the controls that are in place to make sure that they are still effective: for example, if the security measures in place to check visitors' proof of identity are not consistently effective, this may involve reviewing the agreed ways of working in place for allowing visitors to enter the premises and providing further training in this area.

KEY TERM

Hazard: a danger that has the potential to cause harm.

AC2.2 Types of accidents, incidents, emergencies and health and safety hazards that may occur in the workplace

Accidents, incidents, emergencies, and health and safety hazards can happen at any time, but some occur more commonly in health and social care settings. Review your previous learning in AC1.1 in relation to why health and social care settings may be more susceptible to these.

Table 6.3 outlines some examples of different types of accidents, incidents, emergencies and health and safety hazards that may occur in the workplace where care and support are provided to individuals.

Accidents	Incidents	Emergencies	Health and safety hazards
Slips, trips and falls may be caused by the workplace and its contents not being maintained, or because individuals' conditions such as poor mobility or vision loss make them more prone to falls. They may cause fractures, cuts and bruises.	**Damage to property** may be caused by an environmental emergency such as a fire or a flood. They may cause damage to the building and/or its contents.	**Environmental emergencies** may be caused by fires, gas leaks and floods. They may cause damage to the building and/or its contents and to those in the workplace.	**Hazards in the workplace related to the building**, such as worn carpets and dirty bathrooms and kitchens, may be caused by poor maintenance and cleaning routines. They may cause accidents, incidents and emergencies.
Lifting and handling accidents may be caused by workers not following safe lifting and handling practices (see AC4.3 for more information) when supporting individuals and moving items. They may cause back injuries and fractures.	**Spillages** may be caused by an accident, such as a worker accidentally spilling a cleaning fluid when using it, or a faulty fixture such as a water pipe bursting in the kitchen or bathroom. They may cause damage to the building and/or its contents.	**First aid emergencies** may be caused by different types of accidents and sudden illnesses (see below) that may occur in the workplace. They may cause severe bleeding, fractures, burns. They require immediate attention when they occur.	**Hazards in the workplace related to** high risk activities, such as **needle stick injuries**, may occur accidentally when being used or when being disposed of. They require urgent medical attention.
Physical assaults may be caused by individuals' health conditions such as dementia and mental ill-health. They may cause cuts, bruises and **stress**.	**Security incidents** may be intentional and caused by intruders who cause criminal damage to the building and/or property. Security incidents can also include bomb scares, missing persons and breaches in data protection (when personal information is accessed by an unauthorised person).	**Sudden illnesses** require urgent attention when they occur. They may be caused by medical conditions such as **diabetes**, **asthma** or **heart disease**, or by poor working practices when moving, lifting and handling people and items in the workplace which can lead to back injuries and sprains.	**Hazards in the workplace related** to health and social care settings, such as visitors accidentally leaving their bags unattended or in areas where they may cause trips and falls. They require immediate and safe removal.

▲ Table 6.3 Workplace accidents, incidents, emergencies and health and safety hazards

KEY TERMS

Needle stick injury: a stab wound from a needle or another sharp object that can result in exposure to the blood of another person.

Stress: the body's physical and emotional reaction to being under too much pressure.

Diabetes: a health condition that occurs when the amount of glucose (sugar) in the blood is too high because the pancreas does not produce enough insulin or because the body cannot effectively use the insulin it produces.

Asthma: a lung condition that causes breathing difficulties that can range from mild to severe.

Heart disease: includes conditions that narrow or block blood vessels (this is known as coronary heart disease). This can lead to a heart attack, angina and some strokes. Heart disease also covers conditions that affect the heart's muscle, valves or cause abnormal rhythms (known as arrhythmias).

AC2.3 The importance of risk assessment in the identification of hazards related to the work setting or activities

As you will know, there are many different types of hazards related to both the workplace and work activities that occur in health and social care settings. Using the risk assessment process to identify these hazards is important because it:

- raises everyone's awareness of the hazards that there are in the work setting and work activities
- enables potential and actual dangers to be identified, as well as their associated risks of causing harm or illness, so that controls can be put in place to either eliminate or reduce these risks
- enables workers, individuals and others in health and social care settings to comply with current health and safety legislation, as well as maintain their responsibilities to protect everyone from danger and harm.

RESEARCH IT

Research HSE's website and their published leaflet 'Risk assessment A brief guide to controlling risks in the workplace' available on this link:

www.hse.gov.uk/pubns/indg163.pdf

Discuss with someone you know why risk assessment plays an important role in identifying workplace hazards.

AC2.4 Responsibilities for carrying out, recording and following risk assessments for work activities

Every work setting will have health and safety procedures or agreed ways of working in place that set out everyone's responsibilities for ensuring the safety of the workplace and all work activities.

Carrying out risk assessments

- Responsibilities for carrying out risk assessments for work activities will depend on your job role, the setting where you work and the work activities you are responsible for.
- For example, if you are a **personal assistant**, the individual employing you to provide care and support is your employer, and they will be responsible for carrying out risk assessments for your work activities to ensure that they are safe before you carry them out. You will also be responsible for carrying out your work activities safely, so you will also be responsible for carrying out risk assessments as part of your working practice – you must always report any actual or potential hazards as soon as you have identified them.
- You will learn more about the difference between formal recorded risk assessments and those that are carried out routinely as part of working practice in AC2.5.

Recording risk assessments

- Responsibilities for recording risk assessments for work activities will again depend on your job role, the setting where you work and the work activities you are responsible for.
- For example, if you are a care worker in a **residential care home** then the manager or a senior member of the team will be responsible for recording risk assessments.

  This doesn't mean that as a care worker you will not be involved in the process; the person responsible for recording risk assessments for work activities will want to discuss these with everyone involved to ensure that they contain accurate and factual information. If you have any questions about any aspect of the risk assessment process you must raise this.

You will find it useful to refer to AC2.5, as it provides more information about different types of risk assessments.

Following risk assessments

- Responsibilities for following risk assessments are essential for complying with health and safety legislation and the employer's health and safety procedures.
- Everyone is responsible for following risk assessments that are in place. It doesn't matter if you are a worker, an individual or a visitor to a health and social care setting; if you are made aware that a risk assessment has been put in place, you must follow it as not doing so may put you, workers, individuals and others in danger.
- In addition, if you do not understand any aspect of the risk assessment, you must raise this with the manager or employer so that they can guide you and assist you with understanding how to follow it.

KEY TERMS

Personal assistant: a worker who provides care and support to an individual in their own home and is employed directly by the individual.

Residential care home: a care setting for individuals who require assistance with their daily activities such as washing, dressing and meal preparation.

AC2.5 The difference between formal recorded risk assessments and those that are carried out routinely as part of working practice

Assessing risks in the workplace is a legal requirement. Risk assessments can be formally recorded or undertaken routinely as part of working practice. Both types are important and essential for safeguarding everyone's health and safety. Table 6.4 shows the differences between the two types.

Formal assessment	Routine assessment
Usually planned by a designated person, specific to an individual or work activity and written down (such as the one included in the case study below).	Usually completed visually during practice and can be completed by workers. They can include more general health and safety checks.
Often used for new work activities or work practices that have not been assessed, so that any potential danger or harm can be assessed before they take place.	Used in addition to the formal recorded risk assessment. Can be useful for assessing work activities and practices as they are happening.
Completed when there are changes to either work activities or work practices. For example, an individual's condition may improve and therefore the previously identified risk may no longer be relevant. The risk assessment needs to be reviewed and updated to reflect this, to ensure the care and support provided are relevant.	Used to inform the recorded risk assessment because this is when improvements to and/or difficulties for individuals and or work activities are noticed during day-to-day practice.

▲ Table 6.4 Differences between formal and routine risk assessments

CASE STUDY

Julio and his family live in Swansea, and have recently started fostering children through a local fostering service. At present Julio and his family have been fostering Dylan, who is 14 years old, for a few days every month to enable Dylan's mother, who is unwell, to rest and have a short break.

Julio would like to involve Dylan in the outdoor climbing activities he and his family enjoy, but is not sure whether this is too risky and whether or not he needs to complete a risk assessment.

Discussion points:

- What are the benefits of completing a risk assessment?
- What are the consequences of not completing a risk assessment?
- Where could Julio and his family go for additional support and guidance?

AC2.6 The importance of reporting concerns or incidents that have or may be likely to occur

All workers in health and social care settings have a duty of candour, which means that they have a legal responsibility to be open and honest when care or support goes wrong. We explored this concept in Units 001/002.

When incidents have occurred or you have concerns that an may be likely to occur, more commonly referred to as **near misses**, it is important to report these:

KEY TERM

Near misses: incidents that have the potential to cause harm.

- It means you are acting responsibly and fulfilling your duty of candour. This will mean that individuals, your colleagues, employer and others such as individuals' families will trust you and feel reassured that you are doing your job to the best of your ability.

 For example: reporting that an individual's medication was administered late.

- Not doing so will mean that the potential hazard and associated level of risk cannot be assessed or acted on, and could therefore lead to actual harm and a failure in your legal requirement to safeguard individuals from danger, harm or neglect.

 For example: not reporting that an individual's medication was administered late may make the individual feel anxious and/or may prevent further action being taken if their condition worsens.

- You will be able to reflect on what could be improved and/or what can be put in place to reduce the likelihood of the danger occurring.

 For example, reporting that an individual's medication was administered late will help with understanding why this happened and how to prevent it happening again.

REFLECT ON IT

Reflect on an occasion something went wrong because of your actions.

- What happened?
- How did you feel?
- Did you tell anyone?

Looking back over this occasion, is there anything you could have done differently? Why?

L03 KNOW HOW TO PROMOTE FIRE SAFETY IN WORK SETTINGS

AC3.1 Key legislation that relates to fire safety

AC3.2 The responsibilities of the employer, worker and others for fire safety in the work setting

Knowing about the legislation that relates to fire safety is important for understanding your responsibilities as a worker and the responsibilities of your employer and of other people such as visitors to work settings, in relation to promoting fire safety in the workplace. Everyone's health and safety will depend on how well they work together in promoting fire safety.

Table 6.5 provides you with information about the key fire safety legislation, its purpose and how it relates to work settings in terms of employers, workers and others' responsibilities.

Legislation	Purpose of the legislation	How it relates to the work setting
The Health and Safety at Work Act 1974	To promote and ensure the safety of everyone in work settings.	It ensures work settings have fire safety procedures in place that set out employers', workers' and others' key duties and responsibilities. For example: • for employers to provide fire safety training • for workers and others to follow fire safety procedures.
The Regulatory Reform (Fire Safety) Order 2005	To reduce the risks of fires in work settings.	It requires employers to: • complete fire risk assessments • provide fire safety training • provide fire equipment – fire extinguishers as well as fire escape routes and exits. Workers and others are required to attend fire safety training and know what to do in the event of a fire.
COSHH 1999 Hazardous Waste	To reduce the risks associated with **hazardous substances** in work settings.	It requires employers to: • carry out risk assessments • provide information, training and supervision around the use of hazardous substances that, if not used correctly, may lead to a fire starting. It requires workers and others to use safe working practices when using hazardous substances, such as: • following manufacturer's instructions when using hazardous substances • wiping all spillages immediately.
The Provision and Use of Work Equipment Regulations (PUWER) 1998	To reduce the risks associated with **equipment** in work settings.	It requires employers to: • provide training, supervision • ensure work equipment has visible warning signs. It requires workers to understand the safety precautions to take when using work equipment; not doing so may result in a fire.

▲ Table 6.5 Fire safety legislation

Legislation	Purpose of the legislation	How it relates to the work setting
The Electrical Equipment (Safety) Regulations 1994	To reduce the risks associated with electricity including electrical equipment in work settings.	It requires employers to ensure electrical equipment is safe to use and well maintained. It requires workers and others to use safe working practices including reporting faulty equipment; not doing so may result in a fire starting.
The Management of Health and Safety at Work Regulations 1999	To reduce health and safety risks by carrying out risk assessments in work settings.	It requires employers to: • carry out risk assessments • have emergency procedures in place, such as in the event of a fire • inform everyone about these procedures. It requires workers and others to follow emergency procedures.
Workplace (Health, Safety and Welfare) Regulations 1992	To reduce health and safety risks, promote safety and good working conditions in work settings.	It requires employers to provide a safe work setting. Buildings and equipment that are clean, maintained and safe to use will reduce the likelihood of a fire occurring. It requires workers and others to use the facilities provided.

▲ Table 6.5 Fire safety legislation *(continued)*

KEY TERMS

Hazardous substances: in health and social care settings, they can include cleaning substances, used PPE or dressings that have come into contact with body fluids such as blood, faeces, urine, sputum and vomit.

Equipment: in health and social care settings, this can include cleaning equipment.

RESEARCH IT

Research a fire that you may have read or heard about that has occurred in a health or social care setting. Find out:
● what caused the fire
● whether anyone failed in their responsibility to promote fire safety.

Think about the importance of complying with fire safety legislation in the workplace.

AC3.3 Practices that prevent fires from starting and spreading

Practices that prevent fires from starting

Knowing how to prevent fires from starting, as well as the correct actions to take to prevent fires from spreading, will ensure you fulfil your responsibilities to promote fire safety in the work setting and reduce the likelihood of danger and harm.

Fires start when heat, fuel and oxygen come together. This is known as the fire triangle:

● Heat can be caused by an unattended cigarette or an electrical heater that is faulty and has overheated.
● Fuel can be any item that can burn, such as a solid, liquid or gas.
● Oxygen is present in the air and can be given off by some chemicals.

If one of these elements is not present then the fire will not start; this is known as breaking the fire triangle.

Fires can be prevented from starting by following safe working practices such as:

● being vigilant when working and reporting any potential fire hazards that you notice – such as an overloaded electric socket; an electric appliance such as a heater that becomes very hot when switched on; and loose wires in plugs.
● ensuring that anything flammable that may cause a fire is removed – such as an unattended cigarette; clothes being dried in front of an open oven door; hazardous and flammable substances.
● following your employer's fire safety training and procedures – such as keeping your fire safety knowledge up to date and attending training, for example, in relation to potential fire hazards; following procedures such as who to report fire hazards to, when and how.

Practices that prevent fires from spreading

Your employer's fire safety procedures will also include guidance on the practices to follow in the event of a fire starting, to prevent it from spreading and causing further damage and harm. Table 6.6 contains a list of dos and don'ts for preventing the spread of fire.

REFLECT ON IT

Reflect on how you might feel if you came across a fire in the workplace.
- What would you do?
- What wouldn't you do? Why?
- Where could you access further guidance and support?

Do	Don't
Know your responsibilities in relation to maintaining fire safety equipment such as fire alarms and smoke detectors in good working order; doing so will ensure they work effectively when a fire starts and raise the alarm to stop it spreading. Your responsibilities may include testing that they are working and reporting any faults.	Don't ignore potential fire indicators or avoid saying anything in case you are mistaken, such as the smell of burning or an electric failure. Reporting all potential fire indicators, however small, will minimise the risk of a fire spreading.
Carry out health and safety checks while you are working, such as checking that fire equipment such as fire alarms, fire extinguishers, smoke detectors, fire blankets are not obstructed with other items. Make sure that they can be accessed quickly in the event of a fire to prevent it from spreading.	Don't open windows and doors in the event of a fire; keeping them closed will contain the fire and prevent it from spreading.
Know what to do in the event of a fire: participate in fire drills and attend fire training, so that you can respond quickly in the event of a fire to prevent it from spreading.	Don't try and deal with a fire yourself unless you have been trained to do so. If you delay calling for help, this could lead to the fire spreading.

▲ Table 6.6 Dos and don'ts for preventing fires from spreading

AC3.4 The importance of knowing about and following fire evacuation procedures

Your employer's fire safety procedures will include details about what to do in the event of a fire.

It is important that you read and understand these so that you can respond quickly in the event of a fire and safeguard yourself and others from danger and harm. Your responsibilities will depend on your job role and your workplace, but most fire safety procedures will include following these safe practices:

1 Raise the alarm: sound the fire alarm and alert a senior member of staff by shouting out 'FIRE'. It is important to do this as soon as possible to minimise the risk of the fire spreading and causing more harm. Check your responsibilities with raising the fire alarm, as in some workplaces fire alarm systems automatically dial the fire brigade, and in others only designated staff members can contact the fire brigade.

2 If it is your responsibility to do so, call the emergency services or inform someone else to do this. Again, you must do this immediately so help can arrive quickly.

3 Ensure the safety of others by moving them away from any danger. It is important you know how to do this as this will vary depending on individuals' conditions and your responsibilities. For example, if some individuals are likely to get distressed or they are unable to mobilise easily, it may be safer for them to remain in their rooms until help arrives.

4 Only attempt to put out the fire if you have been trained to do so safely, such as placing a fire blanket over a small fire in the kitchen caused by an overfilled pan of cooking oil.

5 When leaving the workplace, close all doors behind you so the fire doesn't spread. Walk calmly to reassure others, and don't run as this may cause

others to panic, leading to slips and falls. Don't stop to take any personal belongings with you as this will delay you from leaving the building.

6   Go to the assembly point. Workplaces have designated areas and you must know where yours is for your own and others' safety.

7   Once you've left the building, do not return until you've been told it's safe to do so; doing so will mean you may place yourself in danger as others may not be aware that you have re-entered the building.

AC3.5 The importance of maintaining clear exit routes at all times

Every workplace will have designated fire escape routes that enable you and others to exit safely in the event of a fire. It is important that you know where these are so that you will know the safest and quickest way to exit the building, thus ensuring your own and others' safety.

Fire evacuation or exit routes must also be:

- safe to use
- clearly signposted
- be well-lit
- fitted with fire safety equipment such as fireproof doors and fire extinguishers.

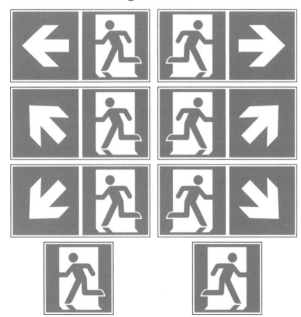

▲ Figure 6.2 Do you know what these fire escape signs mean?

Maintaining clear exit routes at all times is also very important because:

- It will be easier to escape the building if exit routes are clear with no obstructions (such as boxes of PPE, wheelchairs or other equipment). Not doing so may prevent people escaping from the fire and could result in fatalities.
- The likelihood of people slipping or falling over is reduced when they are trying to escape in the event of a fire. Not doing so may lead to people having accidents and sustaining injuries when exiting the building.
- Exit routes will remain wide enough to enable more people to exit the building safely and quickly in the event of a fire. Not doing so may lead to panic and some people not being able to exit safely.

CASE STUDY

Zee has just arrived to start his work shift at the day care centre. As he enters the building, the painter, who is decorating one of the rooms, asks Zee whether it's okay for him to leave his painting and decorating materials for ten minutes or so by the fire escape door in the room he'll be decorating. At the same time, Zee is approached by his manager who asks whether he can see him urgently for five minutes before he begins his shift.

Discussion points:

- Who should Zee prioritise in this situation – the painter or his manager? Why?
- What should Zee say to the painter? Why?
- What should Zee say to his manager? Why?

Check your understanding

1 Give two reasons why it is important to raise concerns about unsafe practices.

2 Name two accidents and two incidents that may occur in the workplace.

3 Describe in one sentence what risk assessment means.

4 Describe two practices that prevent fires from starting and spreading.

Question practice

1 What key piece of legislation requires employers to carry out risk assessments in the workplace?

a Management of Health and Safety at Work Regulations (MHSWR) 1999

b Workplace (Health, Safety and Welfare) Regulations 1992

c Provision and Use of Work Equipment Regulations 1998

d Lifting Operations and Lifting Equipment Regulations 1998

2 Whose responsibility is it to report accidents and incidents to the HSE?

a the worker

b others

c the employer

d all three of the above

3 Which of the following is TRUE?

a Risk assessments identify hazards only.

b Risk assessment is a three-step process.

c Risk assessments must continue to be reviewed and updated to be effective.

d Employers with ten or more employees are required to record their risk assessments.

4 Why is it important to report a concern that an incident is likely to occur?

a to reduce or eliminate the risk of it causing harm

b to increase the risk of it causing harm

c to prevent others in the workplace from doing so

d to save time

5 Which of the following describes the purpose of the Regulatory Reform (Fire Safety) Order 2005?

a to reduce the risks of fires in work settings

b to reduce the risks associated with equipment in work settings

c to reduce the risks associated with electricity in work settings

d to reduce health and safety risks

6 Which of the following actions must you not take when following fire evacuation procedures?

a Raise the alarm immediately.

b Close all doors behind you when leaving the building.

c Run out of the building as quickly as possible.

d Do not re-enter the building until you have been told it is safe to do so.

LO4 KNOW THE KEY PRINCIPLES OF MOVING AND HANDLING AND MOVING AND POSITIONING

AC4.1 The terms 'moving and handling' and 'moving and positioning'

The term 'moving and handling' is a general term, and refers to work activities that involve the moving of objects or people. It can include lifting, lowering, pushing, pulling and carrying. In health and social care settings:

● moving and handling objects can involve moving large pieces of play equipment, lifting a laundry bag or carrying a box full of PPE
● moving and handling people can involve supporting a young person to get in and out of a swimming pool or using a hoist to move an individual with care and support needs from their bed to an armchair.

The term 'moving and positioning' is more commonly used when referring to the support required by individuals to move and position from one position to another. It can include:

● supporting the individual with a verbal prompt
● providing reassurance
● lifting and carrying babies and children
● physically assisting the individual by giving them a supporting arm, or through the use of equipment such as a **stand aid**.

KEY TERM

Stand aid: a piece of equipment that supports an individual to stand up from a sitting position.

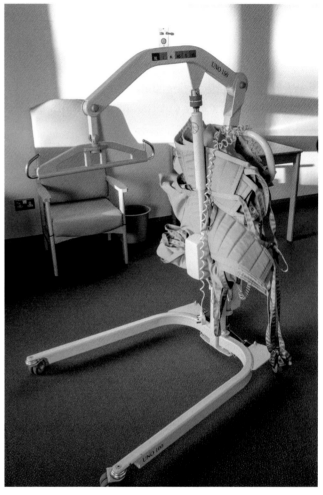

▲ Figure 6.3 Do you know how moving and handling equipment is used in health and social care settings?

AC4.2 Key legislation that relates to moving and handling, and what this means in practice

There are three key pieces of legislation to ensure that safe practices are followed when carrying out moving and handling in the workplace. You will also find it useful to review your learning in AC1.1 in relation to health and safety legislation.

Manual Handling Operations Regulations 1992 (as amended) (MHOR)

These regulations define manual handling as transporting or supporting a load. This could be an object (such as a box) or a person, and applies to a range of moving and handling activities in the workplace including lifting, putting down, pushing, pulling and carrying.

These regulations set out measures for dealing with risks that arise from moving and handling activities by requiring employers to do the following:

1 Consider whether the need for moving and handling can be avoided.
2 Assess the risk of injury from moving and handling that cannot be avoided.
3 Reduce the risk of injury from any hazardous moving and handling.

In practice, employers are also required to provide information, training and supervision to employees in relation to safe moving and handling techniques.

Employees are required to:

- read and understand the information that their employer provides in relation to moving and handling
- attend training
- follow safe moving and handling procedures in their workplace
- only carry out moving and handling activities they've been trained in
- use equipment provided correctly
- inform their employer of any unsafe moving and handling activities they identify.

Provision and Use of Work Equipment Regulations 1998 (PUWER)

These regulations are in place to prevent or control risks to health and safety from equipment used in the workplace. In relation to moving and handling work, equipment used in health and social care settings could include hoists, **bath lifts**, **lifting cushions** and **bariatric equipment**.

Employers are required to ensure that equipment:

- is safe for use
- is maintained in a safe condition
- is monitored to ensure it is in good working order
- is suitable for the intended use
- includes protective devices, such as an emergency stop device, visible markings and warning signs
- is used only by those who have been trained to use it.

In practice employees must:

- only use equipment that they have received information, instruction and training in
- comply with their employer's safe working procedures when using equipment.

KEY TERMS

Bath lift: this assists individuals to get in and out of the bath.

Lifting cushions: these assist individuals to get up from the floor or bath.

Bariatric equipment: aids specifically manufactured to assist individuals who are obese with moving and positioning.

Lifting Operations and Lifting Equipment Regulations 1998 (LOLER)

These regulations are in place to ensure that lifting equipment used in the workplace is suitable for the work task, safe for use and maintained in good working order (the requirements of the Provision and Use of Work Equipment Regulations 1998 apply here).

Employers are required to:

- plan all work activities that require lifting
- supervise workers when they are carrying out lifting activities
- use workers that are competent
- arrange for yearly inspections of lifting equipment and maintain records for this.

Employees are required to:

- only use lifting equipment if they have been trained to do so

- follow their employer's procedures and the manufacturer's instructions
- report any unsafe practices or faults with equipment.

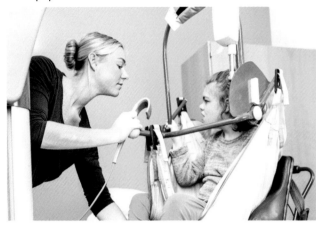

▲ Figure 6.4 Do you know your employer's safe moving and handling procedures?

REFLECT ON IT

Reflect on the responsibilities of employers and employees when moving and handling in the workplace.

Think about the consequences on the employer, employees, individuals and others of not fulfilling these responsibilities.

AC4.3 Principles and techniques related to safe moving and handling

AC4.4 Potential implications of poor practice in relation to moving and handling

A wide range of moving and handling equipment is used in health and social care settings, including lifting equipment such as:

- mobile hoists that lift and lower individuals from, for example, their bed to an armchair
- moving and handling equipment, such as transfer boards that enable individuals to slide across from their wheelchair into an armchair
- moving and handling aids, such as walking frames that assist individuals when walking.

Good practice rules or principles and techniques are in place to enable you to follow safe moving and handling practices in the workplace; your workplace's procedures will provide you with more information.

Table 6.7 sets out some of the main safe principles and techniques, as well the implications of poor practice when moving and handling. Can you think of any others?

Safe moving and handling principle/technique	Examples in practice
Follow your workplace's moving and handling procedures to ensure you're complying with them.	• Read your workplace's moving and handling procedures and carry out your activities in line with them. For example, check the hoist before using it that it is clean, fully charged and safe to use. • If you read your employer's procedures and there is something you don't understand, then ask. Not doing so may lead to you carrying out unsafe practices. For example, what should you do if you're about to use the hoist and it develops a fault?
Follow the moving and handling guidelines that are in place for individuals to promote their safety and well-being.	• Read through the guidelines in place for each individual before you carry out any moving and handling, to ensure your practices are up to date and nothing has changed. For example, check the individual's condition, and the risk assessment. • If you can't follow the guidelines, then stop what you are doing and report this immediately, so that the correct actions can be taken.

▲ Table 6.7 Safe moving and handling principles and techniques and implications of poor practice

Safe moving and handling principle/technique	Examples in practice
Complete health and safety checks before using moving and handling equipment, to ensure it is safe to use and avoid any accidents.	• Complete your health and safety checks by visually checking the equipment you are about to use to check it is, for example, clean and in working order. Not doing so can lead to accidents happening. • If the equipment is dirty, worn or has developed a fault, do not use it and report this immediately so the correct actions can be taken. The equipment will also have to display an 'Out of order' sign on it to prevent others from using it and becoming injured.
Prepare for all moving and handling activities carefully to ensure you are carrying these out safely and reducing the risk of harm and injury to you, your colleagues, individuals, and others.	• Plan all moving and handling activities by first checking whether you have all the necessary equipment in place and that there is sufficient space to use it. Some hoists can be quite large and may be difficult to use in a small area such as a bathroom. Not doing so may lead to delays, and the incorrect equipment and techniques being used. • If the individual's guidelines state that two people are required to assist them to move from one position to another, ensure that there is another person to assist you who is also trained and competent to do so. Not doing so may place you and the individual in danger.
Report any concerns you have in relation to moving and handling to reduce the risk of harm and injury to you, your colleagues, individuals, and others.	• Report any concerns you have, however small, with immediate effect to the person responsible – your employer or manager. For example, you notice that a bed lift sounds noisy when being operated. This could indicate that it is not working correctly, so reporting it could prevent it from being used unsafely. • If you notice a work colleague not using safe moving and handling practices, such as not following an individual's guidelines, you must report this. Not doing so may mean that your colleague continues to practise unsafely (they may not know that they are doing so) and cause unnecessary harm or injury to the individual.
Communicate clearly with all those involved when moving and handling. Not doing so may result in errors happening and unsafe practices that could lead to harm and injury to you, your colleagues, individuals, and others.	• Communicate clearly with the individual involved in the move. For example, explain how you plan to support them before the move and how they can be involved in the move, and check with them that they are not in any pain. • Not communicating with the individual may result in them not co-operating with being moved, because they may be unsure about what's happening. • Communicate clearly with your work colleagues when moving and handling. For example, you can check with your colleague your role and theirs in the move, decide who's going to lead the move, where you're both going to stand, how you are going to agree when to move the individual, such as on the count of 1, 2, 3. • Not communicating with your work colleagues may mean that you or they become injured, and this could lead to the individual being injured.
Maintain a safe posture when moving and handling.	Use a safe posture when moving and handling: • Keep your legs and feet slightly apart and your knees slightly bent. • Keep your shoulders facing in the same direction as the hips. • Keep your head up and look ahead. • Do not stoop or twist. • Keep the object or person as close to your body as possible. Not maintaining a safe posture may lead to you: • injuring your back by overstretching and twisting • causing your back irreversible damage • not being able to continue with the move, which may cause distress to the individual.

▲ Table 6.7 Safe moving and handling principles and techniques and implications of poor practice *(continued)*

RESEARCH IT

Research the moving and handling procedures for one health or social care setting. Read them and write down the principles and techniques they include for safe moving and handling.

- How do they compare to the ones you've just learnt about?
- What are the similarities and differences?

Produce an information handout with your findings.

As you will have read in Table 6.7, the potential implications of poor practice in relation to moving and handling can cause accidents, injuries and harm to you, your work colleagues and individuals. It is also important to remember that as a health or social care worker, you also have health and safety responsibilities and a duty of care that involves not putting yourself, your work colleagues, individuals and others at risk of danger or harm. Doing so may result in your employer taking action against you for failing in your duty and responsibilities, the loss of your job and at worst not being able to work in the health or social care sector again.

Check your understanding

1 What safe practices/principles must be followed when using equipment to move an individual?

2 What are the consequences of poor practice when using moving and handling equipment?

CASE STUDY

Alaw is a care worker in a care home and is assisting Brangwen, who is 90 years old, with having a bath this morning. Alaw reads through Brangwen's care plan and checks that there have been no changes to her risk assessment or moving and handling guidelines.

After checking with Brangwen that she is ready to have a bath, Alaw then prepares the bathroom, ensuring it is warm, comfortable and that all necessary toiletries, towels and clothes are in the bathroom. As Alaw assists Brangwen to sit on the bath lift and begins to operate it so that she can be lowered into the bath, the bath lift stops working.

Discussion points:

- Could Alaw have done anything differently to prevent this situation from happening? Why?
- How do you think this situation affected Brangwen? Do you think it affected Alaw? How?

Question practice

1 Which of the following pieces of legislation relates to moving and handling?

a Personal Protective Equipment (PPE) at Work Regulations 1992

b Workplace (Health, Safety and Welfare) Regulations 1992

c Control of Substances Hazardous to Health Regulations (COSHH) (2002)

d Provision and Use of Work Equipment Regulations 1998 (PUWER)

2 Which of the following is not a safe moving and handling technique?

a completing health and safety checks before using equipment

b following individuals' moving and handling guidelines

c communicating only with your colleagues when moving and handling

d maintaining a safe posture, with your legs and feet slightly apart and your knees slightly bent

LO5 KNOW THE MAIN ROUTES OF INFECTION AND HOW TO PREVENT THE SPREAD OF INFECTIONS IN THE WORKPLACE

GETTING STARTED

Preventing the spread of infections in workplaces including in health and social care settings is everyone's responsibility because infections can affect everyone by making them feel unwell; in some cases, they can even result in fatalities. For example, in November 2020 it was reported that 15 individuals at the Llangollen Fechan Care Home died in a three-week period following a COVID-19 outbreak, and a total of 56 individuals and 33 staff members tested positive for the virus.

Think about:

- how the spread of COVID-19 in workplaces in Wales affected everyone
- the precautions that helped to reduce the spread of the virus.

AC5.1 The differences between bacteria, viruses, fungi and parasites

AC5.2 Common illnesses and infections caused by bacteria, viruses, fungi and parasites and the potential impact of these

Infections can range from being mild to severe. They are caused by harmful disease-causing germs referred to as pathogens that can be found everywhere, including inside our bodies and in the air, and can be spread from person to person.

There are many different types of pathogens, but the two main types are bacteria and viruses. Knowing about these and their associated illnesses and infections is important when reducing their spread and supporting individuals and others who may become unwell.

Bacteria

Bacteria reproduce in large numbers to cause infections and can multiply outside the human body. Bacterial infections can usually be treated with antibiotics.

Examples of infections caused by bacteria include:

1 Gastroenteritis – a relatively common infection of the stomach and/or bowel that causes diarrhoea and vomiting.
2 Tuberculosis – an infection which is rarely found in the UK but is still found in South-East Asia. It mainly affects the lungs but can also affect other parts of the body. It causes breathlessness that gradually worsens and a persistent cough that lasts more than three weeks.
3 Cellulitis – a serious infection affecting the deeper layers of the skin and tissue. It causes the skin to become painful, hot and swollen.

There are some infections caused by bacteria that are known to mainly affect people who are staying in healthcare settings such as hospitals; you will learn more about why some people are more at risk of infections in AC5.6:

- MRSA (Methicillin-resistant Staphylococcus aureus) is commonly referred to as a super bug, because it is resistant to some antibiotics and therefore can be more difficult to treat.
- MRSA is a bacteria that can affect the skin and can get deeper into the body. It can cause swelling, pain, dizziness and confusion.

Viruses

Viruses are smaller in size than bacteria and reproduce in small numbers to cause infections. Viruses can only multiply within the human body and cannot be treated with antibiotics.

Examples of infections caused by viruses include:

1 Influenza – an infection of the respiratory system that causes a sudden high temperature and an aching body.
2 Measles – a highly infectious illness that causes sore red eyes and a red-brown blotchy rash on the body.
3 Chicken pox – a highly infectious disease that mostly affects children and causes red spots that can blister and a fever.

A particularly serious viral infectious disease of the respiratory tract, that has led to many deaths and continues to be a risk to life, is COVID-19, which is caused by the virus SARS-CoV-2. This virus has led to many fatalities, with older people and those with health conditions in particular being at high risk. For example, CIW reported that between 1 March and 20 November 2020, they were notified of 934 care home resident deaths with suspected or confirmed coronavirus.

The main symptoms of COVID-19 are:

- a high temperature – you will feel hot to touch on your chest or back
- a new, continuous cough – coughing for more than an hour, or three or more coughing episodes in 24 hours
- a loss or change to your sense of smell or taste.

At the time of writing, further research is also being undertaken to explore the longer term effects of COVID-19, such as an illness referred to as Long Covid that affects some people who have had the virus and recovered, but are still experiencing symptoms 12 weeks after becoming infected. Symptoms include:

- breathing difficulties
- extreme fatigue
- impaired ability to carry out day-to-day tasks
- anxiety and depression.

Cardiff and Vale Health Board is the first in Wales planning to open a multi-disciplinary rehabilitation service that will treat the physical and mental health symptoms associated with Long Covid.

Fungi

Fungi are more complex than bacteria and viruses. They appear in the form of moulds or yeasts, and can multiply both inside and outside the human body.

Examples of infectious diseases caused by fungi include those that affect the skin only, such as ringworm, and those that can affect the whole body, such as thrush.

1 Ringworm is caused by a fungus called the dermatophyte fungus that lives on dead skin, hair and nails. It can appear on:
   - the feet as itchy, red, scaly patches in between the toes, commonly known as athlete's foot
   - the scalp as sore, scaly patches that can lead to hair falling out
   - nails, causing them to become thick, discoloured and brittle.

It can easily spread through the use of shared bathrooms and damp towels and mats.

2 Thrush is caused by a fungus called yeast candida that can affect the mouth, the armpits and groin. Thrush causes:
   - itching
   - irritation
   - a painful rash
   - white/yellow discharge.

Thrush is harmless but can be uncomfortable and keep reoccurring, even after treatment.

Parasites

Parasites can multiply both inside and outside the human body; about 70 per cent are not visible to the human eye. Examples of conditions that are caused by parasites are head lice, scabies and threadworms.

1 Head lice are parasites that live in human hair and whose bites can become infected if excessively scratched. Children are particularly vulnerable to head lice as these parasites spread:
   - mainly through close head-to-head contact
   - indirectly when clothing and grooming equipment is shared among children.
2 Scabies are parasites that live in the skin and are very infectious. Symptoms:
   - begin with intense itching (usually at night)
   - develop into a rash (usually starts between the fingers) and tiny red spots that can spread across the whole body (apart from the head).

3 Threadworms are parasites that infect the large intestine and in the UK are common in children under the age of 10. Symptoms:
- itching around the anus and vagina (usually at night)
- threadworms on bedclothes, sheets or in stools

Potential impact

Common illnesses and infections caused by bacteria, viruses, fungi and parasites impact negatively on individuals as they cause unpleasant symptoms and serious illnesses and infections.

In health and social care settings, the potential impact of an outbreak of an infection can have disastrous consequences, leading to individuals, workers and others developing similar signs and symptoms and becoming unwell, and can even lead to fatalities. It is very important to recognise any changes in individuals and/or workers promptly, so that potential outbreaks of infections can be managed quickly by putting infection prevention and control measures in place. You will learn more about these measures in ACs 5.9, 5.10, 5.11 and 5.12.

The potential impact on health and social care workplaces and employers must also be remembered. For example, the reporting in the media of care homes that had outbreaks of COVID-19 during the initial stages of the pandemic in 2020 led to some individuals' families removing their relatives from these settings, and others deciding to care for their relatives themselves at home where they felt they were safer. This had an immediate financial impact on these settings and also damaged their reputation for being safe environments for individuals to live in and be cared for.

These outbreaks of COVID-19 infections also led to a government policy of not allowing individuals' families and friends to visit in order to safeguard individuals from the virus. The impact of this on individuals has been far-reaching, and has led to:

- individuals feeling isolated and becoming withdrawn
- their families and friends feeling anxious about their relatives and frustrated that they are unable to visit.

Similarly, employers have experienced financial losses during the COVID-19 pandemic in terms of:

- seeing a loss in demand for their services
- having to buy additional equipment such as PPE for their workers
- recruiting additional and new workers to support existing workers with individuals' care and to replace workers who have become unwell.

Infection outbreaks can therefore affect everyone in the setting, and lead to anxiety and low morale.

CASE STUDY

Common illnesses and infections

You work in a children's centre and you have been asked by your manager to produce a short presentation to the rest of the team about the common illnesses and infections associated with bacteria, viruses, fungi and parasites. Your manager would like you to do this as it will help the team recognise what these are so that they can prevent their spread.

You can think about examples of common illnesses and infections you have learnt about, including their symptoms.

AC5.3 The terms 'infection' and 'colonisation'

AC5.4 The terms 'systemic infection' and 'localised infection'

Understanding commonly used terms when learning about infections in the workplace is essential for developing your knowledge in this important area. Here are some of the main ones:

- **Infection** refers to harmful pathogens such as bacteria, viruses, fungi and parasites (see AC5.2 for more information about these) that cause disease. Infection can affect any organ, such as intestine or lungs, or any system of the human body, such as the digestive system, respiratory system.
  Cross infection refers to the spread of infection from person to person, equipment or within the body and can cause people to feel unwell. It can range from being very mild to very serious, and sometimes can cause death.

- **Colonisation** refers to when harmful pathogens multiply on or in a person without harming them (for example, some people have reported that they have no symptoms of COVID-19 despite testing positive for the virus). That person – commonly referred to as a carrier – can however pass these harmful pathogens onto another person who may then develop an infection.
- **Systemic infection** affects all of the human body. An example is influenza: it affects the respiratory system but also causes a high temperature and an aching body.
- **Localised infection** affects one specific area of the human body. For example, athlete's foot will lead to red and itchy skin in between your toes, but will not make you feel generally unwell.

AC5.5 Ways in which infections are transmitted and poor practices that may lead to this

How are infections spread?

Understanding how infections are transmitted is essential for preventing the spread of infections in workplaces such as health and social care settings. Infections spread through six key stages, often referred to as the 'chain of infection'.

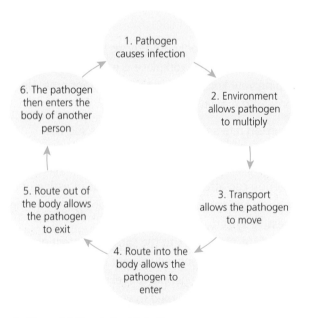

▲ Figure 6.5 The chain of infection

1 **Stage 1:** The chain begins when a harmful pathogen (bacteria, virus, fungus, parasite) causes an infection.
2 **Stage 2:** In the correct environment, harmful pathogens can grow and multiply very quickly. For example, for bacteria to grow they require moisture (damp conditions), warmth (the human body's temperature), food (such as leftover food), time to multiply, acidity levels, and sometimes but not always, oxygen. Only when these conditions are present will bacteria grow and multiply.
3 **Stage 3:** Harmful pathogens then need transport to move around from place to place. This process is called transmission. Harmful pathogens can be transported in different ways, including through:
   - water; example: the bacterial infection **typhoid**
   - food; example: the bacterial infection **salmonella**
   - animals and insects; example: the disease **malaria**
   - air and dust; example: the infection **whooping cough**
   - droplets when coughing and sneezing; example: the viral infection COVID-19
   - contaminated objects with bodily fluids such as PPE, towels; example: the fungal infection athlete's foot
   - directly from person to person; example: viral diseases **Human Immunodeficiency Virus (HIV)** or **Hepatitis B**.
4 **Stage 4:** Harmful pathogens can also enter into the human body by different methods including through the:
   - respiratory route (mouth and nose)
   - digestive route
   - genital route
   - blood route – such as wounds from cuts, surgical procedures, bites, tattoos
   - touch – such as hands
   - bodily fluids.
5 **Stage 5:** Harmful pathogens can also exit out of the human body before entering the body of another person, through the routes described in stage 4.
6 **Stage 6:** Harmful pathogens can then enter the body of another person and spread from person to person; a process referred to as cross infection. Harmful pathogens are transported both directly (through actual physical contact with an infected person) and indirectly (through objects, food and bodily fluids expelled from the human body).

KEY TERMS

Typhoid: a bacterial infection that can affect the whole body, and causes high temperature, aches and pains.

Salmonella: a bacterial infection that affects the intestinal tract, and causes fever, abdominal cramps and vomiting.

Malaria: a disease spread by infected mosquitoes that can affect the whole body, and causes high temperature, feeling hot and shivery, and vomiting.

Whooping cough: a bacterial infection that affects the lungs and respiratory tract, and causes a worsening cough and breathing difficulties.

Human immunodeficiency virus (HIV): a virus that damages the cells in the immune system and therefore impairs the body's ability to fight off infections and diseases. Flu-like symptoms may be experienced initially but the symptoms may disappear, although the virus continues to damage the cells in the immune system.

Hepatitis B: an infection of the liver caused by a virus that is spread through blood and body fluids. It may not cause any symptoms.

What poor practices can lead to the spread of infections?

In workplaces such as health and social care settings, cross infections can be prevented and controlled by avoiding the use of poor practices such as:

- **Poor cleaning practices** – not checking that equipment such as hoists and wheelchairs are clean before and after use can lead to these objects being contaminated with harmful pathogens that can spread indirectly to another person.
- **Poor maintenance practices** – not checking that surfaces such as bathroom floors and kitchen worktops are clean and free from dirt such as bodily fluids and leftover food before supporting individuals with their personal hygiene and preparing food. This can lead to indirectly contaminating all those who use them with harmful pathogens.
- **Poor hygiene practices** – not washing your hands before and after supporting individuals with eating, drinking or washing may lead to harmful pathogens present on your hands spreading to other individuals and workers who you come into contact with. You will learn more about good personal hygiene and hand washing techniques to prevent the spread of infection in AC5.10 and AC5.11.
- **Poor working practices** – not following your employer's and workplace's procedures for infection prevention and control can lead to the spread of infections. For example, not wearing PPE when you carry out tasks where bodily fluids may be present (such as when changing bed linen) or disposing of waste (such as used dressings) may lead to you and others becoming infected with harmful pathogens.

As well as these poor practices, remember that poor or out-of-date knowledge of how to prevent the spread of infections can also increase the likelihood of infections spreading in the workplace. Attending your employer's training on infection prevention and control, and reading information provided by your employer, are two good ways of keeping your knowledge and therefore your practice up to date.

> ### REFLECT ON IT
>
> Reflect on the sources of information and support that workers can use to keep their knowledge and working practices in relation to infection prevention and control up to date.

CASE STUDY

Poor practices

Read the following three scenarios and for each one, identify the poor workplace practices that may lead to cross infections, and explain why.

1. Pryce is a community carer. Because he wants to arrive at each of his clients on time, he always wears gloves and an apron but does not always have time to wash his hands before and after each client.

2. Eddie is a residential care worker. When using lifting equipment at work, such as hoists, although he checks it is working correctly, he does not clean it before each use but always cleans it afterwards.

3. Matilda works in a creche. Although she is not feeling well, she decides to go into work because she does not want to let her manager and the children down.

AC5.6 Key factors that make it more likely that infections will occur

As you have read, the conditions required for harmful pathogens to multiply as well as poor working practices are contributory factors for the spread of infections in workplaces. There are other factors too that make it more likely that infections will occur in places where care and support are provided. Below are some of the key factors:

1 **Individuals' susceptibility to infections** – some individuals are more susceptible to infections than others. For example:
   - Babies and children have immature **immune systems**, which means that as they are not fully developed, they will have less protection against infection.
   - Older individuals' immune systems become less effective with age and therefore their bodies will be more susceptible to infections.
   - Individuals who are unwell will have weakened immune systems that have been damaged through illness such as cancer or treatment such as chemotherapy, and therefore their immune systems will be less effective in fighting off infections.

2 **Communal environments** – places such as hospitals, GP surgeries and care homes that are shared by people who have immature, ineffective or weakened immune systems can be perfect breeding grounds for harmful pathogens to multiply very quickly. Infections can be spread directly via individuals and workers but also through shared areas such as living areas and bathrooms.

3 **High risk work activities** – many work activities in health and social care settings can be high risk in terms of making it more likely that infections will occur. For example:
   - In a hospital where an individual is having a surgical operation, the open wound could be an entry route into the body for a harmful pathogen.
   - In an individual's home where a carer is assisting an individual with personal care tasks such as washing, dressing, grooming, they will come into close contact with the individual and their bodily fluids.

Always be vigilant and report any changes you may notice in the individuals you provide care and support to; doing so may prevent infections spreading. Take care of your own health too and do not continue working if you are unwell. Above all, follow your employer's infection prevention and control procedures: remember, it is your duty of care to safeguard individuals from danger and harm.

KEY TERM

Immune system: the body's natural defences that work together to fight disease and infections.

AC5.7 Key legislation and standards related to infection prevention and control

Key legislation

The key legislation related to infection prevention and control include the Control of Substances Hazardous to Health Regulations (COSHH) (2002), as well as the health and safety legislation you learnt about in AC1.1.

RESEARCH IT

Review your learning in AC1.1 of health and safety legislation. For each piece of legislation, find out how it relates to infection prevention and control. Discuss your findings with someone you know.

In March 2020, due to the threat of danger and harm to life posed by the COVID-19 pandemic, the Welsh Government introduced the Coronavirus Act 2020 (Commencement No. 1) (Wales) Regulations 2020.

This Act gave public authorities legal duties to prevent and control risks to people's health and well-being from the spread of the COVID-19 infection in Wales.

Restrictions imposed under the Act included:

- restricting how many people and households could meet up together indoors
- prohibiting people from entering or leaving Wales
- requiring people and those who come into contact with them who test positive for coronavirus to isolate from others

- requiring places where people come together, such as shops, to put in place safety measures such as limiting contact with others by maintaining a distance of 2 metres from others, wearing face coverings over the nose and mouth, and maintaining hygiene and cleaning procedures.

Over time the rules may be updated as knowledge develops though the pandemic.

Standards

In addition to legislation, there are also recognised published standards or codes of practice and guidance that have been put in place to prevent and control the spread of infections. Table 6.8 provides information about examples of some of these.

Standard	How it relates to infection prevention and control
NICE Quality Standard 6.1 Infection Prevention & Control April 2014	This quality standard is for the prevention and control of infection for people receiving healthcare in settings such as hospitals, GP surgeries, dental clinics, care homes, individuals' own homes, schools, prisons and care delivered by the ambulance service and mental health services. This quality standard is needed because healthcare-associated infections affect people of all ages including those with and without clinical conditions and those that care for individuals, such as workers, individuals' families. The purpose of this quality standard is to: • reduce infection rates for healthcare-associated infections • prevent people dying unnecessarily • ensure people have a positive care experience and are treated and cared for in a safe environment where they are safeguarded from harm. The standard is available at: **www.nice.org.uk/guidance/qs61/resources/infection-prevention-and-control-pdf-2098782603205**
WHO Clean Care is Safer Care: Five Moments for Hand Hygiene	This guidance produced by WHO is for the prevention and control of infection and applies to all care settings. The purpose of this guidance is to set out the five moments or steps involved in good hand hygiene. The guidance defines the five moments for hand hygiene as: 1 before contact with individuals 2 before any work task 3 after any task where you've come into contact with bodily fluids 4 after contact with individuals 5 after contact with the individual's environment, for example, items, furniture belonging to the individual. The guidance is available at: **www.who.int/gpsc/tools/Pocket-Leaflet.pdf?ua=1**
Standard Infection Control Precautions (SICPS) Public Health Wales (2013)	This guidance sets out the essential infection prevention and control measures that need to be in place to reduce the spread of infections. This guidance applies to all care settings at all times to all individuals, whether or not they have an infection, to safeguard everyone who lives, works in or visits care settings. This guidance sets out measures in relation to: • assessing infection risks • hand, respiratory and cough hygiene • PPE, care equipment, care environment, linen • blood and body fluid spillages • safe disposal of waste (including **sharps**) • prevention and exposure to risks management including sharps. The guidance is available at: **Chapter 1 Standard Infection Control Precautions (SICPs) - Public Health Wales** **https://phw.nhs.wales/services-and-teams/harp/infection-prevention-and-control/nipcm/chapter-1-standard-infection-control-precautions-sicps/**

▲ Table 6.8 Infection prevention and control standards

Standard	How it relates to infection prevention and control
Welsh Healthcare Associated Infection Programme procedure No 6 – management of blood and bodily fluid spillages (WAG 2009)	This guidance is for all those involved in the provision of care. It sets out the key infection prevention and control practices and procedures to be followed across nine areas. Procedure 6 provides guidance on the safe practices to follow when managing blood and bodily fluid spillages. This procedures provides guidance in relation to: • training and vaccinations of staff (such as hepatitis B vaccination) • dealing with spillages (immediate, safe disposal of waste) • use of PPE • cleaning practices. The guidance is available at: **www.wales.nhs.uk/sites3/documents/379/PHW_SpillPolicy_20100322_V1.pdf**
All Wales NHS Dress Code, Free to Lead, Free to Care (2007) (as amended 2010)	This code of practice is for all NHS staff. It is aimed at ensuring NHS staff present a professional, smart image that inspires confidence and at the same time controls the spread of infections. The code includes key principles to follow, including: • ensuring clothes worn in the workplace are clean and tidy • not wearing wrist watches or false nails (which can harbour harmful pathogens) • not wearing an NHS uniform outside of the workplace when socialising • wearing short sleeves (to enable effective hand washing) • comfortable clothing and footwear. The code of practice is available at: **https://gov.wales/sites/default/files/publications/2019-03/all-wales-nhs-dress-code-free-to-lead-free-to-care.pdf**

▲ Table 6.8 Infection prevention and control standards *(continued)*

KEY TERM

Sharps: equipment that is sharp and may cause an injury by cutting or pricking the skin, such as needles and syringes.

CASE STUDY

Infection control standards

Martine works in a homeless shelter and is updating the workplace guidance for the prevention and control of infections. She wants to include useful codes of practice and standards.

Discussion points:

- Discuss an example of a relevant code of practice.
- Discuss an example of a relevant standard.
- Discuss an example of a relevant piece of guidance.

AC5.8 The roles and responsibilities of employers, workers and others for infection prevention and control

In your workplace you, your employer and others have a vital role to play in preventing cross infections and controlling their spread.

Employers' roles and responsibilities

1 **To provide information on infection prevention and control to workers, individuals and others who visit.** For example:
   - by displaying hand washing posters above sinks
   - providing information leaflets on infection prevention to workers and visitors
   - maintaining accurate records of any infection outbreaks.

2 **To provide education to workers, individuals and others who visit.** For example:
- developing infection prevention and control procedures and ensuring these are followed
- training staff on recognising the symptoms of illness such as COVID-19, and the actions to take if a person in the workplace develops symptoms
- providing updates on changes to legislation (such as when the Coronavirus Act made the use of face masks a requirement when providing care to an individual)
- monitoring work practices to ensure they are safe and comply with legislation and guidance in place.

3 **To provide free of charge equipment and facilities.** For example:
- making available PPE such as face masks, gloves and aprons to workers
- testing workers for COVID-19
- providing access to hand washing facilities and hand sanitisers.

Workers' roles and responsibilities

1 **To follow the employer's agreed ways of working.** For example, reading and understanding:
- the workplace's infection prevention and control procedures, such as those in relation to the use of PPE and the safe disposal of waste
- changes or updates to legislation, such as those in relation to the Coronavirus Act 2020.

2 **To attend training provided by the employer.** For example:
- learning from the training provided
- applying learning from training received to day-to-day work practices, to comply with the employer's procedures and set a good example to others in the workplace.

3 **To record and report.** For example:
- recording all potential and actual infection hazards and risks immediately (such as a broken sharps waste bin that cannot be used)
- reporting all potential and actual infection hazards (such as reporting if you become unwell with an infection such as COVID-19).

Others' roles and responsibilities

1 **To follow the employer's agreed ways of working.** For example:
- reading and understanding the workplace's infection prevention and control procedures, such as those in relation to hand washing and visiting.

During the COVID-19 pandemic, individuals' families were unable to visit their relatives in care settings to reduce the risk of spreading the virus.

2 **To have an up-to-date knowledge of infection prevention and control.** For example:
- asking the employer for information and guidance
- asking questions if there is something they do not understand.

3 **To report all potential and actual infection hazards and risks immediately.** For example:
- if they observe a worker or visitor not using an effective hand washing technique
- if they or someone they have come into contact with has been unwell. By everyone working together, infections can be prevented.

AC5.9 Ways of maintaining a clean environment to prevent the spread of infection

As you will have learnt earlier in this unit, the perfect breeding grounds for harmful pathogens include damp and dirty environments. Maintaining a clean environment removes harmful pathogens and therefore reduces cross infections.

Maintaining a clean environment in the workplace includes cleaning the building, the furniture and fixtures, as well as other work equipment you and others may use. You can maintain a clean environment and prevent the spread of infection by:

- **carrying out regular maintenance** – maintain and keep clean the building's doors, windows, lights, chairs, tables, wall shelves and cupboards.

- **having in place cleaning schedules** – prevent a build-up of dust and dirt by following weekly and monthly cleaning schedules for cleaning rooms, toilets, bathrooms, kitchens, dining areas; vacuuming carpets; mopping floors.
- **increasing cleaning when needed** – when there is a spillage on the floor, or after an individual has used the shower, toilet or hoist.
- **maintaining cleaning equipment** – regularly change cloths, washing and changing mop heads; clean vacuum brushes and change their filters; colour-code equipment according to the area it has been used in, such as kitchen, bathroom, bedroom, laundry area.
- **following manufacturers' instructions** – when using cleaning detergents, follow the instruction to mix it with warm or hot water, or to rinse off after it is used.
- **using decontamination techniques** – **clean** a bathroom floor using hot water and detergent; rinse the detergent off afterwards and leave the floor to air dry; **disinfect** a commode by using a chemical cleaning agent as per the manufacturer's instructions; **sterilise** babies' bottles using heat (boiling water or steam).

KEY TERMS

Decontamination: cleaning to a high standard, to remove or reduce harmful pathogens and therefore the spread of infection.

Clean: the decontamination technique used for low infection risk items, such as floors and furniture.

Disinfect: the decontamination technique used for medium infection risk items, such as bedpans and bottles.

Sterilise: the decontamination technique used for high infection risk items, such as medical instruments used for surgery.

AC5.10 The importance of good personal hygiene to prevent the spread of infection

Maintaining your personal hygiene to a good standard and supporting individuals to do the same is not only more pleasant for everyone but is also essential to prevent the spread of infection. Table 6.9 gives examples of good personal hygiene.

Area of personal hygiene	Procedures to avoid spread of infection
Hair care	• Regularly wash and brush hair • Tie back long hair when supporting individuals and carrying out work activities such as preparing food, to prevent unwanted hairs from falling into food or spreading infection.
Hand and nail care	• Keep nails clean and short. • Do not wear rings and bracelets that may harbour dirt. • Do not wear nail varnish or nail extensions as they may come off. • Use essential hand washing techniques as described in AC5.11.
Oral care	Brush teeth regularly to avoid mouth fungal infections such as oral thrush and halitosis (bad breath).
Body care	• Wash, shower or bathe every day. • Regularly clean and change clothes to prevent unpleasant body odour and the spread of infection to others.
Skin care	• Keep your skin moisturised, so that it does not become dry and flake off. • Treat and cover skin wounds and rashes to reduce the risk of infection.
Clothing/uniform	• Keep work clothes clean: wash regularly at the correct temperature to destroy harmful pathogens. • Do not wear work clothes outside work to prevent the spread of infection to others. You will find it useful to refer to the All Wales NHS Dress Code, Free to Lead, Free to Care (2007) (as amended 2010).

▲ Table 6.9 How personal hygiene can avoid the spread of infection

AC5.11 Hand washing techniques used to prevent the spread of infection

A key part of good personal hygiene and one of the most effective ways of preventing the spread of infection in health and social care settings is through good **hand washing techniques**. The NHS recommends that you should follow the following steps when washing your hands and that you should wash your hands for the amount of time it takes to sing 'Happy Birthday' twice (around 20 seconds):

1 Wet your hands with water (it should be warm – if it is too hot or too cold, you are less likely to wash your hands for the recommended duration of 20 seconds).
2 Apply enough soap to cover your hands, back and front.
3 Rub your hands together (palm to palm).
4 Use one hand to rub the back of the other hand and clean in between the fingers. Do the same with the other hand.
5 Rub your hands together and clean in between your fingers.
6 Rub the back of your fingers against your palms.
7 Rub your thumb using your other hand. Do the same with the other thumb.
8 Rub the tips of your fingers on the palm of your other hand. Do the same with other hand.
9 Rinse your hands with warm water (having warm water will ensure that you rinse your hands fully).
10 Dry your hands completely with a disposable towel.
11 Use the disposable towel to turn off the tap (to reduce the risk of transferring pathogens on the taps to your hands).

(NHS, *Healthy body: How to wash your hands*, March 2020)

This NHS guidance is also accompanied with a video titled 'How to wash your hands' and can be accessed on this page:

www.nhs.uk/live-well/healthy-body/best-way-to-wash-your-hands/

In health and social care settings, it is also recommended that hand washing must take place:

- before and after you start work
- before and after contact with every individual
- before putting on and after disposing of PPE
- before and after handling raw foods such as meat and vegetables
- before and after handling food
- before and after eating
- before and after treating a cut or wound
- after contact with your own or individuals' and others' bodily fluids
- before changing a nappy
- before and after smoking
- after going to the toilet or changing a nappy
- after coughing, sneezing or blowing your nose
- after disposing of waste or handling used or soiled linen
- after coming into contact with clinical waste (that contains bodily fluids)
- after touching pets, their food and cleaning their beds or cages (individuals living at home may have pets).

KEY TERM

Hand washing techniques: techniques that meet current national and international guidelines; for example, *Clean Care is Safer Care: Five Moments for Hand Hygiene*, published by WHO.

AC5.12 The use of PPE used to prevent the spread of infection

In health and social care settings, PPE refers to equipment that is worn by workers to protect against the spread of infection. PPE can prevent the spread of infection because it:

- protects individuals from infections you may be carrying
- protects you from infections individuals may be carrying
- creates a barrier between the infection and you, which means that it cannot spread from you to others or vice versa, or from a surface or piece of equipment touched by you or others.

To be effective in the spread of infection, you must use PPE correctly. You can do this by:

- reading and following your employer's procedures for using PPE
- reading and following the manufacturer's instructions when using PPE
- washing your hands before using and disposing of PPE.

Tables 6.10 and 6.11 provide you with additional information about why, when and how to use the three main examples of PPE used in health and social care settings.

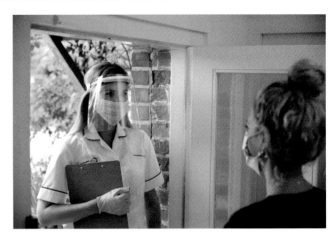

▲ Figure 6.6 How can PPE prevent the spread of infection?

Type of PPE	Why use it	Examples of when to use it
Disposable gloves	To provide a barrier from contact with pathogens and to reduce the risk of passing on any pathogens you are carrying on your hands.	When dealing with an accident, because you will come into contact with bodily fluids such as blood and vomit.
Disposable plastic aprons	To provide a barrier for the pathogens that can be spread on clothing.	When handling food, because you will come into contact with both raw and cooked foods.
Surgical face masks	To provide a barrier for the pathogens that can be spread through breath from your nose and mouth.	When supporting individuals with personal care, because you will come into close contact with them.

▲ Table 6.10 Why and when to use PPE

Type of PPE	Putting it on	Taking it off
Disposable gloves	• Ensure the gloves are the correct size. If they are too tight, they may tear; too loose and they may come off. • Wash your hands before putting them on.	• Remove one glove at a time. • Hold the outside of the glove with your opposite gloved hand and peel it off so it turns inside out and place it balled in your gloved hand. • Then, taking care not to touch the outside of the glove, place your finger tip inside the other glove and peel this one off so the first glove ends up inside it. • Dispose of the gloves in the allocated bin. Wash and dry your hands.
Disposable plastic aprons	• Wash your hands before putting them on, to prevent harmful pathogens getting onto the apron. • Place the apron over your head and then tie it round your waist to prevent the transport of pathogens from/onto your clothing.	• Unfasten or break the ties round the waste. Remove the apron by pulling it away from your neck and only touching the inside of the apron while doing so. • Roll up the apron and dispose of it in the allocated bin. Wash and dry your hands.
Surgical face masks	• Wash your hands before putting them on to prevent harmful pathogens getting onto the mask. • Place the mask over your nose and mouth, and minimise any gaps between the mask and your face. • Avoid touching the front of the mask. Use the ear loops to put it on.	• Remove the mask by using one ear loop at the time and moving the mask away from your face. Avoid touching the mask. • Dispose of the mask in the allocated bin. Wash and dry your hands.

▲ Table 6.11 How to use PPE

Remember that some individuals may not understand why you are using PPE. They may think it looks frightening, or that you think they are dirty.

So, it is important to explain to every individual why it needs to be worn and how it prevents the spread of infection.

CASE STUDY

Mina is a care worker and has been recruited by a local home care agency to provide support to Hari, who lives in his own home. Previously Mina has worked as a care worker in residential care homes, and is aware of the infection prevention and control procedures to follow for this type of environment, but is unsure how to prevent and control the spread of infection when someone lives in their own home.

Discussion points:

- Imagine you are the manager of the local home care agency and you are responsible for providing Mina with information and guidance on infection prevention and control. What guidance would you give her in relation to infection control? Why?
- Do you think there may be any differences between working practices in relation to the spread of infection in a residential care home and in an individual's home? How would you prevent the spread of infection at home?

LO6 KNOW HOW TO IMPLEMENT FOOD SAFETY MEASURES

GETTING STARTED

One of the environments that harmful pathogens can exist and multiply in is food. Knowing about food hygiene and how to implement food safety measures is therefore very important for preventing cross infections.

Think about an occasion when you or someone you know had **food poisoning**. What caused it?

KEY TERM

Food poisoning: an illness affecting the stomach and illness, caused by eating food that has been contaminated with harmful pathogens. Symptoms include nausea, vomiting, diarrhoea.

AC6.1 Key legislation for food safety

Table 6.12 sets out the key legislation for this area.

Legislation	Explanation
Food Safety Act 1990	This is the main piece of legislation that governs the safety of food. It requires: • good personal hygiene when preparing and cooking, serving meals and supporting individuals with eating • keeping records of where food is from, so it can be traced if needed • keeping records of when unsafe food has been removed.
Food Hygiene (Wales) Regulations 2006	This sets out the legal responsibilities of employers and workers for food safety, including having food safety procedures in place, such as: • carrying out and recording temperature control checks to prevent harmful pathogens from developing • following food hygiene requirements • keeping records. Failure to comply with these regulations could result in a fine or imprisonment.
Food Information (Wales) Regulations 2014	These regulations set out the labelling requirements for food that is sold, including information about additives, allergies and nutritional information. Being aware of food labelling when supporting individuals with eating and drinking and, in some cases, preparing and cooking meals is important for their health and safety.
Food Standards Agency (FSA)	This is an independent agency responsible for food safety and food hygiene in England, Wales and Northern Ireland to safeguard the public from harm from food. In 2010, the FSA established the Food Hygiene Rating Scheme to provide information to the public about food hygiene standards in businesses, including in health and social care settings.

▲ Table 6.12 Key legislation for food safety

AC6.2 The roles and responsibilities of employers and workers for food safety

AC6.3 The importance of implementing food safety measures

Food safety is the joint responsibility of both employers and workers in the workplace. Having food safety measures in place and implementing these is essential for complying with the law and safeguarding people from danger and harm by keeping food safe.

Table 6.13 sets out some of the main roles and responsibilities of employers and workers for food safety, and why it is important to implement them.

Role and responsibilities of employers	Role and responsibilities of workers	Importance of implementing food safety measures
Having food safety procedures in place in relation to preparing, cooking, reheating, cooling and storing food – such as in relation to defrosting food – and making sure these are provided to and understood by workers.	Complying with the employer's food safety procedures – such as placing food in the fridge to defrost.	Harmful pathogens can grow in food that is not defrosted thoroughly. Placing food in the fridge ensures food is defrosted at a safe temperature.
Having food hygiene procedures in place in relation to preparing, cooking, reheating, cooling and storing food – such as provision of hand washing facilities, equipment, ventilation, bins.	Complying with the employer's food hygiene procedures, such as: • washing hands before and after touching or handling food • wearing clean clothes and PPE such as apron and gloves • not coughing or sneezing over food • covering cuts with a dressing.	Good personal hygiene (see AC5.10 and AC5.11 for more information) is essential for preventing the spread of infection, and preventing individuals and others from becoming unwell.
Having a system in place for carrying out and recording food safety and hygiene checks completed – keep records of safe practices such as • temperature control checks • when practices go wrong and the actions taken • maintenance checks of equipment such as fridges and freezers.	Complying with the employer's food safety and hygiene checks, such as: • carrying out hourly temperature checks of food items • cleaning equipment before and after use • reporting any faults with equipment to your employer immediately.	Ensuring that employers and employees are complying with the law and following safe methods. Implementing these food safety measures will be reflected in the food hygiene rating that must be displayed in Wales at the entrance of the building where it can be seen. Following an inspection from the FSA, a rating will be given, ranging from 5 where hygiene standards are very good, to 0 where urgent improvement is required.

▲ Table 6.13 Employers' and workers' responsibilities for food safety and their importance

---

REFLECT ON IT

Reflect on the importance of implementing food safety measures in the workplace as well as the consequences of not doing so.
- Who could be affected?
- How are they affected?

AC6.4 Food safety hazards that can occur through the preparation, serving, clearing away and storing of food and drink

AC6.5 Reasons for keeping surfaces, utensils and equipment clean for food preparation

AC6.6 When PPE should be used

Maintaining good hygiene in kitchens and other areas where food is handled (including keeping surfaces, utensils and equipment clean and wearing PPE) will prevent harmful pathogens from being transmitted between surfaces, equipment and people.

When safe practices are not implemented in terms of food safety and hygiene, there is a risk that harmful pathogens can multiply and spread when food and drink are being prepared, served, cleared away and stored, causing illnesses such as food poisoning.

Examples of these safe practices include:

- preparation
- serving
- clearing away
- storing.

Preparation

- Wash your hands before and after preparing food.
- Wear PPE such as an apron, hair covering and gloves.
- Follow instructions on food packaging when preparing food, such as rinsing all salads and vegetables under cold water.
- Ensure prepared food is within the sell-by and use-by-date as per the packaging, to reduce the risk of harmful pathogens.
- Ensure separate utensils such as knives and other items such as chopping boards are used for different foods such as meat, fish and vegetables, to avoid contamination with harmful pathogens.

- Always follow cooking and thawing instructions for all frozen foods.
- Ensure food, including pre-cooked and frozen meals, has been cooked at the correct temperature to ensure it is hot all the way through, so that harmful pathogens are destroyed.
- Do not reheat leftover food or meals more than once, so as to destroy harmful pathogens and prevent illness such as food poisoning.

Serving

- Wash your hands before and after serving food.
- Wear PPE when serving food, such as an apron and gloves to protect your clothes, and the food and drink from harmful pathogens.
- Do not cough or sneeze over food and drink you're serving.
- Let your employer know if you feel unwell, to avoid the spread of infection.

Clearing away

- Wash your hands before and after clearing away.
- Wear PPE when clearing away food and drink, such as an apron and gloves, to prevent transmission of harmful pathogens.
- Wipe clean any spillages and safely dispose of leftover food or drink items in waste bins.
- Use the recommended cleaning agent for keeping kitchen surfaces and food trays clean, to avoid contamination with harmful pathogens.
- Wash all used utensils, cups, plates, glasses in the dishwasher in a residential care home, or in the sink with hot water and detergent in an individual's home.

Storing

- Wash your hands before and after storing food and drink, and wear PPE.
- Clean the inside and outside of fridges and freezers, and carry out regular temperature checks to prevent dirt and harmful pathogens from multiplying.
- Cover all food and drink placed in the fridge to avoid spillages onto other items.
- Ensure cooked food is cool before storing it in the fridge or freezer, to reduce the likelihood of harmful pathogens growing.

- Store foods such as meat on the bottom shelf in the fridge to avoid it contaminating other food, by meat juices dripping onto other items.

See AC6.7 for more information on safe practices for storing food.

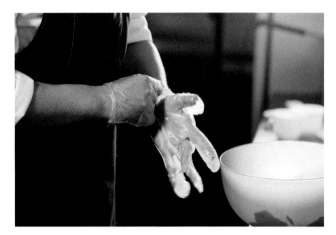

▲ Figure 6.7 Food safety and hygiene

RESEARCH IT

Food poisoning can have severe consequences for individuals who have immature or weakened immune systems such as babies, children, older individuals and individuals who are unwell. Research the dangers and their consequences.

AC6.7 Safe storage of food and drink

Contamination of food with harmful pathogens is also likely to take place if food and drink are not stored safely.

- Keep all storage areas such as cupboards, fridges, freezers clean and free from dirt, leaks/spillages. This will prevent the growth of harmful pathogens and infestations of pests such as rats and cockroaches that can carry harmful pathogens.
- Store food items and drinks in containers intended for their use. Make sure they are not damaged or broken, otherwise they could become contaminated with air, pests that carry diseases and harmful pathogens.
- Regularly rotate all food items and drinks, with oldest dates to the front so that these are used first. Check for the expiry of sell-by and used-by dates, to prevent contamination with harmful pathogens.

- Store all food items and drinks in the correct conditions and as per the manufacturer's instructions – such as in a cool, ventilated area, away from sunlight, in the fridge, in the freezer, at room temperature. Not doing so may mean that the items become contaminated with harmful pathogens. (See also AC6.4 for more information.)

AC6.8 Safe disposal of food waste

Contamination of food waste can also occur if it is not disposed of safely. Follow these guidelines:

- Clear away and dispose of leftover food waste in the bin.
- Do not leave leftover food waste on surfaces such as kitchen worktops and floors, where it can contaminate equipment and people who come into contact with these surfaces.
- Empty bins regularly to avoid food waste overflowing onto the floor and contaminating the area with harmful pathogens.
- Always wash your hands after disposing of food waste.

CASE STUDY

Marco is working as a kitchen assistant in the hospital and has received a complaint from a patient that the meal they were served was cold in the middle and was served on a dirty food tray. Marco is very upset because he usually has very high standards, but thinks his work standards may be affected because he has not been feeling very well.

Discussion points:
- What are the food safety hazards of this situation?
- What actions could be taken to address these?

Check your understanding

1 Name two differences between bacteria and viruses.
2 Name two poor practices that can lead to the spread of infections in the workplace.
3 Give two examples of how to store food and drink safely.

Question practice

1 What is the meaning of a systemic infection?

   a an infection that affects all of the human body

   b an infection caused by bacteria

   c an infection caused by viruses

   d an infection that affects one specific area of the human body

2 Which of the following does not help to prevent the spread of infection in the workplace?

   a hand and nail care

   b good hand washing techniques

   c not taking precautions when supporting individuals with their pets

   d wearing and using disposable gloves

3 What is the main piece of legislation for food safety and hygiene?

   a The Food Safety Act 1980

   b The Food Safety Act 1990

   c The Food Safety Act 2006

   d The Food Safety Act 2014

4 When should PPE be used?

   a when preparing food only

   b when preparing and serving food only

   c when preparing, serving, clearing away and storing food only

   d when preparing, serving and clearing away food only

LO7 KNOW HOW TO STORE, USE AND DISPOSE OF HAZARDOUS SUBSTANCES SAFELY

GETTING STARTED

Think about cleaning agents you use that may be a danger to your health if you don't follow their instructions and use them correctly.

How can they affect your health?

AC7.1 The term 'hazardous substances'

AC7.2 The term 'Control of Hazardous Substances'

AC7.3 Types of hazardous substances that may be found in the workplace

Health and care settings are environments where different types of substances can become a hazard to people's health if they are not stored, used and disposed of safely. Knowing the safe practices to follow means you will be safeguarding individuals, workers and others in the workplace from danger and harm.

Hazardous substances are substances that have the potential to cause harm and illness to others. Examples of types of hazardous substances that can be found in health and social care settings include:

- cleaning agents
- cleaning materials such as cloths
- medication
- bodily fluids
- used dressings
- PPE
- towels
- clothes
- bed linen that has come into contact with bodily fluids.

The term 'Control of Hazardous Substances' refers to the management systems that must be put in place by employers and the procedures that must be followed by employees for the safe storage, use and disposal of hazardous substances, to prevent incidents and ill-health in the workplace.

RESEARCH IT

The Control of Substances Hazardous to Health Regulations (COSHH) (2002) that you learnt about in AC1.1 requires employers to control hazardous substances. It classifies hazardous substances into different types depending on the dangers they pose – toxic, very toxic, corrosive, harmful or irritant.

- Research the meaning of these types.
- Design a poster with your findings.

AC7.4 Safe practices for storing, using, dealing with spillages and disposing of hazardous substances

COSHH (2002) requires employers to have procedures in place for storing, using, dealing with spillages and disposing of hazardous substances safely and employees to comply with these. Table 6.14 includes examples of safe practices to follow

Safe practices	Precautions to take for hazardous substances
Storing substances	• Check *where* they are stored. For example, medication needs to be locked away securely so individuals cannot access it and harm themselves. • Check *how* they are stored. For example, cleaning agents need to be stored at a cool temperature and in a ventilated area, as they may be highly flammable and could cause a fire. • Check they are stored in line with the manufacturer's instructions. For example, store cleaning agents in their original containers, labelled correctly and with their safety lids on, so that individuals do not accidentally mistake them for a drink and swallow them.
Using substances	• Check the information supplied. For example, check the label of the hazardous substance for the COSHH hazard symbol, the **COSHH file** for the precautions to take, and the employer's procedures before using it, so you will use it safely and avoid harm to yourself and others. • Check how to use them. For example, whether PPE must be worn when using the hazardous substance to avoid skin rashes and or burns; whether the hazardous substance must be diluted before use. • Check you are using them securely. For example, medication must not be left unattended, to prevent individuals swallowing it or passing it on, which can lead to illnesses and fatalities; make sure you are not interrupted or distracted when using hazardous substances, to ensure safe practices are followed.
Spillages	• Check the information supplied. For example, check the COSHH file and the employer's procedures for what to do if there is a spillage involving a hazardous substance, including how to record and report it to ensure safe practices are followed. • Check how to deal with the spillage. For example, check how it must be cleaned, with what cleaning agent and who must clean it, to ensure you are working within your responsibilities. • Check you are dealing with spillages. For example, know how to alert others with a warning sign when there is a spillage, and how to maintain the area securely to avoid slips and accidents.
Disposing	• Check where to dispose of them. For example, sharps in a sharps box to prevent needle stick injuries; waste that contains body fluids in a clinical waste bag separate to the general waste in a care home to avoid contamination; waste that contains body fluids double-bagged in the general waste in an individual's home to prevent cross infection. • Check how to dispose of them. For example, wash your hands after disposal of hazardous substances such as soiled bed linen; wear PPE to prevent harmful pathogens being transported from one place/ person to another. • Check you are disposing of them safely. For example, check what actions must be taken if you or others are exposed to them; and how to report and record what has happened.

▲ Table 6.14 Safe practices for hazardous substances

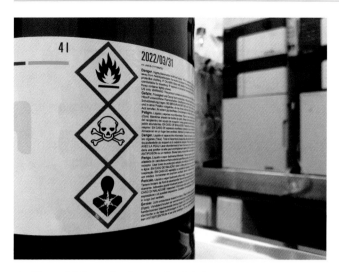

▲ Figure 6.8 Example of a warning label

KEY TERM

COSHH file: the records that must be kept by employers in relation to the storage, use and disposal of hazardous substances.

REFLECT ON IT

Reflect on the importance of following safe practices in health and social care settings when spillages of hazardous substances happen.

CASE STUDY

Gwen works in a care home and is administering medication this morning to individuals. As Gwen gives an individual their tablets in a medication cup, her colleague runs down the corridor calling for help, as a visitor has fallen over in the corridor. Gwen immediately leaves the individual with their medication and the unlocked medication trolley in the corridor, and goes to help her colleague.

Discussion points:

- Has Gwen followed safe practices when administering medication?
- What are the consequences of Gwen's actions?
- What actions should Gwen have taken?

LO8 KNOW HOW TO MAINTAIN SECURITY IN THE WORK SETTING

GETTING STARTED

Think about an occasion when you visited a workplace and you were asked who you were – your name, the purpose of your visit.

- Why was this necessary?
- What could have been the consequences of not doing so?

AC8.1 Potential risks to security in the work setting

Health and social care settings are workplaces as well as environments where individuals live and people visit. It is important to be aware of the potential risks to security to ensure these settings are kept safe for everyone.

Examples of potential risks to security in the work setting include:

- bogus visitors claiming to be workers or contractors but whose intentions are to steal or cause harm to property and/or people
- security breaches of people's personal information that may lead to unauthorised people having access to sensitive information
- aggressive behaviour from members of the public, which could involve damaging property and causing physical or emotional harm to others.

RESEARCH IT

Research a security breach you have read or heard about in a health or social care work setting in Wales.

- What happened?
- Who did it affect?

AC8.2 Safe practices used to maintain security in the work setting

Maintaining security in the work setting by following safe practices means that you are safeguarding individuals, workers and others from potential harm and danger. Table 6.15 shows the dos and don'ts for maintaining security in the work setting.

Do	Don't
Ask visitors to sign in with their full name, the company they are from, the date and purpose of their visit before they enter the building, checking visitors' proof of identity. Make individuals aware of the precautions to take too.	Don't allow visitors access to the premises if they have not signed in and/or confirmed who they are.
Ask the person requesting information what their role is and why they require the information. Only share information if you have permission to do so.	Don't allow visitors to walk through the premises unescorted, so that they cannot access areas and/or individuals without authorisation.
Follow the employer's procedures for maintaining security in the work setting, such as locking doors and windows, reporting any windows/doors that are broken, keeping door codes and key safe codes safe. In some work settings, visitors may be required to wear a badge so that others are aware of who they are.	Don't carelessly share information with others, such as: - leaving written records unattended in a public area where they can be read by others - speaking to others such as family and friends outside the work setting.
Check with the employer if you are unsure what information about an individual you can share. For example, you may be required to share information about an individual's medical condition with a GP or nurse.	

▲ Table 6.15 Dos and don'ts for maintaining security in the work setting

Lone working

Lone workers are those workers who work by themselves without close or direct supervision, such as people who:

- work from home
- work alone for long periods
- work outside normal working hours
- visit other premises, including care and support workers who visit individuals in their own homes.

Employers are required to have procedures in place to ensure the safety of lone workers. These involve:

- Following the employer's lone working procedures – such as carrying a personal alarm to call for help, phoning when you arrive at and leave an individual's home so that people know where you are.

- Telling other people where you are – this is important in the event of an emergency such as a fire, but also in case your assistance is needed by another worker.
- Access to work settings – such as signing in and out every time you enter and leave the building, informing a named person if you are working outside office hours, the address of where you'll be and the time you will finish.
- Dealing with incidents of aggressive behaviour from members of the public – such as following the employer's procedures and training in the event of aggressive behaviour, keeping yourself and others safe, calling for help, and reporting and recording all incidents.

Gracie is a lone worker, providing care and support to older people who live in their own homes. At the end of her last call, Gracie receives a message from one of her clients explaining that when she visited her this morning she forgot to give her a very important letter to post and wondered whether Gracie could post it for her this evening. As Gracie is only ten minutes' drive away, she decides to quickly pop into this client's house and post the letter for her. As this will not take long, Gracie decides to not let the office know what she is doing.

Discussion points:

- Do you agree with Gracie's actions? Why?
- What are the potential consequences of Gracie's actions?
- What should have Gracie done in this situation? Why?

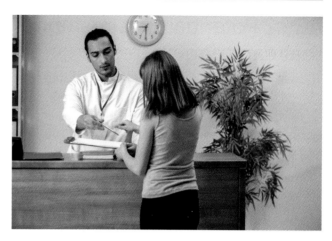

▲ Figure 6.9 What are ways to maintain security in a work setting?

L09 KNOW HOW TO MANAGE STRESS

GETTING STARTED

Think about an occasion when you or someone you know felt stressed.

- What was the cause of the stress?
- What changes did you notice, both emotionally (such as feeling sad and tearful) and physically (such as not sleeping or eating less)?

AC9.1 Common signs and indicators of stress

Stress can happen at any time and to anyone, at work or outside work. Stress affects everyone differently, but being able to recognise the common signs and indicators of stress in yourself is important so that you can get help, and in others so that you can support them.

- **Physical signs and indicators** of stress can include: rapid heartbeat, high blood pressure, being tense, dizzy, nausea, diarrhoea or constipation, headaches and migraines, developing cold sores.

- **Emotional signs and indicators** of stress can include: low moods, feeling irritable, anxiety, unhappiness, anger, an overwhelming sense of being unable to cope.
- **Mental signs and indicators** of stress can include: difficulties with concentration and memory, having radical thoughts such as believing that others around you want to hurt you, being unable to think logically.
- **Behavioural signs and indicators** of stress can include: being unable to sleep or sleeping too much, eating more than usual or eating much less, withdrawing from situations, particularly those that involve speaking with and socialising with others.

RESEARCH IT

- Research what happens in your body when you are stressed; this is commonly referred to as the body's 'fight or flight' response.
- Discuss your findings with someone you know.

AC9.2 Potential circumstances that can trigger stress

The main way of preventing stress developing into something more serious is by being aware of the circumstances that can trigger stress in yourself and others so that you and others are prepared and able to deal with this. This skill is often referred to as resilience.

Examples of potential circumstances that can trigger stress include:

- **changes in financial circumstances** – such as losing your job, being given reduced hours, having unexpected expenditure
- **changes in personal circumstances** – such as being bereaved, divorced, separated
- **changes in work** – such as working longer hours, reduced staff, illness and conditions to manage in individuals
- **ill-health** – such as becoming unwell, supporting others who have become unwell
- **life events** – such as moving house, taking exams, starting a new job.

> **REFLECT ON IT**
>
> Reflect on a situation that makes you stressed. Why is this a trigger to your stress?

AC9.3 Ways to manage stress
AC9.4 The importance of recognising stress and taking action to reduce it

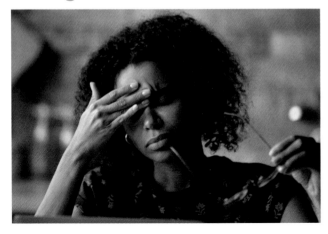

▲ Figure 6.10 Know the signs of your stress

Once you can recognise the indicators and triggers of stress, you can begin to look for ways to manage stress for yourself and others in different circumstances.

Doing so will help you avoid unhelpful ways of managing stress, such as 'comfort' eating, drinking excessive amounts of alcohol and smoking heavily. These can lead to ill-health and illness such as heart attacks and liver cancer.

Recognising stress and taking action to reduce it is important for staying in good physical and mental health. Positive ways of managing stress can include:

- **Being active physically and mentally** – for example, by going for a walk or reading a book after a long shift at work. Both activities can help with reducing your body's stress levels by making you feel calmer and able to think clearly again.
- **Staying positive** – thinking about what positive things have happened rather than what has gone wrong will help you feel more in control and therefore more able to deal with difficult circumstances. If someone close to you has died, think about how they would have wanted you to live your life without them.
- **Being in contact with others** – meeting up and socialising with family and friends can prevent you from becoming isolated. You may be able to share how you are feeling with others.
- **Helping others** can lead to feeling good and positive about yourself, and less likely to think about your own stress.
- **Learning to say 'no'** – by not taking on too much at work or in your personal life, you can remain in control of your limits and reduce your stress.
- **Making time for yourself** – you can feel calmer and put things into perspective by taking time out for yourself to stop and think.
- **Asking for help** – seeking help from others when you need it is a brave thing to do, and can prevent your stress from worsening. You will learn more about what help is available in AC9.5.

AC9.5 Where to access additional support if experiencing stress

Sometimes, no matter what you do, you may still experience the ill-effects of stress. Don't ignore it – get help because stress doesn't just go away.

- At work, you may be able to talk to your employer, manager or someone else who knows you well. They can be good sources of information and suggestions for ways of managing your stress based on their own and others' experiences.
- Your supervision and appraisal meetings with your manager can be positive ways of assessing and reflecting on work situations you've managed well, the techniques you've used and other skills that you can learn. This may help you to manage these situations better or differently.
- External agencies and counsellors can provide help and support over the telephone and in person.
- People who you feel close to and who know you well, such as your family and friends, can also provide you with much needed practical and emotional support. All these sources are excellent ways of reducing your stress and remaining in control of how you think and feel.

Check your understanding

1 Describe two practices for the safe disposal of hazardous substances.
2 Name two security breaches that could happen in the work setting.
3 Describe two practices for safe lone working.
4 Give two examples of sources of support if you are feeling stressed.

Question practice

1 Before using hazardous substances, what information must you check?
   a the label of the hazardous substance only
   b the COSHH file only
   c the employer's procedures only
   d all of the above

2 What checks must you carry out when storing hazardous substances?
   a the temperature that they can be stored at only
   b that the storage area is secure only
   c that you have read the manufacturer's instructions only
   d all of the above

3   Which of the following are safe practices to follow when receiving visitors?

   a   Ask the visitor for their name only.

   b   Ask the visitor for their name, signature and purpose of their visit.

   c   Ask the visitor for the purpose of their visit only.

   d   Ask the visitor for their name and signature only.

4   Which of the following are unsafe practices to follow when sharing information?

   a   Check the identity of the person requesting the information.

   b   Speak to others about an individual when out shopping.

   c   Write records in a private office.

   d   Maintain records in a locked cupboard.

5   Which of the following are common signs and indicators of stress?

   a   dizziness, unable to concentrate, feeling anxious only

   b   not sleeping, feeling unable to cope, low moods only

   c   eating less, being unable to think logically, nausea only

   d   all of the above

6   Which of the following can be a positive way of managing your stress?

   a   not talking to anyone

   b   comfort eating

   c   making time for yourself

   d   keeping busy by working hard

FURTHER READING AND RESEARCH

Books and booklets

Health and Safety Executive (2020), *Protecting lone workers: How to manage the risks of working alone.*

(2014), *Health and safety in care homes* (HSG220-2nd edition)

(2014), *Risk assessment: A brief guide to controlling risks in the workplace.*

(2012), *Manual handling at work. A brief guide.*

Weblinks

CIW website for reports on the safety of care services in Wales:
www.careinspectorate.wales

The FSA website for information on food safety and hygiene:
www.food.gov.uk

NHS Wales' website for the e-manual for National Infection Prevention and Control and information about SICPS:
https://phw.nhs.wales/services-and-teams/harp/infection-prevention-and-control/nipcm/

The Welsh Government's website for information about current and relevant health and safety, legislation including the Coronavirus Act 2020, and food safety legislation:
www.wales.nhs.uk

Glossary

Abuse when someone is mistreated in a way that causes them pain and hurt.

Accidents unexpected and unintentional events that cause damage or personal injury, such as a fall.

Accurate records contain factually correct information.

Active listening a communication technique that involves understanding and interpreting what is being expressed through verbal and non-verbal communication.

Active monitoring monitoring the condition but not treating unless proven that condition is worsening.

Active offer providing a service in Welsh without someone having to ask for it.

Active participation the Code of Professional Practice for Social Care defined active participation as a way of working that regards individuals as 'active partners in their own care rather than passive recipients. Active participation recognises each individual's right to participate in the activities and relationships of everyday life as independently as possible'.

Advance care planning the plan an individual will create stating the care they wish to receive at the end stage of life.

Advance directive also referred to as a living will, this is a legal document detailing the actions to take at the end stage of life.

Advocacy a service which provides representation to people for purposes relating to their care and support.

Aggressive behaviour may range from verbal to physical abuse, and cause physical or emotional harm to others.

Agreed ways of working the policies and procedures set out by your employer for your work setting.

Allegations when an individual or another person tells you that they are being abused or that abuse is happening.

Alleged abuse when an individual says that they are being abused, without you knowing whether or not this is true.

Anaemic a decrease of haemoglobin in the blood.

Anosmia loss of smell.

Anxiety a feeling of fear or worry that may be mild or serious and can lead to physical symptoms, such as shakiness.

Aphasia a condition that affects a person's speech, understanding and use of language. This condition can cause difficulties in putting words together to form sentences.

Arts music, dance, drama, painting, drawing, sculpture, photography and crafts.

Asperger's syndrome a disability that affects how individuals interact with others. They may have difficulty understanding and relating to other people, and taking part in day-to-day activities.

Assessing the risks identifying dangers with the potential to cause harm, deciding on the level of risk and putting in place processes for reducing or controlling these risks.

Assessment a way of finding out what help and support a person needs. This will be different for each person.

Assistive technology aids, devices and equipment that can support an individual with disabilities to actively participate in their lives.

Asthma a lung condition that causes breathing difficulties that can range from mild to severe.

Asylum seeker a person who escapes from their home country because of fear or danger and seeks refuge and safety in another country.

Autistic spectrum disorder a lifelong condition that affects how a person perceives the world and interacts with others. For example, they may have difficulties interacting and socialising with others or expressing emotion.

Bariatric equipment aids specifically manufactured to assist individuals who are obese with moving and positioning.

Bath lift this assists individuals to get in and out of the bath.

Building rapport establishing a connection with someone. This usually takes place at the start of a relationship. It is based on mutual trust and involves finding common ground. Showing you understand someone and listening to them establishes rapport.

Care and support plan this is developed by a social worker, the individual who needs support and their family/carer. It identifies what matters to the individual, and what help the individual needs in order for them to be as independent as possible, to ensure their well-being, achieve personal outcomes and support their development.

Carer a person who provides or intends to provide care for an adult or disabled child. For the purposes of the Act, the person is not a carer if they provide care under a contract or as voluntary work.

Cerebral palsy a condition that causes lifelong conditions affecting movement. It is caused by a problem with the brain before, after or during birth.

Child-centred care and support making sure children and young people receive care and support that meets their individual needs.

Child development the sequence of language, physical, emotional and thought changes that occur from childhood to adulthood.

Clean the decontamination technique used for low infection risk items, such as floors and furniture.

Communication how we interact with others.

Communication methods different ways of communicating, such as verbally, in writing, non-verbal communication, using digital technologies.

Compassion this is central to keeping individuals' personal information secure, as doing so shows your kindness towards individuals in upholding their rights to dignity, respect and being taken seriously.

Competence to effectively apply the knowledge, skills and behaviours you have learnt.

Complete records contain full details and all the information that is necessary.

Compulsorily detained this means being held in hospital and given treatment, whether or not you agree with it, because of concerns for own safety and/or that of others.

Confidentiality to keep something private or secret.

Consent when someone agrees to something. You will need to obtain 'consent' or permission from an individual, or their representative if the individual is unable to.

Continence the ability to control movements of the bowels and bladder. A continent individual knows when they need the toilet and uses it.

COPD (chronic obstructive pulmonary disease) a group of lung conditions that result in long-term breathing difficulties.

COSHH file the records that must be kept by employers in relation to the storage, use and disposal of hazardous substances.

COVID-19 pandemic also known as the coronavirus disease pandemic. It is caused by a virus that was first identified in 2019 and spread globally around the world.

Cultural needs the particular traditions, customs and values shared by a group of people or society.

Cyber bullying bullying carried out through computers, phones and other electronic devices.

Deafblind manual alphabet a method of spelling out words on an individual's hand by using signs and certain places on the hand.

Deafblindness a combination of hearing and sight loss which affects the individual's ability to communicate, impacts on their mobility and reduces their access to information.

Decontamination cleaning to a high standard, to remove or reduce harmful pathogens and therefore the spread of infection.

Dementia a group of symptoms that affect how you think, remember, solve problems, use language and communicate. These occur when brain cells stop working properly and the brain is damaged by disease.

Dementia friendly community the local community sharing the responsibility for ensuring that people with dementia feel understood, valued and able to contribute.

Depression a medical condition causing low mood that affects your thoughts and feelings. It can range from mild to severe, but usually lasts for a long time and affects day-to-day living.

Diabetes a health condition that occurs when the amount of glucose (sugar) in the blood is too high because the body cannot use it properly.

Digital literacy the ability to read, write, find and evaluate information on any digital platform, such as computers, mobile phones, audio and other technology. It also involves keeping yourself safe online.

Dignity this focuses on the value of everybody as an individual. It involves respecting people's choices and opinions, and not making decisions for people.

Disclosure and Barring Service (DBS) the Government service that makes background checks, for organisations, on people who want to work with adults, children and young people with care or support needs.

Disclosure of abuse when a person tells you that abuse has happened or is happening

Disinfect the decontamination technique used for medium infection risk items, such as bedpans and bottles.

Diversity individual differences we have from each other, such as religious belief, race, gender.

Domains of health physical, emotional, occupational, spiritual, social, environmental and intellectual areas of health.

Domiciliary care workers provide care and support to people in their own homes.

Down's syndrome a genetic condition that causes physical and mental development delays.

Duty of candour being honest when something goes wrong.

Duty of care a moral and legal obligation to ensure the safety and well-being of others.

Dwarfism a medical or genetic condition causing short stature.

Dysphasia a condition that affects how a person understands language. It is a less severe form of aphasia. For example, they may have difficulties listening to and understanding what another person is saying.

Electronic assistive technology equipment that can be used to overcome difficulties for accessing and using computer technology. It also refers to environmental control systems to operate equipment in their environment (such as heating or lighting) using alternative technology.

Emergency a situation that causes immediate danger, such as a first aid emergency.

Empathy being able to see things from another person's point of view in order to understand their situation and feelings.

Employer in the case of foster carers or adult placement/shared lives carers, this is the agency. In the case of personal assistants, this is the person employing them to provide care and support.

Empowerment supporting people to take control over their own lives and make their own decisions.

Epilepsy a central nervous system disorder which causes seizures, unusual behaviour or sensations.

Equipment in health and social care settings, this can include cleaning equipment.

e-safety being safe on the internet.

Experiential learning the process of learning through experience.

Fact a fact is something that is true. It can be proven and measured using evidence or documentation. Fact relies on observation or research.

Female genital mutilation (FGM) a practice where the female genitals are deliberately cut, injured or changed, which might be done because of cultural beliefs.

Fine motor skills skills that require the smaller muscles in the body, especially the hands and fingers.

Food poisoning an illness affecting the stomach and illness, caused by eating food that has been contaminated with harmful pathogens. Symptoms include nausea, vomiting, diarrhoea.

Furloughed when employers tell their staff not to come into work for a fixed period of time because there is not sufficient work for them to do.

Gross motor skills skills that require the large muscles in the body.

Haemoglobin protein found in red blood cells that carries oxygen round the body.

Hallucinations a person experiencing something that isn't really there but feels real to the person. Hallucinations could be visual and involve seeing something such as a fire, or auditory and involve hearing something that isn't really there, such as a voice.

Hand washing techniques techniques that meet current national and international guidelines; for example, *Clean Care is Safer Care Five Moments for Hand Hygiene*, published by WHO.

Harm any type of abuse or neglect that can have a negative effect on an individual's well-being.

Hazard a danger that has the potential to cause harm.

Hazardous substances in health and social care settings, they can include cleaning substances, used PPE or dressings that have come into contact with body fluids such as blood, faeces, urine, sputum and vomit.

Health and Safety Executive (HSE) the regulator for workers in England, Scotland and Wales, and also for individuals in Scotland and Wales.

Health Inspectorate Wales (HIW) reviews and inspects NHS and independent healthcare organisations in Wales.

Hearing impairment hearing loss, which could be in one or both ears. It may be a partial loss or a full loss.

Heart disease a condition that affects your heart and can lead to mild chest pain or a heart attack.

Heel prick test a small sample of the newborn baby's blood is taken from the heel to carry out testing for rare but serious health conditions.

Hepatitis B an infection of the liver caused by a virus that is spread through blood and bodily fluids.

Hoist equipment used to support and carry an individual as they are moved from one place or position to another.

Honour-based violence domestic violence committed in the name of perceived immoral behaviour, that is seen as having brought shame to a family or community.

Human immunodeficiency virus (HIV) a virus that damages the cells in the immune system and therefore impairs the body's ability to fight off infections and diseases. Flu-like symptoms may be experienced initially but the symptoms may disappear although the virus continues to damage the cells in the immune system.

Hydration ensuring the body absorbs enough water to keep hydrated.

Hypogeusia loss of taste.

Hypoesthesia reduced sense of touch.

Immune system the body's natural defences that work together to fight disease and infections.

In confidence when sharing information, this means to trust that it will be kept confidential.

Incidents unexpected events that cause damage to property, such as a broken window.

Informed consent when an individual decides to consent when they have been fully informed about the benefits, risks and consequences.

Judgement a decision which takes everything into account. You look at the facts and people's opinions and then make your own judgement.

Lack capacity when an individual is unable to make a decision for themselves because of a learning disability or a condition, such as dementia or a mental health need, or because they are unconscious.

Language talking and understanding – it is not only verbal.

Lasting power of attorney (LPA) covers decisions relating to health and care, finances or both. An individual would set up a lasting power of attorney to ensure they will be supported if they lose capacity in the future. The LPA agreement states the decisions (health- and/or finance-related) that individuals are happy for other people to make on their behalf, and also who they want to make those decisions.

Legible records are written in a way that can be easily read and understood.

Lifting cushions these assist individuals to get up from the floor or bath.

Literacy includes reading, writing, summarising information, using grammar and correct spelling and punctuation. It also includes the ability to speak and listen effectively to ensure effective communication.

Makaton a method of communicating that uses symbols, signs and speech to help people with communication difficulties. It is often used with people with learning disabilities and children.

Malaria a disease spread by infected mosquitoes that can affect the whole body, and causes a high temperature, feeling hot and shivery, and vomiting.

Medical model of disability a way of providing care and support that focuses on the medical condition.

Mental capacity the ability to make an informed decision, and to be able to weigh up the options and consequences.

Mouth care oral hygiene and maintaining good oral health through different oral health techniques.

Musculoskeletal disorders injuries, damage or disorders of the joints or other tissues in the upper and lower limbs or the back.

Near misses incidents that have the potential to cause harm.

'Need to know' you should only pass on information when it is absolutely necessary in order to protect an individual's privacy and ensure their safety.

Needle stick injury a stab wound from a needle or another sharp object that can result in exposure to the blood of another person.

Neglect a failure of others to care for and meet an individual's needs which results in harm being caused to the individual. An individual can also cause harm to themselves if they fail to care for themselves, such as by not taking prescribed medication or not eating and drinking healthily.

Non-verbal communication communicating without talking, using body language, eye contact, gestures and facial expressions.

Numeracy the ability to understand and work with numbers, such as adding, subtracting, working out percentages and multiplying figures.

Nutrition a healthy and balanced diet with the correct nutrients.

Open questions starting a question off with 'Why ...?', 'What ...?' or 'How ...?' encourages the person to share facts, opinions, feelings and emotions. It encourages conversation as opposed to a closed question, such as 'Did you ...?' The answer here is likely to be 'yes' or 'no'.

Opinion a person's view of something which may or may not be true. Their view may be different from another person's view about the same thing.

Oral health care the care we give to our oral health.

Over the counter medication usually refers to non-prescription medication that you can buy in a pharmacy.

Pathway plan this is drawn up between a social worker and a young person leaving care or transitioning to adult services. It defines what help the person needs and how they will be prepared for this transition.

Perinatal the short period of time immediately before and after birth, usually a few weeks.

Personal assistant a worker who provides care and support to an individual in their own home and is employed directly by the individual.

Personal identity the concept we develop about ourselves over time; for example, I am smart/funny/kind.

Personal information information that is personal to the individual such as their name, date of birth, weight, care needs.

Personal plan this looks in detail at what support a person needs in order to achieve their goals.

Policies and procedures policies describe how an organisation plans to carry out its services. Procedures set out how an organisation expects its employees to put their policies into action on a day-to-day basis.

Positive approaches these are based upon the principles of person-centred care. Their aim is to support the individual's well-being and prevent the need for more restrictive practices.

Positive risk taking supporting people to take risks which results in them having a better quality of life.

Preventative services these include services which will help people to be as independent as possible, or to prevent a situation from getting worse, for example, dietician involvement for somebody with an eating disorder. Preventative services aim to reduce the amount of help and support people might need in the future

Processing information recording, using, storing and sharing information.

Regulator an organisation that supervises a particular sector.

Residential care home a care setting for individuals who require assistance with their daily activities such as washing, dressing and meal preparation.

Resilience the ability to cope with problems.

Respect this means taking into account other people's feelings, rights and wishes. It is about being thoughtful, courteous and compassionate to the other person.

Responsibilities the legal and moral duties and tasks that you are required to do as part of your job role. Examples include writing information in an individual's record book clearly, only noting factual information, completing records fully and accurately so that they can be read and understood.

Restraint an intervention when a person is trying to harm themselves or others. It involves preventing, restricting or subduing the movement of the body, or part of the body of another person.

Restrictions interventions used to prevent a person harming themselves or others such as restricting a person's freedom of movement. They are only used for as long as is necessary and as a last resort.

Restrictive practice a wide range of activities that stop individuals, children and young people from doing things that they want to do, or encourage them to do things that they don't want to do. They range from limiting an individual's choices, to physical interventions which restrict their movements in an emergency situation.

Rights-based approach ensuring that individuals' rights are upheld in their day-to-day lives.

Rights legal entitlements to something; for example, to have the information held about you by an organisation kept secure.

Risk assessment a process used in workplaces for identifying hazards, assessing the level of risk and reducing or controlling the risks identified.

Rooting a baby's natural reflex to root for their mother's milk.

Safeguarding protecting an individual's health, well-being and human rights; enabling them to live free from harm and abuse.

Salmonella a bacterial infection that affects the intestinal tract, and causes fever, abdominal cramps and vomiting.

Self-esteem the value a person places on themselves – what they think and feel about themselves. Low self-esteem refers to a person not feeling very positive about themselves or their abilities.

Sensory loss mostly used to describe sight loss, hearing loss and deafblindness, but can also relate to a loss or impairment of any of the senses including sight, hearing, taste, smell and touch.

Shared Lives carer someone who opens up their home and family life to include someone with support needs so that they can participate and experience community and family life. The individual may stay with them for the weekend, or they may even go on holiday together.

Sharps equipment that is sharp and may cause an injury by cutting or pricking the skin, such as needles and syringes.

Significant others important people, other than family, in a child or young person's life.

Signs something that can be seen by others, such as bruises, sores and malnutrition. Signs can also include changes in behaviours and moods.

Social bullying bullying carried out without the individual knowing, designed to harm the individual's reputation.

Social identity the self-concept we have of ourselves based on social groups; for example, I am a teacher/ Muslim/parent.

Social model of disability a way of providing care and support that focuses on the individual

Social prescribing connecting people to community services to support their health and well-being.

Speech the expression of words, thoughts and feelings by articulate sounds.

Spina bifida a birth defect caused when the spine and spinal cord do not form properly.

Stand aid a piece of equipment that supports an individual to stand up from a sitting position.

Standards these tell you how you should work to ensure quality and implement the legislation. They are the minimum requirements, and may include codes of conduct and practice and regulations.

Stereotyping a set idea that may be widely held about what someone or something is like.

Sterilise the decontamination technique used for high infection risk items, such as medical instruments used for surgery and catheters that are inserted into the body.

Stress the body's physical and emotional reaction to being under too much pressure.

Stroke a life-threatening medical condition that occurs when the blood supply to part of the brain is cut off.

Supervision a worker, usually a manager, working with another worker in order to support them to meet organisational, professional and personal objectives.

Suspected abuse when you notice signs, or are told by someone about signs, that make you think that abuse may be happening.

Symptoms these are experienced by individuals. They are an indication that something is wrong, for example, feeling upset, angry, scared or alone. Symptoms could be the result of an illness or abuse.

Tongue-tie a condition where the bottom of the tongue is tethered to the floor of the mouth by a short, tight or thick band of tissue.

Typhoid a bacterial infection that can affect the whole body, and causes a high temperature, aches and pains.

Up to date records contain information that reflects the current situation.

Valid consent informed agreement to an action or decision in relation to a person's treatment in an NHS setting. The process of establishing consent will vary according to a person's assessed capacity to consent.

Values ideas that form the system by which a person lives their life; often a person's beliefs can develop into their values.

Vetting and barring scheme this ensures that any person who is not fit or appropriate to work with adults, children and young people does not do so.

Vision loss severely or partially impaired vision.

Well-being a person's health, happiness and ability to achieve goals and develop.

Whistleblowing exposing any kind of information or activity that is deemed illegal, unethical or not correct.

Whooping cough a bacterial infection that affects the lungs and respiratory tract, and causes a worsening cough and breathing difficulties.

Williams syndrome a rare genetic disorder causing mild learning or developmental challenges.

Worker the person providing care and support or services to individuals

Workplace a setting in which care and support is provided, such as residential child care, individuals' own homes, foster care.

World Health Organization (WHO) an organisation that promotes health across the world by promoting access to health services and medicines and responding to emergencies such as the COVID-19 pandemic.

Index

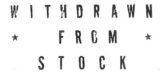
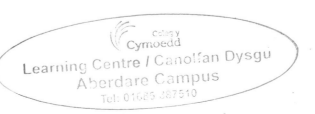